TP14002015
SOS

Functional Foods & Nutraceuticals in Cancer Prevention

Functional Foods & Nutraceuticals in Cancer Prevention

Ronald R. Watson, Editor

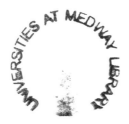

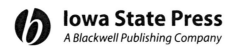
Iowa State Press
A Blackwell Publishing Company

Ronald R. Watson received his B.S. degree in chemistry from Brigham Young University in Provo, Utah, and his Ph.D. degree in biochemistry from Michigan State University, East Lansing. He completed his postdoctoral schooling at the Harvard School of Public Health in nutrition and microbiology, including two years of post-doctoral research in immunology. His research for over 20 years has been related to nutrition and its role in moderating cancer by immune enhancement. He has written and edited numerous books and articles in his field. Dr. Watson initiated and directed the Specialized Alcohol Research Center for 6 years at the University of Arizona College of Medicine. Currently he is a research professor in the University of Arizona College of Public Health and School of Medicine.

Dr. Watson is a member of several national and international nutrition, immunology, and cancer research societies. He has directed a program studying nutritional methods to reduce cancer, funded by the Wallace Research Foundation, for twenty-six years.

Iowa State Press
2121 State Avenue, Ames, Iowa 50014

Orders: 1-800-862-6657
Office: 1-515-292-0140
Fax: 1-515-292-3348
Web site: www.iowastatepress.com

First edition, 2003

Library of Congress Cataloging-in-Publication Data

Functional foods and nutraceuticals in cancer prevention / edited by Ronad R. Watson—1st ed.
    p. ; cm.
Includes bibliographical references and index.
    ISBN 0-8138-1854-0 (alk. paper)
    1. Cancer—Diet therapy. 2. Functional foods—Therapeutic use. 3. Cancer—Prevention. 4. Dietary supplements—Therapeutic use.
    [DNLM: 1. Neoplasms—prevention & control. 2. Nutrition. QZ 200 F979 2003] 1. Watson, Ronald R. (Ronald Ross)

    RC271.D52F86 2003
    616.99'40654—dc21   2003003933

The last digit is the print number: 9 8 7 6 5 4 3 2 1

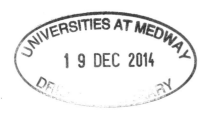

Contents

Contributors

The chapter number is in parentheses after each name.

T. Bermejo Vicedo (1)
Doctor of Pharmacy, Hospital Pharmacist, Practicing Professor, Pharmacy Faculty of the Complutense University of Madrid, Spain.

Antonella Brusamolino (8)
Ph.D., Department of Food Science and Microbiology, Division of Human Nutrition, University of Milan, Italy.

Michael R. Clemens (11)
Forschungszentrum für Psychobiologie und Psychosomatik, Universität Trier, Trier.

Cindy D. Davis (4)
Ph.D., Research Nutritionist at the U.S. Department of Agriculture, Grand Forks Human Nutrition Research Center, Grand Forks, North Dakota; currently, Program Director, Nutritional Sciences Research Group, National Cancer Institute.

Ester Du (3)
Visiting student from Vanderbilt University.

Nancy J. Emenaker (9)
Ph.D., M.Ed., R.D., Columbia University, College of Physicians and Surgeons, Department of Physiology and Cellular Biophysics, New York, New York; Life Sciences Research Office, Bethesda, Maryland.

John W. Finley (4)
Ph.D., U.S. Department of Agriculture, Grand Forks Human Nutrition Research Center, Grand Forks, North Dakota.

Danine Fisher (2)
Member, Minority Undergraduate Medical Research Students, University of Arizona, Tucson.

Tina L. Green (15)
M.S., R.D., Clinical Nutrition Research Specialist, Department of Nutritional Sciences and Arizona Cancer Center, University of Arizona, Tucson.

Hubert T. Greenway (6)
M.D., Assistant Clinical Professor, University of California, San Diego; Director, Cutaneous Oncology, Scripps Clinic, La Jolla, California

Ju-yuan Guo (13)
Ph.D., Post-Doctoral Fellow, Food Science and Missouri University Center for Phytonutrient and Phytochemical Studies, University of Missouri, Columbia.

Debra Hickman (10)
B.S., Member, Minority High School Teacher program, University of Arizona, Tucson.

F. J. Hidalgo Correas (1)
Pharm.D., Hospital Pharmacist, Severo Ochoa Hospital, Leganés, Madrid, Spain.

Destiny M. Hollis (14)
Department of Pathology, South Carolina Cancer Center, University of South Carolina School of Medicine, Columbia.

Paula Inserra (7, 16)
Ph.D., R.D., Louisiana State University Health Sciences Center, Stanley S. Scott Cancer Center, New Orleans, Louisiana.

Bailin Liang (3)
Ph.D., Research Scientist, Centocor, Inc., Radnor, Pennsylvania.

Dennis B. Lubahn (13)
Ph.D., Associate Professor, Child Health, Biochemistry and Animal Sciences; Director Missouri University Center for Phytonutrient and Phytochemical Studies, University of Missouri, Columbia.

Ruth S. MacDonald (13)
R.D., Ph.D., Professor and Chair, Department of Food Science, University of Missouri, Columbia.

Brent P. Mahoney (7, 16)
Ph.D., Tulane University School of Medicine, New Orleans, Louisiana.

Satoru Moriguchi (5)
Ph.D., Graduate School of Health and Welfare, Yamaguchi Prefectural University, Yamaguchi, Japan.

Craig Naugle (6)
M.D., Director, Mohs Micrographic Surgery, Hulston Cancer Center, Springfield, Missouri

Piergiorgio Pietta (12)
Ph.D., Research Director, Institute of Biomedical Technologies, National Council of Research, Italy.

Marisa Porrini (8)
Ph.D., Professor, Department of Food Science and Microbiology, Division of Human Nutrition, University of Milan, Italy.

Steven Pratt (6)
M.D., F.A.C.S., Assistant Clinical Professor, Department of Ophthalmology, University of California, San Diego, and Scripps Memorial Hospital, San Diego, California.

Patrizia Riso (8)
Ph.D., Department of Food Science and Microbiology, Division of Human Nutrition, University of Milan, Italy.

Mary Sharl Sakla (13)
M.D., Graduate Research Assistant, Genetics Area Program, University of Missouri, Columbia.

Nader Shenouda (13)
M.D., Ph.D., Post-Doctoral Fellow, Missouri University Center for Phytonutrient and Phytochemical Studies, University of Missouri, Columbia.

Eiji Shimizu (5)
M.D., Ph.D., 3rd Department of Internal Medicine, School of Medicine, University of Tottori, Yonago, Japan.

Cynthia A. Thomson (15)
Ph.D., R.D., Department of Nutritional Sciences and Arizona Cancer Center, University of Arizona, Tucson.

Ali Reza Waladkhani (11)
Forschungszentrum für Psychobiologie und Psychosomatik, Universität Trier, Trier.

Michael J. Wargovich (14)
Ph.D., Department of Pathology, South Carolina Cancer Center, University of South Carolina School of Medicine, Columbia.

Ronald R. Watson (Editor, 3)
Ph.D., Professor, Health Promotion Sciences in Mel and Enid Zuckerman College of Public Health; Professor, Department of Family and Community Medicine, School of Medicine, and Adjunct Professor, Nutritional Sciences, University of Arizona, Tucson.

Satoe Yamashita (5)
M.S., Graduate School of Health and Welfare, Yamaguchi Prefectural University, Yamaguchi, Japan.

Mary E. S. Zander (14)
Ph.D., Department of Pathology, South Carolina Cancer Center, University of South Carolina School of Medicine, Columbia.

Jin Zhang (3)
Ph.D., Fellow, Vascular Research Division, Harvard Medical School.

Preface

Cancer is a leading cause of death among adults. About 25% of Americans will have cancer in their lifetimes. Treatment usually involves the expensive and often traumatic use of drugs, surgery, and irradiation. Yet, in some populations, the rates of cancer are reduced by lifestyle changes. Nutrition and foods are related to 30% of cancers. Animal studies have shown that a deficiency of any of the 40 nutrients needed for life increases the risk of cancer. Not unexpectedly, any high intake of nutrients can frequently reduce that risk. As a significant lack of precise recommendations exists due to insufficient information, many major clinical trials continue testing nutrient supplementation in humans to treat and prevent cancer. Epidemiology investigations and in vitro tests show the importance of nutrients in reducing cancer.

Increasingly, Americans, Japanese, and Europeans are turning to the use of dietary vegetables, medicinal herbs, and their extracts or components to prevent or treat cancer. It has been known for decades that those populations with high vegetable consumption have reduced risks of cancer. However, which vegetables, how much of them, and which extracts or components are best to prevent which cancers?

This book brings together experts working on the different aspects of nutrient supplementation, foods, and plant extracts in cancer prevention. Their expertise and experience provide the most current knowledge to promote future research. Dietary habits need to be altered, for most Americans. Therefore, the conclusions and recommendations from the various chapters will provide a basis for change.

Plant extracts are now a multi-billion-dollar business, built upon extremely little research data. The FDA is pushing this industry, with the support of Congress, to base its claims and products on scientific research. Therefore, a focus on vegetable extracts will be a key area of dietary herbal medicine in this book. Since common dietary vegetables and over-the-counter extracts are readily available, this book will be useful to laymen who apply it to modify their lifestyles, as well as to the growing nutrition, food science, and natural product community.

This book focuses on the growing body of knowledge on the role of various dietary plants in reducing cancer initiation. The topics range from trace elements to the role of cruciferous vegetables. Most of the expert reviews define and support the actions of bioflavonoids, antioxidants, and similar materials that are part of dietary vegetables, dietary supplements, and nutraceuticals. As nonvitamin materials with health-promoting activities, nutraceuticals are an increasing body of materials and extracts that may have biological activity. Therefore, their role in preventing breast, cervical, and other cancers is a major emphasis, along with discussions of which agents may be the active components.

The goal of this book is to get experts to explore the ways nutritional and dietary changes, particularly nutraceutical supplements or foods, and herbal medicines prevent cancer. The overall goal is to provide the most current, concise, scientific appraisal of the efficacy of key foods and alternative medicines in dietary plants in preventing cancer and improving the quality of life. While vegetables have traditionally been seen to be good sources of vitamins, the anticancer roles of other constituents have only recently become more widely recognized. This book reviews and often presents new hypotheses and conclusions on the effects of different bioactive components of the diet, derived particularly from vegetables, to prevent cancers and improve the health of various populations.

Acknowledgments

This book is a product of the research funded by the Wallace Research Foundation. The work of Alyson Beste, Thom S. Eagan, and Michael Mortensen in typing and communicating with authors was critical to the successful completion of the book and is much appreciated.

Part I

Approaches to Cancer Prevention: Role of Nutrition

1

Antioxidants as Cancer Therapies

T. Bermejo Vicedo and
F. J. Hidalgo Correas

FREE RADICALS IN THE GENESIS OF CANCER

Free Radicals and Reactive Oxygen Species

Some substances that can damage DNA and cause cancer are known as free radical (FR) producers.

FR are charged or uncharged chemical species that have an unpaired electron (e·) in their outermost orbit and are hence highly reactive, causing a chain of chemical reactions that damages cells. Because of this, defense mechanisms need to be established to stop these reactions. This can be achieved by an antioxidant or by the binding of two FR.[1,2]

Many factors are involved in certain processes that lead to mutations and finally to the development of cancer including, among others, **reactive oxygen species** (ROS), lipid radicals, and radicals related to the heme group, which are byproducts of cellular metabolism and respiration.[1,2]

ROS are generated naturally as a result of oxidative phosphorylation reactions. The most common ones are the superoxide anion (O_2^-), hydroxyl radical (OH^-), hypochlorite radical (OCL^-), and nitric oxide (NO^-) radical.[1,2,3,4]

The major reactions where ROS are generated are

$$O_2 + e^- \rightarrow O_2^- \text{(superoxide radical)}$$

$$2\,O_2^- + 2\,H^+ \xrightarrow{\text{SOD}} O_2 + H_2O_2 \text{(hydrogen peroxide)}$$
$$O_2 + 2\,e^- + 2H^+ \rightarrow H_2O_2$$

$$H_2O_2 \xrightarrow{\text{catalase}} 2\,H_2O + O_2$$

$$Fe^{2+} + H_2O_2 \xrightarrow{\text{Fenton's Reaction}} Fe^{3+} + OH + OH^- \text{(hydroxyl radical)}$$
$$O_2 + H_2O_2 + 4\,H^+ \cdot \rightarrow O_2 + H_2O + OH^-$$
$$O_2^- + H_2O_2 \xrightarrow{\text{Haber-Weiss Reaction}} O_2^- + OH^- + OH^-$$

$$ROOH + 2GSH \xrightarrow{\text{Glutathione peroxidase}} ROH + H_2O + GSSG$$

$$O_2 + \text{energy} \rightarrow O \cdot_2 \text{(singlet oxygen)}$$

FR are produced in all aerobic organisms as a result of mitochondrial respiration, which consumes oxygen in the process of generating ATP by coupling the electron transport chain and oxidative phosphorylation. But they may also be generated by exogenous factors such as drugs and environmental toxins. Figure 1.1 shows the cellular organelle and the enzymatic mechanisms involved in FR production.[1,2,3]

FR have a variety of effects on the metabolism of basic nutrients:[2]

- Loss of fluidity and cell lysis as a result of lipid peroxidation of unsaturated lipids in the cell membrane
- Changes in carbohydrates that alter cell functions such as those relating to the activity of interleukins and the formation of prostaglandins, hormones, and neurotransmitters
- Inactivation and denaturalization of thiol groups (-SH) and other proteins
- Changes in nucleic acids (DNA) and cause mutagenesis and carcinogenesis

FR and other oxidants are generated under both physiological and pathological conditions. But while a balance exists between FR generation and neutralization under physiological conditions, an imbalance occurs in certain pathological processes and FR accumulate (either due to excess production or depletion of antioxidant substances). In these circumstances, the administration of agents capable of neutralizing FR or restoring natural defenses is useful to stop organ dysfunction and tissue damage.

Antioxidant defenses are natural compounds found in the aqueous and lipid compartments of the body, which are responsible for inactivating FR. They may be classified into enzymatic and nonenzymatic antioxidants.

Intrinsic antioxidant enzymatic systems protect the cell from cellular damage and include:[1,2,3,4]

- Superoxide dismutase (SOD): destroys the superoxide radical by converting it to hydrogen peroxide
- Glutathione peroxidase (GPX): catalyzes reduction of hydroperoxides to hydrogen peroxide using GSH; also reacts with hydrogen peroxide to form water and oxygen
- Glutathione transferases
- Catalases (CAT): react with hydrogen peroxide to form water and molecular oxygen
- Thioredoxin reductase: reduces superoxide and nitric oxide radicals
- Other enzymes: transferrin, ferritin, ceruloplasmin

These enzymes are the first line of defense against oxidative damage produced by FR and are able to antagonize the initiation of carcinogenesis. These enzyme systems are known to diminish with age and it has been hypothesized that this may be a consequence of increased rate of degenerative and carcinogenic diseases associated with aging.[3,4]

The mitochondrial enzyme Mn-SOD is the enzyme that suffers the largest decrease in some tumors, which has led to it being thought that this enzyme could be a new type of tumor suppressor gene, although the mechanism by which it can reduce the development of cancer remains to be clarified.[4]

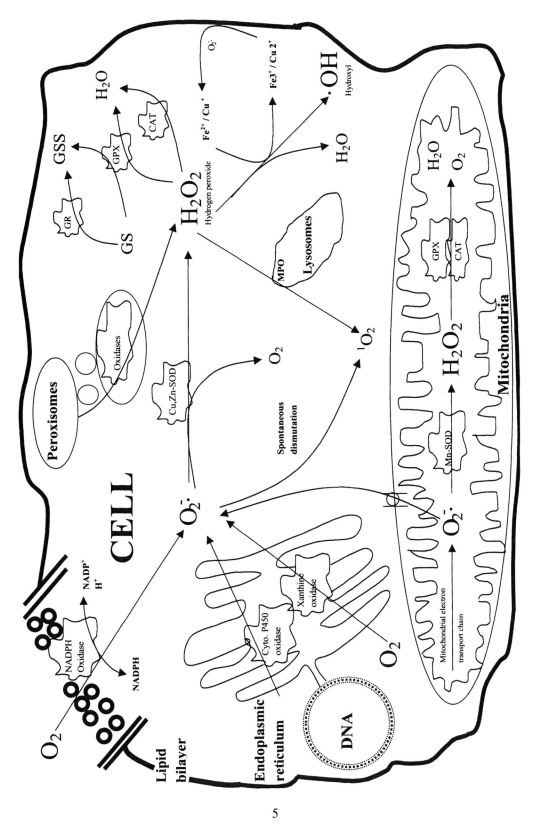

Figure 1.1.   Generation of reactive oxygen species (ROS) and major defense mechanisms against damage caused by ROS.

It has been shown that transition metals such as Mn and Fe are found in very deficient amounts in some tumors, and it has been suggested that a failure in signal transduction may exist in the early stages of carcinogenesis, which could cause the defect in genetic expression of Mn-SOD.

Nonenzymatic antioxidants comprise a wide variety of substances found in the human diet and include vitamin E (alpha-tocopherol), vitamin C (ascorbic acid), vitamin A (retinol and derivatives), carotenoids (chiefly beta-carotenes), glutathione (GSH), and selenium.

Free Radicals in the Genesis of Cancer

FR are capable of inducing changes in the sequence of DNA such as mutations, deletions, gene amplification, and rearrangement, which cause the activation of various protooncogenes and/or tumor suppressor genes.

Damage to DNA can cause multiple lesions such as single- and double-chain ruptures and changes in pyrimidines and purines through various mechanisms:

- Chemical modification of DNA—the simplest (Open purine rings and pyrimidine-ring fragmentation products can block replication.)
- Oxidative damage to specific points of polymerase, which is probably the major contributor to the induction of mutagenesis
- Conformational changes in DNA

Radicals (hydroxyl or singlet oxygen) inhibit DNA replication and transcription by reacting with lipids, proteins, and nucleic acids leading to an accumulation of thymine glycol and 8-hydroxyguanine (by conversion from guanine), which gives rise to mutagenesis when the cell divides. Mutations such as conversion of guanine to thymidine have been found in the p53 gene in carcinomas in smokers and in hepatocellular carcinomas.[3]

Mitochondrial abnormalities are produced in cancerous cells such as structural changes, loss of the electron transport process, alterations in calcium and potassium transport, deficiencies in energy functions, alterations in protein synthesis, and increased respiration. These mitochondrial changes have been linked to the hypoxic state, although other mechanisms have also been suggested, such as a failure in the regulation of calcium or the incorporation of mitochondrial DNA fragments into the nuclear genome.[3]

Most of the alterations that are produced in the mitochondrial genome can increase the generation of ROS because of altered production of essential components (decreased production of antioxidant enzymes) in the mitochondrial respiratory chain responsible for eliminating reactive intermediate products. This genetic mitochondrial damage contributes not only to the process of aging, but also to the development of carcinogenic cells.[3]

Although FR cause a large number of harmful processes in the body, they are also used beneficially to destroy invading bacteria and pathogens. Thus, during infection, neutrophils are cells in the first line of defense, which, when stimulated, are able to take up O_2 to form ROS. Likewise, when stimulated by the action of myeloperoxidase, they can give rise to halogenated species that kill bacteria by phagocytizing them in vacuoles.[1,2]

Free Radicals and Activation of Apoptosis

Homeostasis of cellular metabolism and functions maintains the balance between cellular proliferation and death.[3]

Apoptotic cell death is characterized by controlled self-digestion of cells and is a process that differs from necrosis in various morphological and biochemical events. In the initial apoptotic process, stress-induced damage does not kill the cells directly but rather triggers a series of apoptotic signals that leads to programmed cell death by lipid peroxidation.[4]

Apoptosis can be initiated by a variety of stimuli, including many classes of chemotherapeutic agents, ionizing radiation, and ROS.

The protooncogene Bcl-2 can, in certain contexts, block apoptotic cell death and a mechanism has been proposed by which it causes a regulation of antioxidant processes in sites where radicals are generated. Low doses of hydrogen peroxide are able to induce apoptosis through the generation of hydroxyl radicals and alteration of oxidation/antioxidation mechanisms, and this gene appears to prevent oxidative damage in cellular organelles and lipid membranes and to protect them from oxidative death caused by H_2O_2 and other hydroperoxides.[3,4]

Several lines of research have shown the involvement of oxidative stress as the mediator responsible for apoptosis, as it causes a decrease in intracellular GSH (the main cellular buffer in the redox state) and an increase in ROS. However, the mechanism by which ROS play an important role in cancer inhibition and progression and their ability to induce apoptosis is still not entirely clear.[4]

ANTIOXIDANTS (AO), CHEMOTHERAPY, AND CANCER

The generation of large quantities of ROS intermediates (Fig 1.2) may contribute to induction of mutations in some tumors, inhibition of antiproteases and local tissue damage, and therefore promote tumor heterogeneity, invasion and metastasis. Several recent studies suggest a temporal relationship between oxidative stress, genomic instability and the development of cancer.

In certain types of cancer there is a relationship between a decrease in antioxidant enzyme activity and increased levels of hydroxylated DNA (damaged by oxidative stress); in fact, antioxidant enzymes such as glutathione peroxidase, catalase and superoxide dismutase have been found in lower concentrations in the lymphocytes of patients with lymphoblastic leukemia than in normal subjects. A relationship between reduced levels of Se-glutathione peroxidase (due to low Se levels) and an increased rate of certain tumors has

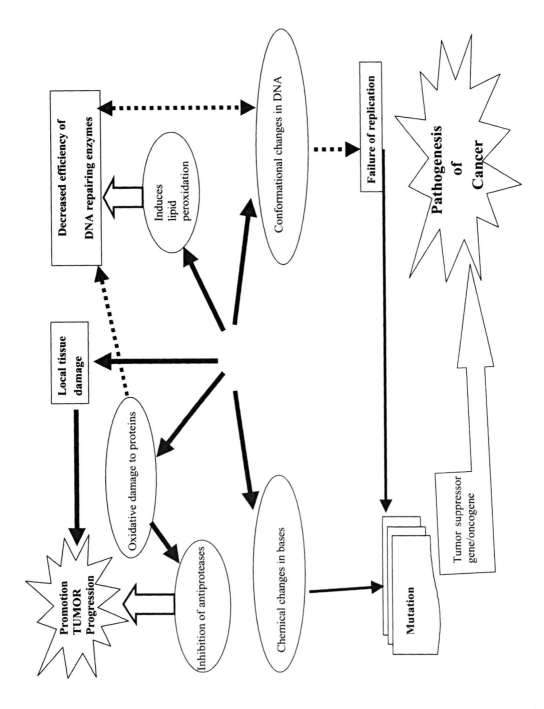

Figure 1.2. ROS and proposed mechanisms for the genesis of cancer.

also been suggested, although it is not known whether this phenomenon is a consequence or causative factor of the disease[4].

The most recently published and relevant data on the role of antioxidants in the prevention of cancer and their use as adjuvants in cancer therapy are discussed below.

Large-scale Clinical Trials (CTs) on the Prevention of Cancer

Starting in 1992, and due to the results of a large number of epidemiological studies on the benefits of the addition of antioxidants to the diet, large-scale randomized CTs including a large number of patients and with several years of follow-up were conducted to evaluate the potential benefits of antioxidant supplementation on cancer incidence and mortality.

The first of these were the Nutrition Intervention Trials, conducted in a population of 30,000 Chinese individuals with a high risk of esophageal and stomach cancer, in whom daily supplementation with alpha-tocopherol 30 mg/day, beta-carotene 15 mg/day, and selenium 50 mcg/day for 5 years significantly reduced overall mortality by 9%, although the protective effect of these supplements was not apparent until 2 years had passed.[5]

The ATBC study (Alpha-Tocopherol Beta-Carotene and Lung Cancer Prevention) was conducted in Finland to determine the effect of antioxidant vitamins on the incidence and mortality of lung and other cancers in 29,000 individuals who were randomized to receive alpha-tocopherol (50 mg/day), beta-carotene (820 mg/day), both, or placebo. Not only was no protective effect on cancer or mortality rates found, but supplementation with beta-carotene also increased the incidence of cancer.[6]

A subsequent study, the Polyp Prevention Study Group study, with beta-carotene, vitamin C, and alpha-tocopherol supplements, showed significant benefits on the incidence of cancer compared to controls.[7]

In 1996, the multicenter CARET (Beta-Carotene and Retinol Efficacy Trial) study, conducted in 18,000 individuals, had to be suspended 21 months after the start of the study because there was a significantly higher incidence of lung cancer in the group receiving beta-carotene plus vitamin A than in the placebo group.[8]

Finally in 1996, the results of the PHS (Physicians Health Study), started in 1982, in which 22,000 physicians participated, indicated that beta-carotene supplementation had no effect on cancer incidence and mortality after 12 years of follow-up.[9] Another study, the Women's Health Study (conducted in 39,876 women aged over 45 years), reached the same conclusions.[10]

The discrepancies in the results of the various studies may be due to various causes such as different study populations (normal or high-risk subjects), different doses of the supplements (nutritionals or higher doses), or different methods of administration. High blood AO concentrations associated with a low risk of disease were also obtained with high dietary intake, but not with high levels of supplementation. AO levels in the principal randomized trials were higher than those found in observational studies to be associated with a low risk of disease.

Finally, high doses of AO have been shown to be pro-oxidants and to have antagonistic effects, since they also lead to the formation of reactive radicals due to the elimination of FR. Furthermore, high doses of AO may have deleterious effects on cellular defense mechanisms and in certain circumstances may facilitate the development of pathological processes such as cancer.

Antioxidants as Adjuvants to Chemotherapy and Radiotherapy in the Treatment of Cancer

A number of studies have been conducted on AO to determine their role in the treatment of various types of cancer as adjuvants to chemotherapy and radiotherapy, since it is thought that they may improve the success of cancer therapy, although this view is controversial. In fact, although this is an area that has been under research for over 30 years, even today there are still many doubts about their definitive role.

Recent studies indicate that chemotherapy and radiotherapy often damage DNA, which subsequently causes apoptosis and necrosis in the cells. Because treatments with AO stimulate apoptosis, there may be a potentially beneficial synergistic effect in the use of AO with chemotherapy and radiotherapy. Some authors also suggest that administration of antioxidants during chemotherapy could prevent certain types of toxicity caused by FR generated by the antineoplastic drugs. Studies carried out in lung cancer patients treated with chemotherapy, radiotherapy, and antioxidants show increased survival time compared to when antioxidants are not administered.

One of the cytotoxic mechanisms proposed for alkylating agents, cytostatic antibiotics and platinum is the formation of FR, which would cause severe cellular damage through reactions with biological macromolecules. Administration of antioxidants could reduce the effectiveness of chemotherapy for this reason; however, side effects such as cisplatin nephrotoxicity, doxorubicin-induced cardiomyopathy, or pulmonary damage by bleomycin are partly due to the formation of free radicals. There may also be a negative interaction between AO and other agents such as tamoxifen and 5-FU.

Chemotherapy causes not only necrosis, but also apoptotic cell death in malignant cells. Antiapoptotic mutations may be the cause of drug resistance, and certain antioxidants such as quercetin have been shown to overcome this antiapoptosis blockade.

Radiotherapy is based on the use of ionizing radiation that causes cell death through the formation of FR by two mechanisms: (1) directly causing cell death within a few hours and (2) inducing failures in mitosis and inhibiting cellular proliferation. It has also been shown that radiation can generate an apoptotic mechanism, apparently through lipid peroxidation.

Chemotherapy, on the contrary, may reduce antioxidant concentrations during treatment of cancer patients. Weijil et al. (1998) studied the effect of cisplatin on plasma concentrations of antioxidants, pro-oxidants, and oxidative damage products in 36 patients with testicular cancer and osteosarcoma, as well as their relationship with nutritional intake during treatment.[11] Plasma antioxidant levels were measured 8 to 15 days from the start of each cycle and compared to pretreatment values. Vitamins C and E and ceruloplasmin decreased significantly, but returned to their baseline values before the start of the next cycle. Vitamin E/cholesterol + triglycerides ratios measured 3 weeks after the start of chemotherapy decreased significantly and remained low compared to pretreatment levels. Daily intake of antioxidants and anthropometric parameters did not change throughout the study period. The authors concluded that chemotherapy with cisplatin induces a fall in plasma antioxidant levels, which may reflect a failure in antioxidant defense mechanisms against oxidative damage, as well as a renal loss of low molecular weight antioxidants.

Antioxidants

Plasma contains a large number of antioxidants, some of which prevent initiation of the oxidation process, while others inhibit the cascade of oxidation reactions. Free radicals are reduced by means of the oxidation of vitamins, which prevents lipid peroxidation in the cell membrane. The nutritional status of cancer patients, especially when antioxidant intake is inadequate, may be a determinant of oxidative damage caused by free radicals in different organs.

Vitamins

Vitamin C (Ascorbic Acid)

Vitamin C is abundant in fruits and vegetables and is found in high concentrations in citrus fruits, tomatoes, cucumbers, green leafy vegetables, and vegetables such as green or red cabbage.[2,12]

It is a scavenger of superoxide and hydroxyl radicals. It eliminates nitric oxide radicals and radicals produced by ozone. It binds to singlet oxygen and inhibits conversion of nitrites to nitrosamides and carcinogenic nitrosamines.

One of its most important functions is to maintain the antioxidant state of vitamin E by reducing the alpha-tocopherol radical.

It inhibits carcinogenesis induced by radiation and by a large variety of chemical agents, including free-radical-producing agents in smokers (rapid depletion of this vitamin occurs in smokers with the consequent increase in free radicals).

Epidemiological studies suggest that an inverse relationship exists between cancer risk and dietary vitamin C intake. In fact, several observational studies have reported a low risk of lung cancer in individuals who consume large amounts of vitamin C (those in the top quartile or quintile) compared to persons who consume less. A relationship has also been observed between vitamin C intake and the risk of colorectal, breast, stomach, oral, and esophageal cancer.[13]

Despite this, the use of vitamin C in cancer therapy remains highly controversial, partly because the studies were carried out with highly questionable methods and partly because very diverse doses were used by the different investigators owing to the wide therapeutic range of this vitamin.

In the study by Pohl and Reidy (1989), oral administration of vitamin C to healthy volunteers was shown to protect against mutagenesis induced by bleomycin chemotherapy.[14] Lymphocyte cultures obtained in 10 volunteers 2 weeks before and 2 weeks after administration of 100 mg or 1 g of vitamin C showed a significant reduction of chromosomal damage, suggesting the administration of high doses of 1 g of vitamin C may reduce the risk of chemotherapy-induced carcinogenesis. This reduction did not occur with the 100 mg dose.

Vitamin C intake was associated with a reduction in the frequency of renal cell cancer in nonsmokers in a case-control study carried out by Lindblad (1997).[15] The type of diet was analyzed over a 20-year period in 379 cases of renal cell cancer and in 350 control subjects. The odds ratio for renal cell cancer from the lowest to the highest quartile for fruit consumption was 0.37 in nonsmokers, and no protective effect was observed in smokers. The odds ratio in nonsmokers corresponding to vitamin C intake (without supplements) was 0.43 (p = 0.04) and 0.37 with supplements, and no protective effect was found in smokers.

Vitamin A (Carotenoids)

Vitamin A encompasses a group of compounds known as carotenoids of which more than 500 have been identified. They are found in fruits and vegetables, mainly in carrots, tomatoes, sweet potatoes, yellow squash, spinach, and cantaloupe.[12]

Beta-carotene is the most important antioxidant carotenoid and the precursor of vitamin A, requiring the presence of vitamin E for its conversion to vitamin A (an excess of vitamin E > 600 IU/day reduces absorption of beta-carotene and its conversion to vitamin A and vice versa). However, while vitamin A is found in limited amounts (its excess can cause toxicity), this does not occur in the case of beta-carotenes.

In addition to beta-carotene, other carotenoids such as lycopenes, alpha-tocopherol, lutein, and zeaxanthin have a certain degree of antioxidant activity. Lycopenes have an antioxidant activity ten times greater than beta-carotenes and have demonstrated anticarcinogenic activity in experimental studies (high lycopene intake with a diet rich in tomatoes was associated with a reduction in prostate cancer in a prospective cohort study), although subsequent studies did not find an association between lycopenes or lycopene-rich products and prostate cancer.[16]

Most studies have been conducted with all-trans retinoic acid (RA) and cis-retinoic acid. RA does not accumulate in the liver and consequently does not cause hepatotoxicity, although continued use can cause other side effects such as headache, lethargy, anorexia, vomiting, and visual disturbances.

Various clinical studies have been carried out on carotenoids and cancer. Although initial studies seemed to show a significant reduction in the incidence of tumors and increased survival, recently Culine et al., after supplementing the diet of hormone refractory prostate cancer patients with oral doses of vitamin A of 45 mg/m²/day, found a low response in only 15% of patients.[17]

In 1993, the coadjuvant effect of high doses of vitamin A was tested in 300 patients with stage I small cell lung cancer.[18] Following curative surgery, the patients were randomized to receive retinol palmitate (300,000 IU/day p.o. for 12 months) or no treatment in the control group. After an average follow-up of 46 months, the number of patients with recurrences or occurrence of a new primary tumor was 56 (37%) in the treatment group and 75 (48%) in the control group. Eighteen patients in the treatment group and 29 patients in the control group developed a second primary tumor. In this study, daily administration of high doses of the vitamin was shown to be effective to reduce the number of new primary tumors related to smoking and to improve disease-free survival time in patients with lung cancer cured after surgery.

Subsequently, Meyskens et al. (1994) determined in a phase III trial that topical administration of trans-retinoic acid reversed moderate but not severe cervical intraepithelial neoplasia II.[19] A group of 301 women with this neoplasia was randomized to receive a cervical cream containing 0.372% beta-trans-retinoic acid or placebo for 4 days in the first month and for 2 days in months 3 and 6. Trans-retinoic acid increased the histologic grade of regression of moderate neoplasia from 27% in the placebo group to 43% in the retinoic acid group (p = 0.04), although this was not the case in severe dysplasia where there were no differences. Adverse effects were more frequent in the retinoic acid group, but they were mild and reversible.

In the study by Romney (1997), women with histopathologically confirmed cervical intraepithelial neoplasia (CIN) were followed for a period of 9 months in a randomized double-blind CT to evaluate the efficacy of beta-carotenes on CIN.[20] The patients received 30 mg/day of beta-carotenes or placebo. Complete remission (absence of dysplasia) occurred in 23% of patients in the treatment group and 47% of patients in the control group, and therefore supplementation did not have beneficial effects on resolution of CIN.

In a case-control study carried out in 974 patients, Shikany (1997) indicated that the frequency of adenomatous polyps of the distal colon detected by sigmoidoscopy was not directly correlated to beta-carotene serum levels.[21] When the data were analyzed, a large percentage of cases occurred in smokers compared to the control group. Because of this, it is possible that carotenoids have a protective effect only in individuals with a high risk of developing polyps, such as smokers.

Fifty patients were assigned to receive beta-carotenes 60 mg/day for 6 months for treatment of oral leukoplakia (precancerous factor) in the study by Garewal (1999).[22] Supplementation produced a response (partial or total) in 26 patients (2 complete and 24 partial responses). Patients who responded were newly randomized to continue receiving beta-carotenes or placebo for 12 months or until disease progression. Elevated plasma beta-carotene levels did not return to baseline levels until 6–9 months after completing active treatment.

Use as a coadjuvant in chemotherapy and radiotherapy. Retinoids are being proposed more often than other AO as adjuvant therapy for standard chemotherapy, where it has been suggested that they enhance cytotoxic effects and reduce toxicity.

The study by Park (1998) with cis-retinoic acid plus radiotherapy plus interferon-α2a in 50 patients with locally advanced carcinoma of the cervix found a tumor response rate of 47% (complete remission in 33%) versus patients treated with chemotherapy and radiotherapy alone, where the tumor response rate was 42% (complete remission in 17%).[23] The main adverse effect in the group receiving combination therapy was fever (60%). These results can be explained by the antiproliferative, immunomodulatory, and antineoplastic properties of the two compounds, which can enhance the cytotoxic effects of radiotherapy.

A CT by Weisman (1998) found that cisplatin and cis-retinoic acid act synergistically in patients with stage IV squamous cell cancer of the head and neck.[24] Patients received daily oral doses of cis-retinoic acid for 7 days. In the phase I CT, 15 patients were treated to determine the maximum tolerated dose of the antioxidant, which was 20 mg/day. At the end of the trial, of 10 evaluated patients, all achieved a complete tumor response in the primary tumor site. The doses used of cis-retinoic acid were well tolerated, but severe toxicity was detected at doses greater than 40 mg/day.

Kalemkerian et al. (1998) carried out a CT to determine the effects of the combination of all-trans-retinoic acid plus cisplatin and etoposide in patients with small cell lung carcinoma.[25] Of 22 treated patients, 1 achieved a complete response and 9 a partial response; the complete response rate was 45%. The study did not demonstrate any beneficial effects with high doses of 150 mg/m^2/day, although they were tolerated. Thirteen patients prematurely discontinued treatment due to mucocutaneous changes and headache.

Due to the poor response of pancreatic cancer to conventional therapy, Recchia et al. (1998) conducted a phase II study to evaluate whether the addition of beta-interferon and retinoids to cytotoxic drugs can improve response and survival in a group of patients with metastatic disease.[26] Two patients were treated with cycles of epirubicin, mitomycin, and 5-fluorouracil. Patients received 1 million IU/m^2 of beta-interferon subcutaneously three times per week and 50,000 IU of vitamin A palmitate orally twice daily between cycles of chemotherapy. A response was achieved in 35% of patients and disease remained stable in another 35%. Although toxicity was severe (hematologic in 60% of patients, gastrointestinal in 40%, and cardiac in 14%), combined chemotherapy, beta-interferon, and retinoids demonstrated activity in metastatic carcinoma of the pancreas.

Vitamin E (Tocopherols)

This term is used to refer to a group of naturally occurring lipid-soluble antioxidants (tocopherols and tocotrienols) that are found in the oil of various plants. Sources rich in vitamin E are vegetable oils, nuts, and grains.[12]

Of the eight types of antioxidants, alpha-tocopherol has the most potent biological activity. It is the main scavenger of lipid free radicals and prevents the initiation and propagation of lipid peroxidation in cellular membranes.

The activity of vitamin E is exerted primarily on peroxyl and alkoxyl radicals generated during peroxidation by eliminating hydroxyl radicals and binding singlet oxygen. It inhibits the cyclooxygenase cycle by reducing the formation of prostaglandins, which have been shown experimentally to play a role in carcinogenesis. It prevents the conversion of nitrites to nitrosamines.

Experimentally, vitamin E inhibits cellular transformation by free radicals such as X rays, ultraviolet light, ozone, and carcinogenic chemicals, which explains its role in the prevention of cancer.

Its antitumor activity is synergistic with selenium since a deficiency of Se can be improved by intake of vitamin E. Vitamin E absorption decreases with a high intake of vitamin A and beta-carotenes.

Observational studies have shown an inverse relationship between vitamin E consumption and the risk of stomach, colorectal, breast, and lung cancer.[13] The study by

Gogos et al. (1998) was designed to investigate the effect of a diet rich in omega-3 polyunsaturated fatty acids plus vitamin E on the status and survival of well-nourished and malnourished patients with generalized malignancy.[27] In this randomized controlled study in 60 patients (well-nourished and malnourished) with solid tumors, patients received fish oil (18 g/day of omega-3 polyunsaturated fatty acids, PUFAs) or placebo until death. PUFAs had a significant immunomodulatory effect by increasing the ratio of T-helper/T-suppressor cells, and they prolonged survival in malnourished patients.

However, in a prospective cohort study (The Zutphen Study) in which 556 men were followed, no relationship was found between vitamin E intake and lung cancer risk.[28] Intake of vitamin E and other nutrients was analyzed by dietary intake of the patients and food composition tables. A weak association was found between lung cancer risk and vitamin C, beta-carotenes, and consumption of fruits and vegetables.

Use as a coadjuvant in chemotherapy. Various authors have investigated the effect of vitamin E on the development of doxorubicin-induced cardiotoxicity, where it was shown to have little or no benefit.[29]

Weitzman et al. (1980) randomized 16 patients to treatment with oral doses of 1800 IU/day of vitamin E or placebo 1 day before and 7 days after chemotherapy.[30] All patients received a cumulative dose of doxorubicin of 250–260 mg/m^2 in combined chemotherapy regimens. Although the combined regimens may have influenced interpretation of patient outcomes, cardiac function and systolic time interval deteriorated in both groups (control and vitamin E), suggesting that vitamin E does not offer any protective benefit against doxorubicin-induced cardiotoxicity.

Legha et al. (1982) administered doses of 2000 IU/m^2/day of vitamin E orally 7 days before and during chemotherapy to 21 metastatic breast cancer patients treated with 5-fluorouracil, doxorubicin, and cyclophosphamide.[31] Cardiac function studies were performed with a cumulative dose of doxorubicin of 250–450 mg/m^2 whenever cardiac failure was clinically evident. Although there was no control group, vitamin E failed to prevent the electrophysiological changes or to reduce the incidence of congestive heart failure, and therefore no benefits were demonstrated for prevention of doxorubicin cardiotoxicity. Vitamin E also failed to prevent myelosuppression or alopecia, had no effect on nausea, vomiting, and stomatitis in the patients treated with chemotherapy, and did not reduce the antitumor activity of doxorubicin.

Lenzhofer et al. (1983) evaluated the acute cardiotoxic effect of doxorubicin (60 mg/m^2) in metastatic breast cancer patients by measuring left ventricular function based on systolic time intervals.[32] The 6 patients who received 200 IU of vitamin E intramuscularly 6 hours before treatment plus nifedipine (60 mg/day p.o.) showed no change in ventricular function. In 6 other patients who did not receive vitamin E and nifedipine, systolic time intervals increased. The results of this study are difficult to interpret because of concomitant use of nifedipine.

Coenzyme Q$_{10}$ (Ubidecarenone)

Coenzyme Q$_{10}$ (CoQ$_{10}$) is an indispensable cofactor in the mitochondrial electron transport chain, where it acts as an electron carrier between the complex of enzymes of the respiratory chain. It is also a lipid antioxidant that eliminates free radicals in biological membranes and plays an important role in preventing damage by lipid peroxidation in mitochondrial membranes.

A potential application of CoQ_{10} supplements is to prevent chronic cardiotoxicity induced by doxorubicin (dose-limiting) during chemotherapy. The mechanism of this complication, which occurs to a greater or lesser degree with all anthracyclines, involves the production of oxidized agents through Fe-dependent processes and the generation of FR in myocardial cells. But the cardiotoxic effect of doxorubicin on the biosynthesis and function of CoQ_{10} in myocardial cells is also due to a reduction in the content of CoQ_{10} in mitochondrial membranes, inhibition of enzymes dependent on CoQ_{10} in the respiratory chain, and inhibition of mitochondrial biosynthesis of CoQ_{10}. This type of cardiotoxicity is nonreversible, associated with congestive heart failure, nonresponsive to digitalis, and not prevented by antioxidants such as vitamins E and C.

Acute doxorubicin-induced cardiotoxicity is a reversible adverse effect that can be attributed to competitive blockade of respiratory enzymes by doxorubicin and CoQ_{10}.

Some authors have demonstrated tumor regression and increased survival associated with oral administration of coenzyme Q_{10}. In an open-label CT in breast cancer patients with lymph node involvement, administration of 90 mg of coenzyme Q_{10}/day with other AO (vitamin C, 2850 mg; vitamin E, 2500 IU; beta-carotene, 32.5 IU; Se, 387 mcg) and 3.5 g of omega-3 fatty acids, combined with conventional therapy, caused a partial remission in 6 of 32 patients; no deaths occurred during the 18 months of the study period and no patient developed metastasis.[33]

Use as a coadjuvant in chemotherapy. CoQ_{10} supplements during chemotherapy have been used to prevent doxorubicin cardiotoxicity.

Iarussi et al. (1994) evaluated the effects of CoQ_{10} on the development of anthracycline cardiotoxicity in children with acute lymphoblastic leukemia or non-Hodgkin's lymphoma.[34] Twenty children were randomized to receive 100 mg of CoQ_{10} orally twice daily (10 children) or no AO treatment (10 children). Both groups received a cumulative dose of 252 mg/m^2 of daunorubicin and adriamycin. The electrocardiographic study performed in the children who received CoQ_{10} only detected a small reduction in left ventricular fractional shortening versus a higher reduction observed in controls.

In a clinical study in 32 patients with breast cancer (aged 48–82 years), therapy with CoQ_{10} or ubidecarenone seemed to be directly related to partial or complete regression of the tumor.[35] Patients received doses of 90 mg of CoQ_{10} and were supplemented with antioxidants and essential fatty acids. Tumor regression was observed in 6 of 32 patients, no patient died, and 6 patients who had an apparent remission of the tumor also required lower doses of morphine. No distant metastases were observed and clinical condition improved significantly. After 1 year with doses of 90 mg of CoQ, blood levels increased from 0.8 to 1.60 mcg/ml. In the same study, CoQ levels increased to nearly 2 mcg/ml in patients who received doses of 300 mg to 390 mg, and no evidence of distant metastases of the tumor was found after 5 months of treatment.

Selenium

Selenium is an essential component of the enzyme glutathione peroxidase (GPX), which is involved in the reduction of hydroperoxides. There are various Se-containing enzymes. Seven isoforms of GPX are known, three iodothyronine 5-deiodinases, three thioredoxin reductases, and selenophosphate synthetase. Another four enzymes contain Se, although their metabolic functions are unknown: selenoprotein P in plasma, selenoprotein W in muscle, and the selenoproteins found in the prostate and placenta. In all of them, Se is incorporated as the amino acid selenocysteine.[36]

Se is provided in the human diet as selenoamino acids (selenomethionine, selenocysteine, and selenocystine) and a small amount of methylated/unmethylated selenium in food. Se is present in cereals, wheat, and most vegetables, primarily as selenomethionine, which has higher bioavailability (85–100%) than the form found in dairy products and meat. Fish has a high content of Se and a relatively high bioavailability (20–50%).[37]

Epidemiological studies have demonstrated that Se is potentially anticarcinogenic, although not all found an inverse relationship between Se status and cancer risk. It is thought that the anticarcinogenic effects of high levels of Se are not entirely related to the action of these enzymes, but may also be due to metabolites of Se, probably methyl selenol, which causes an increase in carcinogenic metabolism, affects gene expression, increases the immune response, alters the cell cycle, promotes apoptosis, and inhibits neoangiogenesis.[36]

The results of the Nutritional Prevention of Cancer (1996,1998) study indicate the Se intake required to achieve effective levels of these anticarcinogenic metabolites, suggesting that plasma Se levels close to 120 mcg/l may be adequate to minimize the risk of cancer, which corresponds to an intake of 1.5 mcg/kg/day of body weight.[38,39] In this randomized, double-blind, placebo-controlled study with a duration of 10 years (1983–1993) and conducted in a total of 1312 patients with a history of squamous and basal cell carcinomas (randomized to receive 200 mcg of selenium or placebo for 4.5 years with a follow-up of 6.5 years), daily oral supplementation with Se was associated with a significant 37% lower incidence of other types of cancer (except skin cancer) and a 45% lower incidence of all carcinomas. A reduction of 6.3% in prostate cancer, 58% in colorectal cancer, and 46% in lung cancer was observed. The mortality rate for lung cancer decreased by 53% and for all cancers by 50%.

Se levels are generally lower in cancer patients than in healthy persons and this may be partly due to the nutrition typically received by these patients. Although the studies are controversial, it can be concluded that relatively low levels of Se in body fluids can be a risk factor for certain types of cancer and that plasma Se determinations and comparison to normal values in the population may be useful to prediagnose this disease.[40]

Some studies demonstrated an inverse relationship between selenium levels and various types of cancer, such as prostate[41,42], liver[43], and esophageal cancers.

Use as a coadjuvant in radiotherapy and chemotherapy.   An open-label CT in 32 patients with refractory brain tumors found that administration of Se (sodium selenite) in doses of 1000 mcg/day i.v. for 4–8 weeks was associated with a slight improvement in 76% of patients, as it decreased the symptoms of nausea, emesis, headache, vertigo, and convulsions. Patients also received chemotherapy, oxygen, vitamins E and A, diet modification, and psychotherapy.[44]

The study by Hu et al. (1997) was designed to investigate the effect of Se on the development of cisplatin nephrotoxicity in 41 patients treated with 60–80 mg/m^2 of cisplatin per cycle.[45] Patients were randomized to receive organic Se in doses of 4 mg/day p.o. in four divided doses for 8 consecutive days, starting 4 days before chemotherapy during the first and second cycles. The results showed that administration of Se confers significant protection against cisplatin nephrotoxicity, while also reducing leukopenia, use of colony-stimulating factors, and the requirement of blood transfusions.

Melatonin

Although it is not considered a standard antioxidant, melatonin, a hormone secreted by the pineal gland in response to the day-night cycle, has exhibited potent free-radical-scavenging properties against hydroxyl and peroxyl radicals.

Several randomized studies have been carried out using melatonin and recombinant interleukin-2 (aldesleukin) in which a high response and increased survival were achieved. The combination of recombinant human interleukin-2 (aldesleukin) given for 5–6 days per week plus oral melatonin in doses of 10 to 50 mg/day caused a partial or complete response in patients with various types of digestive tract and endocrine tumors.[46,47,48,49,50,51]

In addition, a response rate of 33% (complete or partial response) was observed in a noncontrolled CT in previously untreated nephrectomized patients with advanced metastatic renal cell carcinoma who received combination therapy with oral melatonin (10 mg/day) plus intramuscular human lymphoblastoid interferon (3 times per week) for 5 to 12 months. The mean duration of response was 16 months.[52]

Tamoxifen (20 mg/day) plus melatonin (20 mg/day) administered to 25 metastatic solid tumor patients was demonstrated to be beneficial to control the proliferation of cancer and to improve patient status. The patients included in the study had different types of cancer: melanoma, ovarian cancer, small cell cancer, pancreatic cancer, carcinoma of the uterine cervix, hepatocarcinoma, and other unknown primary tumors. A partial response was observed in 3 (12%) patients, disease stabilized in 13 (52%), and disease progressed in the remaining 9 patients. No toxicity was observed.[53]

The addition of melatonin to luteinizing hormone-releasing hormone (LHRH) therapy for prostate cancer improved patient status in patients progressing on LHRH analogs alone. Oral melatonin 20 mg/day added at night 7 days before the next injection of triptorelin (3.75 mg every 28 days) caused a reduction of over 50% in PSA levels in half of the patients and a one-year survival rate of 64% was achieved.[54]

Use as a coadjuvant in chemotherapy and radiotherapy. Melatonin added to chemotherapy regimens for the treatment of metastatic solid tumors reduced toxicity and increased tumor regression and survival time of patients. Daily administration of melatonin during treatment with chemotherapy resulted in a significant reduction in the manifestations of chemotherapy-induced toxicity.

Eighty patients were administered 20 mg/day of melatonin concomitantly with chemotherapy or chemotherapy alone, with the same supportive care for both groups. Thrombocytopenia was significantly lower ($p < 0.006$) in the melatonin group, as well as anemia and leukopenia. Stomatitis, neuropathy, and cardiac complications were also fewer in this group, although there were no differences in the frequency of alopecia, nausea, vomiting, or diarrhea. The antitumor activity of the cytostatic agent was not reduced by coadministration of melatonin.[55] However, in another study no myeloprotective effect was demonstrated with melatonin in doses of 40 mg/day starting 2 days before and continuing during chemotherapy with carboplatin and etoposide in advanced lung cancer.[56]

A randomized CT was designed to administer two different treatment regimens to small cell lung cancer patients: one with melatonin 20 mg/day plus cisplatin plus etoposide, and another with the chemotherapy cycle alone. One-year survival rates were significantly higher in patients who received melatonin as adjuvant therapy (15/34 versus 7/36). A significantly greater tumor response was not detected in patients treated with melatonin (11/34 versus 6/36). Myelosuppression, neuropathy, and cachexia were decreased in patients receiving melatonin.[57]

Two hundred and five patients with metastatic solid tumors were randomized to receive chemotherapy alone or chemotherapy with 20 mg of oral melatonin starting 7 days before chemotherapy and continuing after stopping chemotherapy until disease progression. No patients treated with chemotherapy alone achieved a complete response (with regression of the lesion for at least 1 month), while 6 patients in the melatonin group had a complete response. A partial response was achieved in 15% of the chemotherapy group and in 29% of the melatonin group. One-year survival was higher in the melatonin group ($p < 0.001$). Chemotherapy-induced toxicity was significantly lower in the melatonin group than in the other group. Melatonin did not cause toxicity.[58]

In another phase II study, melatonin in doses of 20 mg/day produced a normalization of platelet count in 9 of 21 breast cancer patients who had thrombocytopenia during treatment with epirubicin; a reduction in tumor size was observed in 5 of 12 patients.[59]

Initial studies using combinations of oral melatonin plus low-dose subcutaneous interleukin-2 caused a normalization of platelet count in 70% of patients with cancer-induced thrombocytopenia. Pretreatment thrombocytopenia was attributed to prior chemotherapy. Beneficial effects were attributed to melatonin-induced neutralization of the macrophage activation system and the effects of interleukin on the reduction of the platelet count.[60]

Other studies have reported increased survival and clinical improvement when oral melatonin plus supportive care was administered versus supportive care alone in patients with non-small-cell lung cancer and metastatic solid brain tumors. However, the study design method as well as other conditions may have affected the result, in addition to the small number of patients.[61,62]

Patients with glioblastoma treated with radiotherapy and melatonin 20 mg/day had increased survival time compared to the patients who received radiotherapy alone. The melatonin group had a higher 1 year survival rate than the group with radiotherapy alone (p < 0.02). The latter group experienced a significant increase in the number of infections compared to the melatonin group (p < 0.025).[63]

Glutathione

GSH is a tripeptide of glutamic acid, cysteine, and glycine considered to be the most important intracellular component localized in the cytoplasm, nucleus, and mitochondria.

Its mechanism of action is both direct and indirect by maintaining other antioxidants in their natural state. It is involved in the metabolic functions of DNA synthesis and repair, protein synthesis, prostaglandin synthesis, amino acid transport, and metabolism of toxins and carcinogenic substances. It increases immune function, prevents oxidative cellular damage, and participates in enzyme activation.[64]

Its main physiological function is to maintain a "reduced" environment in cellular components and to destroy reactive oxygen compounds and free radicals produced during metabolism.

Reduced GSH serves as substrate for two antioxidant enzymes involved in detoxification processes (redox cycle), but also protects against oxidative stress by nonenzymatic mechanisms since reduced GSH can eliminate radicals and peroxides directly by oxidizing to its GSSG form as well as other compounds, and thus protect cellular membranes from lipid peroxidation and its consequent harmful effects.[64]

It also reacts with peroxides and various electrophiles, including carcinogenic expoxide metabolites. Intracellular depletion of GSH in the liver and breast tissue has been shown to promote binding of carcinogenic substances to DNA.

The case-control epidemiological study by Flagg et al. (1994) in 1830 patients investigated the relationship between dietary GSH intake and the risk of oral and pharyngeal cancer and found an inverse relationship between dietary GSH intake and the risk of oral cancer, but only in the cohort that consumed GSH mainly from fruits and raw vegetables.[65] The authors hypothesized that the possible anticarcinogenic mechanisms of GSH include direct antioxidant functions, indirect maintenance of other antioxidants, a possible role in synthesis and repair of DNA, and the ability to bind to cellular mutagens.

Use as a coadjuvant in chemotherapy.   The main use of GSH is for its potential protective effect in cisplatin-induced nephrotoxicity and peripheral neuropathy, possibly due to a chemical interaction between GSH and cisplatin, suggested by the results of various noncontrolled studies using an intravenous infusion of GSH.[29] In all these studies, patients received the usual number of cycles of chemotherapy appropriate for their diagnosis and GSH in doses of 1.5–3 g/m^2 i.v. Neuro- and nephrotoxicity were reduced, and in some patients the dose of cisplatin could be increased up to 175% of the standard dose before toxicity appeared.

In 1987, in a study in 16 ovarian cancer patients treated with cisplatin (90 mg/m^2) and cyclophosphamide, 7 received an intravenous infusion of GSH 1.5 g/m^2 before each infusion of cisplatin.[66] Patients who received GSH did not have nephrotoxicity or myelosuppression, while in the control group only 2 patients developed significant but transient nephrotoxicity.

Subsequently, Smyth et al. (1997) studied in 50 gastric carcinoma patients (25 control and 25 treated with GSH) the chemoprotective effects of GSH 1.5 mg/m^2 i.v. given before each dose of cisplatin (40 mg/m^2).[67] Patients were then treated with GSH 600 mg i.m. In patients receiving GSH neurotoxicity and cisplatin-induced myelosuppression were significantly reduced and a complete remission was observed in 20% of the GSH group versus 12% of the control group. A similar study with lower doses of GSH (2500 mg/m^2) and cisplatin (50–70 mg/m^2) did not find a reduction in renal toxicity. However, tumor response was comparable to that found in a previous study (72–52 control).[68]

A double-blind CT was also designed to study the neuroprotective effect of intravenous GSH (1500 mg/m^2) during treatment with cisplatin for gastric cancer. After 9 weeks, none of the 24 patients who received GSH developed neuropathy, but 16 of 18 patients who received placebo did. A higher tumor response rate (76%–52%) was also observed with GSH.[69]

In a CT in ovary cancer patients, intravenous administration of 3 g/m^2 of GSH for 20 minutes prior to administration of cisplatin (100 mg/m^2) caused a significant reduction in toxicity compared to those receiving cisplatin alone. Tumor response rate was higher in the GSH-treated patients (73%) than in the control group (62%).[70]

REFERENCES

1. Bendich A. Antioxidant nutrients and immune functions-introduction. Advances in Experimental Medicine and Biology 1990;262:1–12.
2. Bermejo T, Hidalgo FJ. Antioxidantes: una terapéutica de futuro. Nutr Hosp 1997;12:108–20.
3. Seidman MD, Quirk WS, Shirwany NA. Reactive oxygen metabolites, antioxidants and head and neck cancer. Head and Neck 1999;31:467–479.
4. Mates JM, Sánchez-Jimenez FM. Role of reactive oxygen species in apoptosis: implications for cancer therapy. Journal of Biochemistry and Cell Biology 2000;32:157–70.
5. Blot WJ, Li JY, Taylor PR, Guo W, Dawsey S, Wang CQ, et al. Nutrition intervention trials in Linxian, China: supplementation with specific vitamin/mineral combinations , cancer incidence and disease-specific mortality in the general population. J Natl Cancer Inst 1993;85:1483–1492.
6. The Alpha–Tocopherol, Beta-Carotene Cancer Prevention Study Group. The Effect of vitamin E and beta-carotene on the incidence of lung and other cancer in male smokers. N Eng J Med 1994;330:10029
7. Greenberg ER, Baron JA, Tosteson TD, Freeman DH, Jr, Beck GJ, Bond JH, et al. For the Polyp Prevention Study Group: A clinical trial of antioxidant vitamins to prevent colorectal adenoma. N Engl J Med 1994;331:141–147.
8. Omenn GS, Goodman GE, Thornquist MD, Balmes J, Cullen MR, Glass A, et al. Effects of a combination of beta carotene and vitamin A on lung cancer and cardiovascular disease. N Eng J Med 1994;331:141–147.
9. Hennekens CH, Buring JE, Manson J, Stampfer M, Rosner B, Cook NR, et al. Lack of effect on long-term supplementation with beta carotene on the incidence of malignant neoplasms and cardiovascular disease. N Engl J Med 1996;334:1145–1149.

10. Lee IM, Cook NR, Manson JE, et al. Beta-carotene supplementation and incidence of cancer and cardiovascular disease: the Women's Health Study. J Natl Cancer Inst 1999;91(24): 2102–2106.

11. Weijil NI, Hopma GD, Wipkink-Bakker A, Lentjes EGWM, Berger HM, Cleton FJ, Osanto S. Cisplatin combination chemotherapy induces a fall in plasma antioxidants of cancer patients. Annals of Oncology 1998;9:1331–37.

12. Borek C. Antioxidants and cancer. Science and Medicine; Nov–Dec 1997:52–61.

13. Hercberg S, Galan P, Preziosi P, Alfarez MJ, Vazquez C. The potential role of antioxidant vitamins in preventing cardiovascular diseases and cancers. Nutrition 1998;14:513–520.

14. Pohl H, Reidy JA. Vitamin C intake influences the bleomycin–induced chromosome damage assay: implications for detection of cancer susceptibility and chromosome breakage syndromes. Mutant Res 1989;224:247–252.

15. Lindblad P, Wolk A, Bergstrom R, et al. Diet and risk of renal cell cancer: a population-based case-control study. Cancer Epidemiol Biomarkers Prev 1997;6:215–223.

16. Mills PK, Beeson WL, Phillips RL, et al. Cohort study of diet, lifestyle, and prostate cancer in Adventist men. Cancer 1989 Aug 1;64(3):598–604.

17. Culine S, Kramar A, Droz JP, Theodore C. Phase II study of all-trans retinoic acid administered intermittently for hormone refractory prostate cancer. J Urol 1999;161:173–5.

18. Pastorino U, Infante M, Maioli M, Chiesa G, Buyse M, Firket P, Rosmentz N, Clerici M, Soresi E, Valente M, et al. Adjuvant treatment of stage I lung cancer with high-dose vitamin A. Clin Oncol 1993 Jul;11(7):1216–22

19. Meyskens FL, Jr, Surwit E, Moon TE, Childers JM, Davis JR, Dorr RT, Johnson CS, Alberts DS. Enhancement of regression of cervical intraepithelial neoplasia II (moderate dysplasia) with topically applied all-trans-retinoic acid: a randomized trial. J Natl Cancer Inst 1994 Apr 6;86(7):539–43

20. Romney SL, Ho GYF, Palan PR, et al. Effects of beta-carotene and other factors on outcome of cervical dysplasia and human papillomavirus infection. Gynecol Oncol 1997;65:483–492.

21. Shikany MJ, Witte JS, Henning SM, et al. Plasma carotenoids and the prevalence of adenomatous polyps of the distal colon and rectum. Am J Epidemiol 1997;145:552–557.

22. Garewal HS, Katz RV, Meyskens F, et al. Beta-carotene produces sustained remissions in patients with oral leukoplakia: results of a multicenter prospective trial. Arch Otolaryngol Head Neck Surg 1999;125:1305–1310.

23. Park TK, Lee JP, Kim SN, et al. Interferon-alpha 2ᵃ, 13 cis-retinoic acid and radiotherapy for locally advanced carcinoma of the cervix: a pilot study. Eur J Gynaecol Oncol 1998;19:35–38.

24. Weisman RA, Christen R, Los G, et al. Phase I trial of retinoic acid and cis-platinum for advanced squamous cell cancer of the head and neck based on experimental evidence of drug synergism. Otolaryngol Head Neck Surg 1998;118:597–602.

25. Kalemkerian GP, Jiroutek M, Ettinger DS, et al. A phase II study of all-trans-retinoic acid plus cisplatin and etoposido in patients with extensive stage small cell lung carcinoma. Cancer 1998;83:1102–8.

26. Recchia F, Sica G, Casucci C, et al. Advanced carcinoma of the pancreas: phase II study of combined chemotherapy, beta-interferon, and retinoides. Am J Clin Oncol 1998;21:275–8.

27. Gogos CA, Ginopoulos P, Salsa B, et al. Dietary omega-3 polyunsaturated fatty acids plus vitamin E restore immunodeficiency and prolong survival for severely ill patients with generalized malignancy. Cancer 1998;82:395–402.

28. Ocke MC, Bueno-de-Mesquita HB, Feskens EJM, et al. Repeated measurements of vegetables,

fruits, beta-carotene and vitamins C and E in relation to lung cancer. Am J Epidemiol 1997;145:358–365.

29. Conklin K. Dietary antioxidants during cancer chemotherapy: impact on chemotherapeutic effectiveness and development of side effects. Nutrition and Cancer 2000;37(1):1–18.

30. Weitzman SA, Lorell B, Carey RW, Kaufman S, Stossel Tp. Prospective study of tocopherol prophylaxis for anthracycline cardiac toxicity. Curr Ther Res 1980;28:682–686.

31. Legha SS, Wang YM, Mackay B, Ewer M, Hortobagyi GN, et al. Clinical and pharmacologic investigation of the effects of alpha-tocopherol on adriamycin cardiotoxicity. Ann NY Acad Sci 1982;393:411–418.

32. Lenzhofer R, Ganzinger U, Rameis H, Moser K. Acute cardiac toxicity in patients after doxorubicin treatment and the effect of combined tocopherol and nefedipine pretreatment. J Cancer Res Clin Oncol 1983;106:143–147.

33. Lockwood K, Moesgaard S, Hanioka T, Folkers K. Apparent partial remission of breast cancer in high-risk patients supplemented with nutritional antioxidants, essential fatty acids and coenzyme Q10. Molec Aspects Med 1994;15:S231–40.

34. Iarussi D, Auricchio U, Agretto A, et al. Protective effect of coenzyme Q10 on anthracyclines cardiotoxicity: control study in children with acute lymphoblastic leukemia and non-Hodgkin lymphoma. Molec Aspects Med 1994;15:S207–12.

35. Lockwood K, Moesgaard S, Folkers K. Partial and complete regression of breast cancer in patients in relation to dosage of coenzyme Q10. Biochem Biophys Res Commun 1994;199:1504–1508.

36. Combs GF. Selenium in global food systems. British Journal of Nutrition 2001;85:517–547.

37. Sanz MS, Diaz FJ, Diaz C. Selenium and cancer: some nutritional aspects. Nutrition 2000;16:376–383.

38. Clark LC, Combs GF, Jr, Turnbull BW, Slate E, Chalker D, et al. Effects of selenium supplementation for cancer prevention in patients with carcinoma of the skin. A randomized controlled trial. The Nutritional Prevention of Cancer Study Group 1983–1993. JAMA 1996;276;1957–1963.

39. Clark LC, Dalkin B, Kongrad A, Combs GF, Jr, Turnbull BW, Slate E. Decreased incidence of prostate cancer with selenium supplementation: results of a double-blind cancer prevention trial. British Journal of Epidemiology 1998;81:730–734.

40. Suzuki K, Takikawa S, Nagaoka T, et al. Serum selenium levels in hepatocellular carcinoma. Biomed Res Trace Elem 1991;2:57.

41. Criqui MH. Selenium, retinol, retinol-binding protein and uric acid associations with cancer mortality in a population based prospective case-control study. Ann Epidemiol 1991;1:385–93.

42. Hardell L, Degerman A, Tomic R, Marklund SL, Berfors M. Levels of selenium in plasma and glutathione peroxidase in erythrocytes in patients with prostate cancer or benign hyperplasia. Eur J Cancer Prev 1995;4:91–5.

43. Yu S, Zhu YJ, Li WH, et al. A preliminary report on the intervention trials of primary liver cancer in high–risk populations with nutritional supplementation of selenium in China. Biol Trace Elem Res 1991;29:289.

44. Pakdaman A. Symptomatic treatment of brain tumor patients with sodium selenite, oxygen, and other supportive measures. Biol Trace Elem Res 1998;62:1–6.

45. Hu Yj, Chen Y, Zhang YQ, et al. The protective role of selenium on the toxicity of cisplatin-containing chemotherapy regimen in cancer patients. Biol Trace Elem Res 1997;56:331–341.

46. Barni S, Lissoni P, Cazzaniga M, et al. A randomized study of low-dose subcutaneous inter-

leukin-2 plus melatonin versus supportive care alone in metastatic colorectal cancer patients progressing under 5-fluorouracil and folates. Oncology 1995;52:243–245.

47. Lissoni P, Barni S, Tancini G, et al. A randomized study with subcutaneous low-dose interleukin 2 alone vs interleukin 2 plus the pineal neurohormone melatonin in advanced solid neoplasms other than renal cancer and melanoma. Br J Cancer 1994;69:196–199.

48. Lissoni P, Barni S, Tancini G, et al. Immunotherapy with subcutaneous low-dose interleukin-2 and the pin indole melatonin as a new effective therapy in advanced cancers of the digestive tract. Br J Cancer 1993a;67:1404–1407.

49. Lissoni P, Brivio F, Ardizzoia A, et al. Subcutaneous therapy with low-dose interleukin-2 plus the neurohormone melatonin in metastatic gastric cancer patients with low performance status. Tumori 1993;79(6):401–404.

50. Lissoni P, Tisi E, Barni S, et al. Biological and clinical results of a neuroimmunotherapy with interleukin-2 and the pineal hormone melatonin as a first line treatment in advanced non-small cell lung cancer. Br J Cancer 1992;66:155–158.

51. Lissoni P, Barni S, Tancini G, et al. Immunoendocrine therapy with low-dose subcutaneous interleukin-2 plus melatonin of locally advanced or metastatic endocrine tumors. Oncology 1995;52:163–166.

52. Neri B, Fiorelli C, Moroni F, et al. Modulation of human lymphoblastoid interferon activity by melatonin in metastatic renal cell carcinoma: a phase II study. Cancer 1994;73:3015–3019.

53. Lissoni P, Paolorossi F, Tancini G, et al. A phase II study of tamoxifen plus melatonin in metastatic solid tumor patients. Br J Cancer 1996;74:1466–1468.

54. Lissoni P, Cazzaniga M, Tancini G, et al. Reversal of clinical resistance to LHRH analogue in metastatic prostate cancer by the pineal hormone melatonin: efficacy of LHRH analogue plus melatonin in patients progressing on LHRH analogue alone. Eur Urol 1997;31:178–181.

55. Lissoni P, Tancini G, Barni S, et al. Treatment of cancer chemotherapy-induced toxicity with the pineal hormone melatonin. Support Care Cancer 1997;5:126–129.

56. Ghielmini M, Pagani O, de Jong J, et al. Double-blind randomized study on the myeloprotective effect of melatonin in combination with carboplatin and etoposide in advanced lung cancer. Br J Cancer 1999;80(7):1058–1061.

57. Lissoni P, Paolorossi F, Ardizzoia A. A randomized study of chemotherapy with cisplatin vs etopiside vs chemotherapy with cisplatin, etoposido and the pineal hormone melatonin as a first-line treatment of advanced non-small cell lung cancer patients in a poor clinical state. J Pineal Res 1997;23:15–19.

58. Lissoni P, Barni S, Mandala M, et al. Decreased toxicity and increased efficacy of cancer chemotherapy using the pineal hormone melatonin in metastatic solid tumor patients with poor clinical status. Eur J Cancer 1999;35(12):1688–1692.

59. Lissoni P, Tancini G, Paolorossi F, et al. Chemoneuroendocrine therapy of metastatic breast cancer with persistent thrombocytopenia with weekly low-dose epirubicin plus melatonin: a phase II study. J Pineal Res 1999;26:169–73.

60. Lissoni P, Barni S, Brivio F, et al. A biological study on the efficacy of low-dose subcutaneous interleukin-2 plus melatonin in the treatment of cancer-related thrombocytopenia. Oncology 1995a;52:360–362.

61. Lissoni P, Barni S, Ardizzoia A, et al. Randomized study with the pineal hormone melatonin vs supportive care alone in advanced non-small cell lung cancer resistant to a first-line chemotherapy containing cisplatin. Oncology 1992;49:336–9.

62. Lissoni P, Barni S, Ardizzoia A, et al. A randomized study with the pineal hormone melatonin vs supportive care alone in patients with brain metastases due to solid neoplasm. Cancer 1994;73:699–701.

63. Lissoni P, Meregalli S, Nosetto L, et al. Increased survival time in brain glioblastomas by a radioneuroendocrine strategy with radiotherapy plus melatonin compared to radiotherapy alone. Oncology 1996;53:43–46.

64. Lomaestro B, Malone M. Glutathione in health and disease: pharmacotherapeutic issues. Ann Pharmacother 1995;29:1263–73.

65. Flagg EW, Coates RJ, Jones DP, Byers TE, Greenberg RS, Gridley G, et al. Dietary glutathione intake and the risk of oral and pharyngeal cancer. Am J Epidemiol 1994;139:453–65.

66. Oriana S, Bohm S, Spatti GB, Zunino F, DiRe F, et al. A preliminary clinical experience with reduced glutathione as protector against cisplatin toxicity. Tumori 1987;73:337–340.

67. Smyth JF, Bowman A, Perren T, Wilkinson P, Prescott RJ, et al. Glutathione reduces the toxicity and improves quality of life of women diagnosed with ovarian cancer treated with cisplatin: results of a doubled-blind, randomized trials. Ann Oncol 1997;8:569–573.

68. Bogliun G, Marzorati L, Marzola M, et al. Neurotoxicity of cisplatin +/-reduced glutathione in the first line treatment of advance ovarian cancer. Int J Gynaecol Cancer 1996;6:415–9.

69. Cascinu S, Cordella L, Del Ferro E, et al. Neuroprotective effect of reduced glutathione on cisplatin based chemotherapy in advanced gastric cancer: a randomized double-blind placebo controlled trial. J Clin Oncol 1995;13:26–32.

70. Smyth JF, Bowman A, Parren T, et al. Glutathione reduces the toxicity and improves quality of life of women diagnosed with ovarian cancer treated with cisplatin: results of a double-blind randomized trial. Ann Oncol 1997;8:569–73.

2

Cancer and Nutrition

Danine Fisher

No treatment of cancer should be focused on treating only the manifestations of the disease. ... Instead, the focus of treatment should be the balanced promotion of the health of the whole body, mind, and spirit.

—Anonymous

Most scientific studies and research show that weight loss drastically increases the mortality rate for most cancer patients while also lowering the response to chemotherapy. Chemotherapy and radiation are sufficient stressors alone to induce malnutrition. Pure malnutrition (cachexia) is responsible for somewhere between 22% and 67% of all cancer deaths; hence, nutrition therapy is essential to arrest malnutrition.[1] Up to 80% of all cancer patients have reduced levels of serum albumin, which is a leading indicator of protein and calorie malnutrition.[26] Dietary protein restriction does not affect the composition or growth of the tumor but does restrict the patient's well-being.

Properly nourished patients experience less nausea, malaise, immune suppression, hair loss, and organ toxicity than patients on routine oncology programs.[21] Antioxidants, like beta-carotene, vitamin C, vitamin E, and selenium appeared to enhance the effectiveness of chemo, radiation, and hyperthermia while minimizing damage to the patient's normal cells.[11]

In a study, a Finnish oncologist found that using high doses of nutrients along with chemo and radiation for lung cancer patients not only cuts tumor recurrence in half but also lowers cytotoxicity levels.[24] Normally, lung cancer is a "poor prognostic" malignancy with a 1% expected survival at 30 months under normal treatment. In this study, however, 8 out of 18 (44%) were still alive 6 years after therapy. This further proves that nutrition is a very promising, low-cost, nontoxic, and scientifically valid approach to improving the outcome from medical treatment of cancer.[32]

VITAMIN C

Studies have shown that large doses of vitamin C increase survival time in individuals being treated for terminal cancers. Vitamin C can reduce the formation of nitrosamine in the intestinal tract and potentially reduce the incidence of stomach and esophageal cancers.[25] Tumor-bearing mice fed high doses of vitamin C (antioxidant) along with adriamycin (pro-oxidant) had a prolonged life and no reduction in the tumor killing capacity of adriamycin. The mice also experienced an increased tolerance to radiation therapy.[16] Lung cancer patients who were provided antioxidants prior to, during, and after radiation and chemotherapy had enhanced tumor destruction and significantly longer life span.[15]

VITAMIN K

In simplistic theory, vitamin K might inhibit the effectiveness of anticoagulant therapy (coumadin); actually vitamin K seems to augment the antineoplastic activity of coumadin. Patients with mouth cancer who were pretreated with injections of K-3 prior to radiation therapy doubled their odds (20% versus 39%) for 5-year survival and disease-free status.[11]

FISH OIL

EPA improves tumor kill in hyperthermia and chemotherapy by altering cancer cell membranes for increased vulnerability. EPA increases the ability of adriamycin to kill cultured leukemia cells. Tumors in EPA-fed animals are more responsive to Mitomycin C and dexorubicin (chemo drugs). EPA and GLA were selectively toxic to human tumor cell lines while also enhancing the cytotoxic effects of chemotherapy.[8]

VITAMIN A AND BETA-CAROTENE

Beta-carotene and vitamin A together provide a significant improvement in outcome in animals treated with radiation for induced cancers. Vitamin A deficiency is known to impair antibody response and lymphocyte mitogenesis, and decrease natural killer cell activity and interferon-gamma production. In lung cancer patients receiving high doses of vitamin A, enhanced T cell mitogenesis and reversal of postoperative immunosuppression was documented.[32]

Beta-carotene is the principal carotenoid in the human diet. Beta-carotene functions as an antioxidant. Researchers have speculated that it is likely that fruits and vegetables contain other factors that are necessary in combination with or supportive of beta-carotene for its prophylic properties; hence, it is best to obtain carotenoids from a diet rich in fruits and vegetables, rather than from supplements.[32]

VITAMIN E

Vitamin E protects the body from potentially damaging effects of iron and fish oil. Deficiency in vitamin E, common in cancer patients, will accentuate the cardiotoxic effects of adriamycin. Studies have shown that the worse the vitamin E deficiency in animals is then the greater the heart damage from adriamycin. Patients undergoing chemotherapy, radiation, and bone marrow transplant for cancer treatment had markedly depressed levels of serum antioxidants, including vitamin E.[31] Vitamin E supplements prevented the glucose-rising effect of a chemo drug, dexorubicin, while improving the tumor kill rate of the drug.

NIACIN

Niacin supplements in animals were able to reduce the cardiotoxicity of adriamycin while not interfering with its tumor killing capacity. Niacin combined with aspirin in 106 bladder cancer patients receiving surgery and radiation therapy provided for a substantial improvement in 5-year survival (72% versus 27%) over the control group.[29] Niacin also seems to make radiation therapy more effective at killing hypoxic cancer cells. Loading radiation patients with 500 mg to 600 mg of niacin has been shown to be safe and one of the most effective agents known to eliminate acute hypoxia in solid malignancies.[30]

SELENIUM

Selenium is a trace mineral that can have antitumorigenic effects. Found in brown rice, seafood, enriched white rice, whole wheat, and Brazil nuts, it is a powerful antioxidant. Selenium is also a component of glutathione peroxidase, an antioxidant enzyme that helps to protect against free radical damage.

Much of the world's soil is deficient in selenium, which leads to low selenium intake. This accounts for an increased risk in regions of many kinds of cancer, including breast and colon cancer. For example, people in selenium-depleted north-central China suffer some of the world's highest rates of esophageal and stomach cancer. However, these rates declined when some inhabitants were given selenium and vitamin E.[27]

People need very little selenium to protect their health. The RDA for men is 70 mcg (micrograms), and for women it is 55 mcg. Many authorities now advise 200 to 400 mcg per day; however, 700 to 800 mcg a day may be toxic. Chronic ingestion of 5000 mcg a day has been reported to result in fingernail changes, hair loss, nausea, abdominal pain, diarrhea, nerve problems, fatigue, and irritability.[27] Vitamin E increases the possible toxicity because vitamin E enhances selenium; therefore, people taking vitamin E and selenium should be careful.

In 1996, an 8-year-old study by Dr. Larry C. Clarke at the University of Arizona revealed significant reductions in cancer mortality among people taking 200 mcg of selenium daily.[33] Other studies have shown that selenium-deficient animals have more heart damage from the chemo drug adriamycin.[3] Supplements of selenium and vitamin E in humans did not reduce the efficacy of the chemo drugs against ovarian and cervical cancers. Animals with implanted tumors who were then treated with selenium and cisplatin (chemo drug) had reduced toxicity to the drug with no change in anticancer activity. Selenium supplements helped repair DNA damage from a carcinogen in animals. Selenium was also selectively toxic to human leukemia cells in culture.[27]

CARNITINE AND QUERCETIN

Carnitine may help cancer patients by protecting the heart against the damaging effects of adriamycin. Quercetin reduces the toxicity and carcinogenic capacity of substances in the body yet at the same time it may enhance the tumor killing capacity of cisplatin. Quercetin also significantly increases the tumor kill rate in hyperthermia (heat therapy) in cultured cancer cells.[4]

GINSENG

Panax ginseng was able to enhance the uptake of mitomycin (an antibiotic and anticancer drug) into the cancer for increased tumor kill. In both human and animal studies, nutrients improve the host's tolerance to cytotoxic medical therapies while allowing for unobstructed death of tumor cells. Nutrition therapy makes medical therapy more of a selective toxin on the tumor tissue.[21]

FOOD AND NUTRITION FOR CANCER PATIENTS

Certain vitamins, namely A, C, D, and K, folic acid, beta-carotene, and selenium as well as the B complex group are all beneficial in inhibiting carcinogenesis. A major factor involved in the process of carcinogenesis and all degenerative conditions is a high level of cancer-causing, oxygen-scavenging free radicals, which are unstable particles that damage the outer protective membranes of cells and are incrementally self-replicating. Free radicals, when in balance, also serve a beneficial function in helping to kill invading pathogens and thereby preventing inflammation.[15] Vitamins such as A, C, and E are powerful free radical scavengers. These are found in most fruits, vegetables, and whole grains. One of the most powerful, pycnogenol, is highly present in pine bark and grape seeds. It certainly would not hurt to eat a bunch of organic grapes including chewing the seeds when seasonally available. It is recommended for cancer patients to take a daily high dose of pycnogenol that contains 25 mg of grape seeds and 25 mg of pine bark.[9]

Phytochemicals found in a variety of herbs have many ways to offset cancer. First, they stimulate the vital process of detoxification in the body that eliminates carcinogenic factor. Second, they powerfully stimulate and strengthen the body's immune system, which helps it to inactivate, fight, and destroy cancer cells. Last, many herbs have free radical scavenging properties.[21] Sadly, only 1% of the thousands of herbs that have therapeutic value have been researched.

CRUCIFEROUS VEGETABLES

Vegetables in the cabbage family (Cruciferae) contain high amounts of anticancer constituents called indoles and isothiocyanates. They are also high in vitamins A, C, E, beta-carotene, anticarcinogenic minerals, and fiber. These vegetables should always be cooked because when eaten raw they contain a high amount of thyroid lowering agents.[2] Some vegetables in this category include cabbage, collards, kale, broccoli, brussels sprouts, cauliflower, and mustard greens.

DARK LEAFY GREEN VEGETABLES

Dark leafy green vegetables are high in chlorophyll and other anticarcinogenic compounds and should be eaten daily, both raw and cooked. One of the most powerful wild greens, pursland, is high in omega-3 fatty acids, antioxidants, as well as vitamins E, C, K, beta-carotene, glutathione, and psoralens. Psoralens have powerful antioxidant properties, which besides fighting cancer are particularly beneficial for normalizing skin pigmentation.[29]

The greens with a bitter flavor such as dandelion and chicory more powerfully stimulate detoxification, especially from the liver. They are also potassium-rich foods. They can be served steamed or lightly sautéed with a little olive or sesame oil.

FOODS HIGH IN BETA-CAROTENE

Foods high in beta-carotene include yellow-orange vegetables such as carrots, yams, squash, pumpkin, paprika, cayenne, pepper, and turnips. Carotenoids, other than beta-carotene, include canthaxanthin, plytoene, lutein, xanathophylls, and lycopene, many of which, according to herbalist Donny Yance, may offer greater anticarcinogenic effects than beta-carotene.[4] Carotenoids have antioxidant properties, protecting phagocytes, lipids, and the cells against oxidation, strengthen the immune system, increase the production of certain interleukins, and with their special action in the skin, protect against the damaging effects of the sun.

GARLIC AND ONION FAMILY VEGETABLES

In preparing greens one could add chopped garlic, which is high in anticarcinogenic sulfur compounds, including allicin. Other foods that contain similar compounds to a lesser extent include onions, leeks, chives, and shallots.[29]

MUSHROOMS

Edible mushrooms are high in minerals, especially potassium, which is important to regulate intracellular fluid and the absorption of nutrients into the cell. All mushrooms have potent health-giving, anticarcinogenic properties but the most practical one to use is the shiitake mushroom. These can be economically purchased dry, by the pound, in Chinese grocery stores and pharmacies as "black mushrooms." They can then be soaked and reconstituted in water before using. Shiitake mushrooms are high in vitamins B_1, B_2, B_{12}, niacin, and pantothenic acid. B vitamins are necessary for cell energy and hormone production.[4]

They also contain high amounts of protein, enzymes, and eight essential amino acids and have been found to be useful for cancer, heart disease, AIDS, flu, tumors, viruses, high blood pressure, obesity, and aging. Lenient, a polysaccharide found in the root and cell wall of shiitake, has a triple helix structure, a shape considered important for the production of interleukin 1 and 2, known to inhibit the growth of cancers and viruses.[29]

ASPARAGUS

Asparagus is a vegetable that has a cleaning effect through the lymphatic system and the kidneys. It is high in potassium and other anticancer vitamins and minerals but further contains certain protein compounds that, according to Donny Yance, act as "cell growth normalizers" on cancer division. Donny Yance further states that as a form of therapy, asparagus is always cooked and pureed in a blender. It can then be stored in the refrigerator. The dose is 4 tablespoons two or three times daily alone or mixed in hot or cold water.[9]

FRUITS

Apples, grapes (with the seeds), apricots, peaches, and all berries have powerful anticancer properties. They also tend to have a stronger cooling or anti-inflammatory effect so that they are best eaten in the season and climate where they naturally occur. Citrus fruits, more important the peel, contain D-limonene, which has powerful anticancer properties.[4] Always use organic unsprayed citrus fruits, especially if you are going to use the peel. Either orange, tangerine, or lemon rind makes a zesty condiment when mixed into soups, salads, and sauces. They are also very beneficial for digestion and assimilation. A variety of citrus peels is used in teas.

GRAINS

Whole grains provide the most important biochemical balance for health. The most balanced grain is brown rice and should constitute a large part of the diet. Millet, quinoa, whole wheat, corn, oats, and barley are also very beneficial, and contain various anticarcinogenic compounds and properties. Barley contains coixenlide, amino acids, saccharide, and all alkaloids.[29] Coix, a type of barley, is used for a variety of cancers but especially cancer of the breast, larynx, uterus, and stomach. Brown rice also has anticancer and diuretic properties.

BEANS AND VARIOUS LEGUMES

Isoflavones are flavonoid compounds that are commonly found in various legumes including soybeans. One of the most important currently is genistein because of its close molecular resemblance to human estrogen. For this reason it is very important to include beans, especially soybeans, as part of an anticancer diet.[29] Fermented soybean products such as miso, tempeh, and shoyu tamari go through complex chemical processes that are of particular benefit in the prevention and treatment of cancer.

PROTEIN FOODS

Cancer is fundamentally involved with mal-utilization of protein.[30] Oncologists generally agree that the actual cause of death in cancer patients is cachexia, a condition of severe weight loss and wasting associated with protein mal-absorption. In fact, cancer cells are able to grow by making the amino acids of protein available for their growth at the expense of the body as a whole. Meat, especially red meat, becomes a banquet for cancer cells. This emphasizes the use of plant sources of vegetable protein, such as legumes and beans that contain cancer-fighting compounds, should be a prominent part of an anticancer diet.

Legumes and beans supply high-quality protein necessary to rebuild the tissue and maintain a healthy immune system.[30] They are also an important source of insoluble fiber that slows the release of glucose into the bloodstream, keeping blood sugar levels in balance. Sugar speeds up the metabolism and causes tumors to grow at a much faster rate. Fiber is also fermented in the colon mostly by beneficial bacteria that produce short-chain fatty acids (SCFAs), which help prevent colon cancer . Legumes also serve as protease inhibitors, a protein-splitting enzyme, found to be an important source of valuable phytochemicals such as saponins, which tonify the immune system and inhibit the DNA synthesis of cancer cells.[29]

Another important source of protein is from fatty fish, such as salmon, and poultry with the skin removed. Such meats are less-dense red meat, which should be used more often.

JUICES

Cancer patients should have one or two 8-ounce glasses of fresh organic vegetable juice each day. A good combination is carrots, beets, celery, garlic, and, if available, fresh burdock root. For a flavor variation one can add an apple occasionally as desired.[2]

DIETARY FAT

The investigation into the association between dietary fat and cancer has utilized more research dollars than any other single nutrient. Up to this point in time, findings have not been definitive, but trends are suggestive of an increased risk for those people consuming diets high in fat. At this time there appears to be strong epidemiological evidence to support the recommendations for a low-fat diet that limits the amount of red meat, high-fat dairy products, and other high-fat foods to less than 30% of an individual's total fat kilocalories.[10] Populations that consume lower intakes of fat present a lower incidence of a variety of cancers. A greater consumption of animal fat (saturated) and red meat is associated with cancer of the colon, rectum, and prostate.[18]

The exact mechanism involving fat is still unclear, but there are several proposed theories regarding the mechanism. One theory is that dietary fat alters the production of certain hormones, such as estrogen and prolactin, which could be responsible for the promotion of certain cancers. Another theory takes into consideration the type of fat and its negative effect on the cell membranes and prostaglandin synthesis, thereby indirectly involving the immune system. Diets high in linoleic acid and other omega-6 PUFAs have been shown to decrease the immune response in animal models, while omega-3 fatty acids have been shown to exhibit a protective effect against cancer formation; however, researchers are unsure whether this protection comes from the presence of fatty acids or the absence of omega-6 fatty acids, or both.[10]

At this time there is no complete agreement as to what dietary factors protect against or promote the development of colorectal cancer. This type of cancer is among the leading causes of cancer death in the United States. Researchers have reported that fish oils, omega-3 fatty acids, and a low-fat diet may indeed be protective against colon cancer in some instances.[6]

CONJUGATED DIENOIC DERIVATIVE OF LINOLEIC ACID (CLA)

One somewhat unique fatty acid class that may have an anticarcinogenic property is conjugated dienoic derivative of linoleic acid (CLA). As little as 0.5% CLA in the diet of rats may be enough to significantly reduce carcinogen-induced mammary neoplasm development. It is not yet determined how CLA may act to thwart the development of certain cancers; however, it has been speculated that the ois-9, trans-11 CLA isomer thwarts cancer development by integrating into cell membranes and acting as an antioxidant. CLAs are produced by microbes in the rumen of cows and beef and dairy products are the primary providers.[32] Human studies await application of CLA in chemo prevention.

FIBER

Fiber-endowed foods include fruits, vegetables, cereal grains, and other plant-based foods. These foods are generally lower in fat and in addition contain numerous other compounds (phytochemicals) that are protective against cancer.

The majority of investigative evidence supports the notion that a higher fiber diet reduces the risk of colon cancer. The first hypothesis is that fiber increases bulk and in turn dilutes fecal bile acids, which are thought to promote cancer of the colon. Second, dietary fiber may reduce the action of certain colonic bacteria, which are responsible for the transmission of primary bile acids into secondary bile acids. These secondary bile acids are thought to promote tumor genesis in the colon. Third, increased dietary fiber is thought to dilute the contents in the lumen of the colon, which will decrease the exposure of mucosal tissue to potential carcinogens.[24]

The mechanism by which fiber is thought to decrease the risk of breast cancer is less complex. When breast cancer cannot be attributed to genetic predisposition, increased level of circulating estrogen is suspected. Dietary fiber is speculated to bind the estrogen excreted into the digestive tract and block its reabsorption.[10] Also, compounds such as phytoestrogens found in fiber-containing food may compete with estradiol for estrogen receptors in breast tissue and in this manner beneficially affect breast cancer risk. Another proposed mechanism is that fiber may positively influence the formation of mammalian lignan, which are protective against breast cancer tumors.[10]

COFFEE

Research linking coffee to cancer of the bladder, colon, lung, pancreas, and prostate are inconclusive.[22] The link between coffee and breast cancer may stem from the antagonistic impact that caffeine has on fibrocystic breast lumps; however, many studies have found no relationship between caffeine and breast cancer. Even in animal studies, the results are not compelling.[20] For instance, when rats were fed the equivalent of 85 cups of coffee per day for 2 years, no bladder tumors appeared. Many researchers agree that small amounts of coffee may help prevent cancer, while large amounts may have a negative impact on cancer formation. Furthermore, if coffee is to be accused of causing cancer, it is unclear if the caffeine in coffee is to blame for an initiation in cancer or whether it is other known mutagens in coffee, such as chlorogenic acid, atractylocides, and methylglyoxal.

CONCLUSION

It is obvious that nutrition plays a huge role in the recovery and well-being of cancer patients. Fruits and vegetables not only help destroy cancer cells, but also help protect healthy tissue, help maintain a strong immune system, and make medical therapies less irritating to the body. Because "food" (nutrition) is so important, it is crucial for people, especially cancer patients, to eat healthy, nondetrimental foods with beneficial effects.

REFERENCES

1. Albrecht, J. T. Cachexia and anorexia in malignancy. Hematology/Oncology Clinics of North America 10 (4): 791–800, 1996.
2. American Cancer Society. *The American Cancer Society's healthy eating cookbook: a celebration of food, friends, and healthy living.* American Cancer Society, Atlanta, GA., 1999.
3. Andrassy, R. J. Nutritional support of the pediatric oncology patient. Nutrition 14 (1): 124–9, 1998.
4. Bloch, A. S. The role of nutrition during cancer treatment. Journal of Womens Health 6 (6): 671–5, 1997.
5. Bozzetti, F. Nutritional support in patients with cancer of the esophagus: Impact on nutritional status, patient compliance to therapy, and survival. Tumori 84 (6): 681–6, 1998.
6. Bradlow, L. H., Fisherman, and Osborne, M. P., eds. *Cancer: Genetics and the environment.* New York Academy of Science, New York, NY., 1997.
7. Braga, M. Early postoperative enteral nutrition improves gut oxygenation and reduces costs compared with total parenteral nutrition. Critical Care Medicine 29 (2): 242–8, 2001.
8. Brownson, R. C., Remington, P. L., and Davis, J. R., eds. *Chronic disease epidemiology and control,* 2nd ed. American Public Health Association, Washington, DC, 1998.
9. Bulger, E. M. Nutrient antioxidants in gastrointestinal diseases. Gastroenterology Clinics of North America 27 (2): 403–19, 1998.
10. Heber, D., and Kritchevsky, D., eds. *Dietary fats, lipids, hormones, and tumorigenesis: New horizons in basic research.* Plenum Press, New York, 1996.
11. Hensrud, D. D. Diet, nutrients, and gastrointestinal cancer. Gastroenterology Clinics of North America 27 (2): 325–46, 1998.
12. Heys, S. D. Enteral nutritional supplementation with key nutrients in patients with critical ill-

ness and cancer: A meta-analysis of randomized controlled clinical trials. Annals of Surgery 229 (4): 467–77, 1999.

13. Jatoi, A. Nutritional determinants of survival among patients with breast cancer. Surgical Clinics of North America 79 (5): 1145–56, 1999.

14. Latifi, R., and Merrell, R. C., eds. *Nutritional support in cancer and transplant patients.* Landes Bioscience, Georgetown, 2001.

15. Laviano, A. From laboratory to bedside: New strategies in the treatment of malnutrition in cancer patients. Nutrition 12 (2): 112–22, 1996.

16. McCallum, P. D. *The Clinical Guide to Oncology Nutrition.* The American Dietic Association, Chicago, 1999.

17. Mercadante, S. Parenteral versus enteral nutrition in cancer patients: Indications and practice. Supportive Care in Cancer 6 (2): 85–93, 1998.

18. Moyad, M. D., and Pienta, K. J. *ABC's of advanced prostate cancer.* Sleeping Bear Press, Chelsea, MI, 2000.

19. Murphy, G. P., Morris, L. B., and Lange, D. *Informed decisions: The complete book of cancer diagnosis, treatment, and recovery.* Viking, New York, 1997.

20. Ose, T. [The importance of nutrition for cancer patients.] Tidsskrift for Den Norske Laegeforening 118 (22): 3466–70, 1998.

21. Quillin, P. *Beating cancer with nutrition.* Nutrition Times Press, Inc., 2001.

22. Rock, C. L. Nutritional factors in cancer prevention. Hematology/Oncology Clinics of North America 12 (5): 975–91, 1998.

23. Senkal, M. Early postoperative enteral immunonutrition: Clinical outcome and cost-comparison analysis in surgical patients. Critical Care Medicine 25 (9): 1489–96, 1997.

24. Shike, M. Nutrition therapy for the cancer patient. Hematology/Oncology Clinics of North America 10 (1): 221–34, 1996.

25. Sikora, S. S. Role of nutrition support during induction chemoradiation therapy in esophageal cancer. Journal of Parenteral and Enteral Nutrition 22 (1): 18–21, 1998.

26. Whitman, M. M. The starving patient: Supportive care for people with cancer. Clinical Journal of Oncology Nursing 4 (3): 121–5, 2000.

27. Wildman, R. E. C., and Madeiros, D. M. *Advanced human nutrition.* CRC Press, Boca Raton, 2000.

28. Wilkes, G. M. *Cancer and HIV clinical nutrition pocket guide,* 2nd ed. Jones and Barlett, Sudbury, MA, 1999.

29. Wilson, R. L. Optimizing nutrition for patients with cancer. Clinical Journal of Oncology Nursing 2 (1): 23–8, 2000.

30. Yen, P. K. Cancer treatment compromises nutrition. Geriatic Nursing 20 (5): 278–9, 1999.

31. Yip, I. Nutrition and prostate cancer. Urologic Clinics of North America 26 (2): 403–11, 1999.

32. Zappia, V., ed. *Advances in nutrition and cancer* 2. Kluwer Academic/Plenum, New York, 1999.

33. Nelson, M. A., Porterfield, B. W., Jacobs, E. T., and Clark, L. C. Selenium and prostate cancer prevention. Seminars in Urologic Oncology 17: 91–96, 1999.

3

Vitamin E in Cancer Prevention and Treatment

Ester Du,
Jin Zhang,
Bailin Liang, and
Ronald R. Watson

INTRODUCTION

Interest in cancer prevention by means of nutritional modification continued to surge in the last decade. Reports have indicated a low cancer incidence with vitamin E supplementation,[1,2] and chemopreventive clinical trials using vitamin E are being carried out in the United States.[3] The results of epidemiological studies on the preventive effects of vitamin E are presently mixed[4,5,6,7,8] and remain to be determined. However, vitamin E is considered to be the most effective antioxidant,[9] more effective, for example, than beta-carotene at relatively higher oxygen partial pressures,[10] and is more selectively distributed to the nuclear fraction as compared with other subcellular fractions.[11] With these observations and the fact that high dosage of vitamin E is not toxic, many researchers have focused on anticancerous properties of vitamin E.[12,13] Vitamin E is a widely distributed, fat-soluble vitamin composed of several tocopherols and tocotrienols, the most biologically active of which is alpha-tocopherol.[14] Alpha-tocopherol is a principal lipid-soluble, chain-breaking antioxidant, protecting cell plasma membranes and lipoproteins from peroxidative damage.[15,16] Its richest sources include vegetable oils and products made from these oils, with smaller, yet appreciable, levels found in nuts, green leafy vegetables, and wheat germ. Meats, fruits, and vegetables seem to have little vitamin E. Absorption of vitamin E in the body is influenced by dietary fat intake, and high levels of polyunsaturated fats may also be required to increase vitamin E uptake, although high intake of omega-3 fatty acid may reduce plasma concentrations of alpha-tocopherol.[17]

Singlet oxygen (an energized form of oxygen) is produced as a result of an oxidation process that can damage cellular components such as cell membranes and chromosomal material as well as produce free radicals (molecules with one or more unpaired electrons). These compounds react very quickly, causing damage to membranes, enzymes, nucleic acids, and inactive essential proteins. Specific damage to a cell's RNA or DNA may result in uncontrolled cellular transformation and cancerous cell growth. By preventing this damage, vitamin E, as a result of its structure, is categorized into a class of compounds known as "antioxidants." Therefore, vitamin E may protect cells from free radicals, reducing carcinogenesis in the body.

Three other possible mechanisms by which vitamin E may be effective in preventing cancer are proposed in a current review.[18] First, vitamin E acts as an immunoenhancer, decreasing CD8[+] T cells and increasing CD4[+]/CD8[+] T-cell ratio, increasing total lymphocyte counts, and stimulating activity of cytotoxic cells, natural killer (NK) cell activity, phagocytosis of macrophages, and mitogen responsiveness.[19,20,21] Second, vitamin E is an activator of the p53 tumor suppressor gene.[22] It not only enhances the expression of the wild type p53 gene product but also diminishes the expression of mutant p53 and other oncogenes. Third, vitamin E inhibits tumor angiogenesis by decreasing the expression of angiogenesis-promoting factors.[23] The immunostimulatory nature of vitamin E does provide a basis for its use in the modulation of various immune cell components and immune functions in humans, and the consequent therapeutic use for cancer. Therefore, vitamin E supplementation may provide a more effective therapeutic approach with other existing medical therapies for treatment of cancer. Indeed, in vitro studies and animal studies have indicated that vitamin E alters cancer incidence and growth, acting as an anticarcinogen in several ways, including (1) inhibiting tumor initiation by altering cell functions, (2) picking up active forms of carcinogens and preventing them from reaching target sites, (3) enhancing the body's defense systems, and (4) inhibiting or reducing progression of previously initiated cancers.

While vitamin E may prevent cancers, the evidence of the mechanism by which vitamin E prevents certain types of cancers remains inconclusive. Information is still relatively limited as to which forms of vitamin E in what concentrations are effective in preventing cancer in humans. Because of the different cells that become cancerous as well as the number of agents that can cause human cancer, preventive measures may be effective for one cancer but not for another.[24]

This chapter is a review of vitamin E related antioxidant and immunoenhancing therapeutic roles in animals and humans, showing how vitamin E supplementation could be a useful therapeutic agent against human cancer.

VITAMIN E AND IMMUNE FUNCTION

Malignant tumors, or cancers, grow in an uncontrolled manner, invade normal tissues, and often metastasize at sites distant from the tissue of origin. In general, cancers are derived from one or only a few normal cells that have undergone a malignant transformation. Cancers can arise from almost any tissue in the body. Those derived from epithelial cells, called carcinomas, are the most common kinds of cancers. Sarcomas are malignant tumors of mesenchymal tissues and fat cells. Solid malignant tumors of lymphoid tissues are called lymphomas, and marrow and blood-borne malignant tumors of lymphocytes and other hematopoietic cells are called leukemia. Hypothetically, a major function of the immune system is to recognize and destroy spontaneously arising malignantly transformed cells before they grow into tumors, by the process of immunosurveillance. In addition, immune responses to malignant cells may be protective even after these cells have grown into tumors. Immune effectors cells, such as B cells, helper T cells, (Th) CTLs, and NK cells are able to recognize tumor antigens and mediate the killing of tumor cells.

Tumor antigens elicit both humoral and cell-mediated immune responses in vitro, and many immunologic effector mechanisms are capable of killing tumor cells in vitro. They include antibody response, CTL, NK cells, and macrophages.[25,26]

Vitamin E supplementation exerts a positive effect upon the immune system, while its deficiency compromises the immune system.[27,28] Vitamin E has been found to stimulate Th cells, NK cell cytotoxicity, CTL activity, antibody response, delayed cutaneous hypersensitivity reaction, macrophage phagocytosis, T- and B-cell mitogen responsiveness, the reticuloendothelial system, and host resistance in animal models.[29,30,31] Prasad demonstrated a significant increase in bactericidal activity in human leukocytes after ingestion of 300 mg of vitamin E as d-alpha-tocopherol daily for 3 weeks.[32] Vitamin E deficiency in dogs leads to depression of lymphocyte activation by mitogens,[33] and a deficiency in vitamin E intake has been shown to suppress the immune response in species ranging from rodents to humans.[34] In elder human subjects, vitamin E has been shown to increase IL-2 production while decreasing that of prostaglandin E_2, to increase the response to delayed hypersensitivity skin testing, and to enhance lymphocyte proliferation in response to mitogens.[35] Recent data also indicate that long-term vitamin E supplementation maintains this immunostimulatory effect in the elderly.[36,37] In a retrospective epidemiological study in an elderly population, there was a statistically significant association with high levels of plasma vitamin E levels and a low incidence of infection.[38] Penn et al. supplemented institutionalized elderly patients with vitamin A, C, and E for 28 days.[39] There was a significant increase in total T cells and Th cells. Furthermore, lymphocyte proliferation response was increased in the treatment group. The notion that vitamin E supplementation can enhance immune responses is strongly supported by findings regarding the immunoenhancing role of vitamin E supplementation in mice. This study also found that a 15-fold increase of oral vitamin E supplementation significantly stimulated T- and B-cell proliferation compared to controls.[40]

Normal function of immunocompetent cells is regulated by a network of soluble polypeptide growth factors termed cytokines. Cytokines are typically of low molecular weight, usually glycosylated, and capable of affecting local or systemic immune and inflammatory responses. Under appropriate stimuli, macrophages and T lymphocytes will secrete cytokines to initiate and augment immune responses or inflammatory reactions.[41] For example, interleukin-2 (IL-2) is a pivotal cytokine in the growth and differentiation of T and B cells, and in the stimulation of CTL.[42] IL-4, IL-5, and IL-6 are responsible for the growth, proliferation, and differentiation of B cells into antibody-producing cells.[43] Interferon-gamma (IFN-γ) activates phagocytosis of macrophages and neutrophil cells and cytotoxicity of NK cells.[42] Cytokines play extremely important roles in the communication network that links inducer and effector cells during immune and inflammatory responses. Thus, modification of cytokine production by vitamin E could have a major consequence in the prevention of cancer development via modulation immune response. A 15-fold increase of oral vitamin E supplementation significantly increased IL-2 and IFN-γ production by ConA-stimulated splenocytes in vitro compared with controls.[31] In vitro, we also found vitamin E at physiological concentrations (1 to 5 mg/ml) significantly stimulated IL-2 and IFN-γ by mitogen-stimulated lymphocytes compared with controls.[44] Also, vitamin E supplementation in mice stimulated IL-4 and IL-5 production by ConA-stimulated splenocytes compared with controls[31]; IL-4 and IL-5 are key cytokines in the regulation of antibody response. Thus, stimulation of these cytokines is expected to contribute to the anticancer property of vitamin E. Consequently, we understand that the immunostimulatory nature of vitamin E does provide a basis for its use in the modulation of the various cell components and immune functions in humans and the consequent therapeutic use in patients with cancers.

VITAMIN E AND OXIDATIVE STRESS

Highly reactive oxygen-containing molecules termed free radicals, including superoxide radicals, hydrogen peroxides, hydroxyl radicals, and their products lipid peroxides, play an important role in human diseases, including cancers.[45,46] Free radicals are produced through the body's normal use of oxygen. In addition, environmental pollution such as smog, radiation, cigarette smoke, pesticides, herbicides, and many drugs can react within the body to cause the production of free radicals.[47] During a normal day, cells take thousands of oxidative hits without damage, apparently because of the wide range of antioxidants and natural detoxification systems that allow the body to excrete chemical and metal oxidants before they can do harm. So, reaching the point of oxidative stress requires an oxidant exposure of some significance. For example, the basic prerequisite to lipid peroxidation is inadequate antioxidant intake accompanied by (1) sufficient polyunsaturated fatty acids (PUFAs) or a particular sequencing of PUFAs in plasma cell membranes, and (2) excessive exposure to an oxidant, or oxidants. Once set into motion, oxidative stress can lead to a variety of damaging effects, as mentioned earlier—not the least of which are structural damage, cell necrosis, DNA cross-linkage, loss of integrity of subcellular organelles, and macromolecular cross-links of connective tissues that are commonly seen in the aging process.[47] Such damages could significantly contribute to the malignant transformation. In addition, adducts including acetaldehyde adducts suppress cytokine production.

There is a growing body of evidence suggesting that increased free radicals may be generated during carcinogenesis. The increase in free radicals and lipid peroxides may play an important role at increasing the development of cancers.[48,49,50] It is considered that a significant event in free-radical-mediated carcinogenesis is extensive oxidative damage to the nuclear fractions,[51,52] which leads to DNA damage such as DNA single-strand breaks and the enhancement of carcinogenesis.[53,54] Cooperative defense systems that can protect the body from free radical damage include certain enzymes and the antioxidant vitamins E, A, and C, and beta-carotene, which protect cell membranes from oxidative damage. Vitamin E, one of the fat-soluble vitamins, is present in the blood as d-alpha-tocopherol and is well accepted as the major antioxidant in lipid body tissue. Vitamin E is considered the first line of defense against cell-membrane damage due to peroxidation. Since vitamin E functions as an antioxidant terminating chain reactions and scavenging free radicals, it confines damage to limited areas of the membrane.[55] Therefore, vitamin E supplementation should prevent normal cells from malignant transformation and slow tumor growth via reducing the burden of free radicals. In addition, in vitro and in vivo it has been shown that vitamin E can compensate for glutathione deficiency, maintain cellular levels of reduced glutathione (GSH) by diminishing the free radical load, and contribute to regeneration of oxidized glutathione (GSSH) to GSH.[56,57,58,59] This finding is supported by another finding that vitamin E supplementation significantly reduces retrovirus-induced increase of free radical and hepatic lipid peroxidation.[60] Furthermore, the decrease in free radicals or lipid peroxidation by vitamin E supplementation during murine AIDS is correlated with the decrease of tumor size and number. In humans with genetic glutathione deficiencies, vitamin E exerts a compensatory effect.[59,61] In addition, vitamin E supplementation increases serum glutathione peroxidase activity and the glutathione levels in erythrocytes and decreases the level of GSSH in plasma.[62,63] Thus, vitamin E supplementation may protect immune cells from the attack of free radicals and disturbance of lipid peroxidation, intensifying immune responses, as well as protect normal cells from malignant transformation.

VITAMIN E AND CANCERS

Cancer is and has remained the second leading cause of death in the United States for nearly a decade and accounts for 10% of the total cost of disease.[64] Approximately 1,040,000 new cancers are diagnosed per year, and it has been estimated that one in three Americans will develop some form of cancer.[65]

In recent years, remarkable progress has been made in the understanding of cancer-causing agents (tumor initiators and tumor promoters), mechanisms of cancer formation, and the behavior of cancer cells. Normally, body cells reproduce themselves in an orderly process, so worn-out tissues are replaced and injuries are repaired. Quite often, when cells become precancerous, the immune system detects this change and destroys the dangerous abnormality. Cells may undergo an abnormal change without detection by the immune system and begin a process of uncontrolled growth and spread. Transformation of a normal cell into a cancerous cell is considered to proceed through the stages of initiation, promotion, and progression. Cancer invades and destroys normal tissues and, if left untreated, is likely to spread throughout the body, eventually resulting in death.[65]

Vitamin E, one of the major fat-soluble vitamins (as discussed before), is present in the blood as d-alpha-tocopherol and is well accepted as the major antioxidant in lipid tissue. Vitamin E not only scavenges free radicals, terminating chain reactions and confining damage to limited areas of the membrane, but at high levels also enhances the body's immune response, which may play a role in cancer defenses. A recent study has proposed one mechanism in which vitamin E may prevent cancerous formation by inhibiting Protein Kinase C (PKC).[66] PKC is involved in many pathways that control cell growth, death, and stress responsiveness. Many studies also agree that oxidative stress increases the activity of signaling pathways involved in growth control and possibly activating PKC.[67,68,69,70,71] Thus, vitamin E inhibits the excess PKC activity that was initiated by oxidative stress.

Both exogenous and hereditary factors are believed to be involved in cancer development. It has been estimated that approximately 75 to 80% of all human cancers are environmentally induced, 30 to 40% of them by diet. Research data have shown that free radicals frequently have a role in the process of cancer initiation and promotion. Results of cell and animal research and limited epidemiological human studies have suggested that vitamin E and the other antioxidants alter cancer incidence and growth through their action as anticarcinogens, quenching free radicals or reacting with their products. The majority of studies show a protective effect for vitamin E in regard to cancer risk and development. A dietary deficiency of the antioxidants enhances the incidence of certain cancers.

Animal Studies

In cell culture studies, vitamin E and selenium have been effective in inhibiting transformation of normal mouse embryo cells to cancerous cells following exposure to chemicals and radiation.[72] A combination of selenium and vitamin E has a greater inhibiting effect than either nutrient alone. The researchers concluded that the results support the concept that appropriate dietary intake can reduce the rate of cancer in humans.[72] Incubation of mouse cancer cells with vitamin E succinate resulted in a change in cell appearance to that of a more normal cell and also inhibited cancer cell growth.[73] In a study of mammary tumors induced in rats, supplementation with vitamin E and selenium had a significant inhibitory effect on tumor production.[74] In a study of induced colon cancer in mice, vitamin E-supplemented animals had a reduced tumor incidence and fewer invasive tumors than controls.[75]

The enhancing effect of chronic alcohol intake on chemically induced esophageal cancer was investigated in a study with mice. In the vitamin E-treated group, there was a significant decrease in the number of mice with tumors and in average tumor size and frequency compared with unsupplemented mice, especially when retrovirus infection increased oxidative damage and suppressed immunity.[76]

Studies of induced oral tumors in hamsters showed that topical vitamin E significantly inhibited tumor formation and led to regression of established oral tumors.[77,78,79] Combined topical application of vitamin E and beta-carotene also resulted in regression of tumors in the hamster buccal pouch.[80,81] Vitamin E-supplemented hamsters showed evidence of immune-mediated destruction of developing tumor cells.

In a study of induced skin tumors in mice, vitamin E, selenium, and glutathione inhibited tumor promotion by TPA and mezerein.[82] Ultraviolet (UV) irradiation of mice induces skin cancer and an immunosuppression that prevents the host from rejecting antigenic UV-induced tumors. The ability of dietary d-alpha-tocopheryl acetate to reduce photocarcinogenesis was tested in a murine model.[83] Skin cancer developed in 67.5% of UV-B-irradiated mice by 31 weeks after the first UV exposure. Supplementation with 100 or 200 IU of d-alpha-tocopheryl acetate per kilogram of diet led to a reduction of the incidence to 46% and 19%, respectively. The latter value was significantly different from that found in mice fed the basal diet. Skin levels of alpha-tocopherol varied with the dietary dose of d-alpha-tocopheryl acetate. According to their results, chronically applied vitamin E can effectively reduce cancer formation induced by UV irradiation. In a related study, hairless

SKH-1 mice received 5.2 mg of vitamin E acetate 30 minutes before or after a single minimal erythemic dose of UV light.[84] Researchers recorded that the mice with vitamin E acetate treatment delayed tumor formation for the first 20 weeks, but this difference was lost by 30 weeks. This study showed that although vitamin E acetate may mitigate some of the initial events associated with UV irradiation such as DNA damage and p53 expression, it has limited potential in preventing UV-induced proliferation and tumor formation.

In another study, numerous large DMBA-induced oral tumors were observed in unsupplemented hamsters, but none of the DMBA-treated, vitamin E-supplemented animals had grossly visible tumors. Vitamin E-supplemented hamsters showed evidence of immune-mediated destruction of developing tumor cells. It was concluded that vitamin E appears to prevent tumor formation by stimulating a potent immune response to selectively destroy tumor cells as they begin to develop into recognizable cancer cells,[85] and the researchers have since proposed three possible mechanisms, as discussed earlier.[18]

Epidemiological Studies

Stimulated by animal research on the inhibitory effects of vitamin E on tumor production, independent prospective studies have correlated lower blood vitamin E levels with a higher subsequent risk of certain cancers.[86] Although controlled human studies on the antioxidants and cancer are limited in number, the majority of available epidemiological evidence suggests that vitamin E and the other antioxidants decrease the incidence of certain cancers.

In a study by Yang et al. on nutrient deficiencies in an area of China with a high esophageal cancer incidence, about half of the population studied had deficient or low levels of alpha-tocopherol in the blood.[87] The significance of this finding is unclear because the study also identified other nutritional deficiencies that might contribute to cancer risk. A recent study in Hong Kong has found that vitamin E supplementation reduces the risk of cancer in Asian men and women.[88] It is unclear whether this phenomenon is due to genetics or diet, but a different study has shown that a group of Caucasians in Hong Kong had significantly higher plasma vitamin in comparison with the Asian population in the same environment (33 and 24 µmol/L, respectively).[89] Another study to determine serum levels of vitamin E and the future risk of cancer in men[90] revealed that the concentration of vitamin E in the blood of cancer cases and controls was similar, but there was a significant difference between subjects whose cancers were diagnosed within a year after collection of the blood sample and the controls (10.0 and 11.5 mg, respectively). Men whose cancers were diagnosed one or more years after the collection of the blood sample did not have a difference in vitamin E levels. This led the researchers to conclude that the low vitamin E levels in the newly diagnosed cancer cases were not a precursor of cancer, but a metabolic result of the disease. However, in a longitudinal study in six geographic areas in Finland, men with higher blood vitamin E levels had a lower risk of subsequent cancer. Adjusted relative risks in the two highest quintiles of blood vitamin E concentrations compared to all other quintiles were 0.7 for all cancers combined and 0.6 for cancers unrelated to smoking.[91] In a study evaluating the risk of subsequent female cancers in Finland, vitamin E levels were measured from sorted serum samples of women diagnosed with cancer during an 8-year follow-up of a sample of women initially free of cancer and controls. Subjects with low serum selenium and vitamin E levels had a significant, tenfold higher risk of breast cancer. According to the researchers, their results suggest that a low serum vitamin E concentration can predict cancer development in women.[92]

The role of vitamin E in cancers of the lung and breast has been studied in human populations. A study reported in 1986 compared the blood levels of vitamins A and E and selenium in 99 people who were later found to have lung cancer with 196 people who did not.[93] The researchers found that the blood of those people who developed lung cancer during the following 8 years contained 12% less vitamin E than that in the blood of the healthy controls. Those whose blood levels were in the lowest 20% were calculated to have a 2.5 times higher risk of developing lung cancer than those people whose vitamin E levels were in the highest 20%. A study to determine nutrient levels in the blood of families of lung cancer patients revealed that vitamin E levels were lower in the family members of patients with certain lung cancers than that in controls (average levels = 11.85 mg/ml and 14.10 mg/ml, respectively), indicating a possible familial link between low levels of some nutrients and later development of lung cancer.[94] The researchers suggested that either altered nutrient metabolism or common dietary habits among families might account for the low levels seen in this study.

At the present time, conflicting data exist in regards to the protective effect of alpha-tocopherol on the breast. Although in vitro,[95] in vivo,[96] and animal studies[97] report an inverse relationship between vitamin E intake and the risk of breast cancer, the epidemiologic analysis on this subject renders this hypothesis inconclusive. Earlier studies reported that 600 IU per day of vitamin E were beneficial in the treatment of fibrocystic breast disease, thought to be a risk for cancer.[98] Wald et al. conducted a study of 5004 women in which blood samples were analyzed from 39 who subsequently developed breast cancer and 78 controls who did not.[99] The results indicated that there was a fivefold increase in breast cancer among women having vitamin E levels in the lowest 20% as compared to those women whose levels were in the highest 20%. Another study found that vitamin E was inversely associated with breast cancer risk among premenopausal women, but not among postmenopausal women.[100] However, in a study of 508,267 Swedish women, no overall association was found between vitamin E intake and breast cancer incidence.[101] Further research needs to be done on the issue of breast cancer and vitamin E to confirm or negate this hypothesis.

In England, men who were diagnosed as having cancer within 1 year after blood collection had significantly lower mean serum vitamin E levels than controls, and women with low plasma vitamin E levels have a significantly increased risk of breast cancer.[90,99] In a follow-up study in the Netherlands, blood micronutrient levels were compared for subjects who subsequently developed cancer with controls. When all cancers were considered together, vitamin E blood levels were significantly lower for subjects who subsequently developed cancer. Subjects with vitamin E blood levels in the lowest quintile had a 4.4-fold higher risk compared to subjects with levels in the highest quintile. Vitamin E blood concentrations were 9% lower for lung cancer patients than controls, but differences were not statistically significant, which was attributed to the small number of lung cancer cases. Based on their results, the researchers suggested that a low vitamin E blood level may be a risk factor for cancer.[102]

Results of another study in the United States showed that newly diagnosed lung cancer patients had significantly lower average serum levels of vitamin E than controls.[103] Mean blood vitamin E levels were also significantly lower in a group of patients in Japan with lung cancer than controls.[94] Mayne et al. reported the vitamin E supplements protected against lung cancer in nonsmokers, but there has been no strong evidence that it could treat cancer.[104] A Finnish study of 29,133 male smokers showed that vitamin E supplementation had no apparent effect on reducing cancer risks.[105]

Results of a study in the United States demonstrated a significant reduction in average plasma vitamin E level in women with cervical dysplasia or cancer compared with the control group.[106] In a study of the relation of diet to risk of invasive cervical cancer, a high dietary intake of vitamin E supplements was associated with a significantly lower risk of cervical cancer. Use of vitamin E supplements was associated with a slight decrease in cervical cancer risk.[107]

In a study in the United States, individuals who took vitamin E supplements had a significantly reduced risk of oral and pharyngeal cancer.[108] In another study in Italy, the risk of gastric cancer increased with increasing intakes of nitrites and protein and decreased in proportion to increased intake of vitamin E.[109] In a study in Japan, healthy relatives of lung cancer patients had significantly lower blood vitamin E concentrations than controls, while lung cancer patients had lower average blood vitamin E and selenium levels than either family members or controls.[94]

SAFETY OF VITAMIN E

Vitamin E is a unique therapeutic approach in that it has little if any toxicity when taken orally.[110] In several species, the oral LD_{50} was found to be $\geq$ 2,000 IU/kg body weight.[111] Frogs, rabbits, cats, dogs, and monkeys can tolerate 200 IU vitamin E per kilogram body weight without apparent toxic signs. In general, deleterious effects have been observed in animals only when daily doses were $\geq$ 1000 IU/kg body weight,[112] and few side effects have been reported with vitamin E supplementation in humans, even with daily doses $\geq$ 2000 IU.[2] No adverse effects were noted from vitamin E supplementation in doses of 800 IU/day and 2000 IU/day (RDA: 15 IU/day for men and 12 IU/day for women) given to elderly patients to assess its effect upon immunity and upon the development of Parkinson's disease.[113,114,115] While it could be a concern that intake of an antioxidant could inhibit the superoxide mechanism of bacterial killing by neutrophils, this would not be a problem since oral supplementation does not allow the attainment of plasma levels of vitamin E sufficient to exert this side effect.

Results from animal studies show that vitamin E is not mutagenic, carcinogenic, or teratogenic.[116] Evidence from animal experiments shows a lack of significant toxicity where control groups received oral vitamin E supplementation up to 6 months. There was no evidence of renal or hepatotoxicity or any pathologic changes in other major organs at the doses that are effective in killing tumor cells.[19,23] In fact, researchers agree that a much higher dosage of vitamin E than that of the RDA is needed to gain maximum benefits. Meydani et al. reported that 200 IU of vitamin E is an optimal dose to improve immune response in the elderly.[117] The conclusion of several comprehensive reviews of literature concerning vitamin E safety is that the use of supplements of vitamin E at dosages from 200–2400 IU/day (about 13–160 times the current RDAs), administered for periods of up to 4.5 years, is safe.[118,119] Thus, vitamin E nutritional supplementation may provide a therapeutic approach for treatment of patients with cancers without additional toxicity.

TREATING CANCER WITH VITAMIN E

There has been a limited number of concluded intervention studies since the confirmation of vitamin E as a therapeutic treatment for cancer patients. So far, these studies provide inconsistent data and suggest that while vitamin E can do wonders for some cancer, it may also have absolutely no effect on others.

A study in Linxian, China, treated a group of Chinese patients with 15 mg beta-carotene, 30 IU vitamin E, and 50 µg selenium for over 5 years.[120] This area of China had a notoriously high incidence of stomach and esophageal cancers. Results showed a 13% lower risk of cancer death among treated patients than untreated, and Linxian County reported a significant reduction in overall mortality (P < 0.03), mainly due to lowered cancer rates, particularly of the stomach. In patients with oral leukoplakia, a premalignant lesion of oral cancer, it has been shown that the administration of vitamin E at a dosage of 400 IU twice daily for 24 weeks resulted in a regression of oral leukoplakia of 65% in 31 patients.[121] Losonczy et al. reported a reduction in cancer deaths among more than 11,000 elderly men and women who took vitamin E supplements.[122]

However, a Polyp Prevention Study, which investigated the effects of 400 IU vitamin E in combination with 1000 mg vitamin C and/or 30 mg beta-carotene on the recurrence of benign adenomas of the colon, found no significant difference between the active and the placebo groups in 864 patients after 4 years.[173] A Finnish trial of 29,000 men who smoked heavily reported no reduction in lung cancer rates after 8 years of taking 50 IU vitamin E and/or beta-carotene, although incidence of prostate cancer was lowered by 35%.[105] This outcome may be explained by the possible mechanisms of vitamin E function, which are still unclear.

Evidently, more studies must be done to get a clearer picture of vitamin E functions. Meanwhile, current studies suggest that vitamin E supplementation may reduce the risk of certain cancer, and the effects of vitamin E may be related to dosage, duration, and the environment.

CONCLUSION

There is increasing research evidence to implicate free-radical-mediated cell damage in development of various degenerative diseases and conditions. Susceptibility of the body to free radical stress and peroxidative damage is related to the balance between the free radical load and the adequacy of antioxidant defenses. Levels of antioxidants shown to be protective against free radical damage in human studies are substantially higher than intakes from normal diets. As research continues on the beneficial effects of vitamin E and the other antioxidants in counteracting peroxidative damage in the body, increased intakes of vitamin E and the other antioxidant nutrients can provide protection from the increasingly high free radical levels present in the environment and associated with current lifestyle patterns.

Other than programs to decrease cigarette smoking or heavy alcohol intake, few areas of research appear as promising to substantially reduce cancer incidence rates as studies of possible dietary inhibitors of cancer promotion. Based on study results to date, vitamin E and other antioxidants merit continued active evaluation, using controlled human clinical trials and epidemiological studies.[124]

Based on the increasing age-adjusted mortality rate associated with cancer, it has been suggested that a shift in research emphasis from treatment to prevention seems necessary if we are to make substantial progress against cancer.[125] Studies currently in progress, as well as planned future research, will, we hope, provide conclusive documentation on the specific role of the antioxidants in cancer risk and prevention.

Cancer prevention relies on the potential for modulation of the processes of cancer initiation and promotion through use of defined chemical agents to reduce cancer incidence in a specific population.[126] The evidence provided by most epidemiological studies and observations in human populations as well as more controlled animal studies suggests that the antioxidants reduce the incidence of certain cancers, although some studies showed a different result on this issue.

REFERENCES

1. Watson, R. R., and Leonard, T. K. Selenium and vitamin A, E, and C: nutrients with cancer prevention properties. *J. Am. Diet. Assoc.* 1986; 86: 505.
2. Vitamin E Research and Information Service. *Vitamin E research summary.* Vitamin E Research and Information Service, LaGrange, IL, September, 1991.
3. Kelloff, G. J., Boone, C. W., Malone, W. F., Steel, V. E. Chemoprevention clinical trials. *Mutant. Res.* 267, 291, 1992.
4. Blot, W., Li, J. Y., Taylor, P. R., et al. Nutrition intervention trials in Linxian, China: supplementation with specific vitamin/mineral combinations, cancer incidence and disease-specific mortality in the general population. *J. Natl. Cancer Inst.* 1993; 85: 1483–92.
5. Taylor, P. R., Li, B., Dawsey, S. M., et al. Prevention of esophageal cancer: the nutrition intervention trials in Linxian, China, Linxian Nutrition Intervention Trial Study Group. *Cancer Res.* 1994; 54 (suppl. 7): 2029S–31S.
6. The Alpha-tocopherol Beta-Carotene Cancer Prevention Study Group. The effect of vitamin E and beta-carotene on the incidence of lung cancer and other cancers in male smokers. *N. Engl. J. Med.* 1994; 330: 1029–35.
7. Mayne, S. T., Janerick, D. T., Greenwald, P., et al. Dietary beta-carotene and lung cancer risk in US nonsmokers. *J. Natl. Cancer Inst.* 1994; 86: 33–38.
8. Greenberg, E. R., Baron, J. A., Tosteson, T. D., et al. A clinical trial of antioxidant vitamins to prevent colorectal adenoma. *N. Engl. J. Med.* 1994; 331: 141–47.
9. Meydani, M. Vitamin E. *The Lancet* 1995; 345: 170–175.

10. Singh, V. W. A current perspective on nutrition and exercise. *J. Nutr.* 1992; 122: 760.

11. Ueda, T., Ichikawa, H., Igarashi, O. A study on the distribution of α-tocopherol to hepatic sub-cellular fractions in rats treated with high doses of vitamin E. *Proc. 2ⁿᵈ Meeting of the Japan Society of Vitamin E Research*, Tokyo, Japan, 1990, 140.

12. National Cancer Institute. *Cancer prevention research: Chemoprevention and diet.* NCI Office of Cancer Communications, Bethesda, MD, 1987.

13. Vitamin E Research and Information Service. *Role of the antioxidants in cancer prevention and treatment.* Vitamin E Research Information Service, LaGrange, IL, September, 1991.

14. Kayden, H. J., Chow, C., Bjornson, L. K. Spectrophometric method for determination of toco-pherol in red blood cells. *J. Lipid Res.* 14, 533, 1993.

15. Burton, G. W., and Traber, M. G. Vitamin E: antioxidation activity, biokinetics, and bioavail-ability. *Ann. Rev. Nutr.* 10: 357, 1990.

16. Packer, L. Protective role of vitamin E in biological systems. *Am. J. Clin. Nutr.* 53, 1050s, 1991.

17. Wander, R. C., Hall, J. A., Gradin, J. L., Du, S. H., Jewell, D. E. The ratio of dietary (n-6) to (n-3) fatty acids influences immune system function, eicosanoid metabolism, lipid peroxidation and vitamin E status in aged dogs. *J. Nutr.* 127: 1198–1205, 1997.

18. Shklar, G., and Oh, S. K. Experimental Basis for Cancer Prevention by Vitamin E. *Cancer Investigation* 18(3): 214–222, 2000.

19. Shklar, G., Schwartz, J. L., Trickler, D., et al. Prevention of experimental cancer and immuno-stimulation by vitamin E (immunosurveillance). *J. Oral Pathol. Med.* 19: 60–64, 1990.

20. Odeleye, O. E., and Watson, R. R. The potential role of vitamin E in the treatment of immuno-logical abnormalities during acquired immune deficiency syndrome. *Prog. Food Nutr. Sci.* 15: 1, 1991.

21. Wang, Y., and Watson, R. R. Is vitamin E supplementation useful agent in AIDS therapy? *Prog. Food Nutr. Sci.* 17: 351, 1993.

22. Schwarz, J. L., Shklar, G., Trickler, D. p53 in the anticancer mechanism of vitamin E. *Oral Oncol. Eur. J. Cancer* 29B: 313–318, 1993.

23. Shklar, G., Schwartz, J. L. Vitamin E inhibits experimental carcinogenesis and tumor angio-genesis. *Oral Oncol Eur. J. Cancer* 32B: 114–119, 1996.

24. Krishnamurthy, S. The intriguing biological role of vitamin E. *J. Chem. Ed.* 60: 465, 1983.

25. Burnet, F. M. The concept of immunological surveillance. *Prog. Exp. Tumor Res.* 13: 1, 1970

26. Herlyn, M., and Koprowski, H. Melanoma antigens: immunological and biological characteri-zation and clinical significance. *Ann. Rev. Immunol.* 6:283, 1988.

27. Bendich, A. Antioxidant vitamins and their functions in immune responses. *Adv. Exp. Med. Biol.* 262: 35, 1990.

28. Wang, Y., and Watson, R. R. The potential therapeutics of vitamin E in AIDS. *Drugs* 48: 327, 1994.

29. Meydani, S. N., Meyani, M., Blumberg, J. B. Antioxidants and the aging immune response. *Adv. Exp. Med. Biol.* 262: 57, 1990.

30. Kline, K., Rao, A., Romach, E. H., Kidao, S., Morgan, T. J., Snaders, B. G. Vitamin E modula-tion of disease resistance and immune responses. *Ann. N. Y. Acad. Sci.* 587: 294, 1990.

31. Wang, Y., Huang, D. S., Liang, B., Watson, R. R. Normalization of nutritional status and immune functions by vitamin E supplementation in murine AIDS. *J. Nutr.* 124: 2024, 1994.

32. Prasad, J. N. Effect of Vitamin E supplementation on leukocyte function. *Am. J. Clin. Nutr.* 33: 606, 1980.

33. Bendich, A. Antioxidant vitamins and their functions in immune responses. *Adv. Exp. Med. Biol.* 262: 35, 1990.

34. Meydani, S. N. Vitamin E enhancement of T cell-mediated function in healthy elderly: mechanisms of action. *Nutr. Rev.* 53: S52–S58, 1995.
35. Meydani, S. N., Meydani, M., Verdon, C. P., Shapiro, A. A., Blumberg, J. B., Hayes, K. C. Vitamin E supplementation suppresses prostaglandin E2 synthesis and enhances the immune response of aged mice. *Mech. Aging Dev.* 34: 191, 1986.
36. Meydani, S. N., Leka, L., Loszewski, R. Long term vitamin E supplementation enhances immune response in healthy elderly. *FASEB J.* 8: A272, 1994.
37. Meydani, M., Meydani, S. N., Leka, L., Gong, J., Blumberg, J. B. Effect of long-term vitamin E supplementation on lipid peroxidation and immune responses of young and old subjects. *FASEB J.* 8: A415, 1994.
38. Chavance, M., Brubacher, G., Herbeth, B., Vernhes, G., Mikstachi, T., Dete, F., Fournier, C., and Janot, C. Immunological and nutritional status among the elderly, in *Lymphoid Cell Function in Aging*, DeWeek, A. L., ed., 1984, 231.
39. Penn, N. D., Purkins, L., Kelleher, J., Heatley, R. V., Mascie-Taylor, B. H., Belfield, P. W. The effect of dietary supplementation with vitamin A, C, and E on cell-mediated immune function in elderly long-stay patients: a randomized control trial. *Age Aging* 20: 169, 1991.
40. Wang, Y., and Watson, R. R. Influence of vitamin E supplementation on nutritional status and immune response in murine AIDS. *Proc. XV International Congress Nutrition*, Adelaide, Australia, Wahlquist, M., ed., Smith-Gordon, UK, 1994, 593.
41. Mosmann, T. R., and Morre, K. W. The role of IL-10 in cross-regulation of Th1 and Th2 responses. *Immunoparasitol. Today*, A49-A54, 1991.
42. Arai, K., Lee, F., Miyajima, A. Cytokines: coordinates of immune and inflammatory responses. *Ann. Rev. Biochem.* 59: 783, 1990.
43. Balkwill, F. R., and Burke, F. The cytokine network. *Immunol. Today*, 11, 299, 1989.
44. Wang, J. Y., Liang, B., Watson, R. R. Vitamin supplementation with interferon-gamma administration retards immune dysfunction during murine retrovirus infection. *Journal of Leukocyte Biology* 58(6): 698–703, 1995 Dec.
45. Staltman, P. Oxidative stress: a radical view. *Semin. Hematol.* 26: 249, 1989.
46. Halliwell, B. Oxidants and human diseases: some new concepts. *FASEB J.* 1: 358, 1987.
47. Harman, D. Free radical theory of aging: the "free radical" diseases. *Age* 7: 111, 1984.
48. Cerutti, P. A. Pro-oxidant state and tumor promotion. *Science* 227: 375, 1995.
49. Cerutti, P. A. Mechanism of action of oxidant carcinogenesis. *Cancer Detec. Pre.* 14: 281, 1989.
50. Marnett, I. J. Peroxy free radicals: potential mediators of tumor initiation and promotion. *Carcinogenesis* 8: 1365, 1987.
51. Hinrichsen, L. I., Floyd, R. A., Sudilovsky, O. Is 8-hydroxy-deoxyguanosine a mediator of carcinogenesis by a choline-devoid diet in rat liver? *Carcinogenesis* 11: 1879, 1990.
52. Stohs, S. J., Shara, M. A., Alsharif, N. A., Wahba, Z. Z., Al-Bayati, Z. A. F. 2,3,7,8-Tetrachlorodibenzo-p-dioxin-induced oxidative stress in female rats. *Toxicol. Appl. Pharmacol.* 106: 126, 1990.
53. Floyd, R. A. The role of 8-hydroxyguanine in carcinogenesis. *Carcinogenesis,* 11: 1447, 1990.
54. Ames, B. N. Endogenous oxidative DNA damages, aging and cancer. *Free Rad. Res. Commun.* 7: 1447, 1989.
55. Fritsma, G. A. Vitamin E and autoxidation. *Ann. J. Med. Tech.* 49: 453, 1983.
56. Gogu, S. R., Bechman, B. S., Rangan, S. R. Increased therapeutic efficacy of zidovudine in combination with vitamin E. *Biochem. Biophys. Res. Commun.* 165: 401, 1989.

57. Hishinuma, I., and Nakamura, T. Alpha-tocopherol and inhibition of cytolysis in glutathione-depleted hepatocytes in primary culture. *J. Nutr. Sci. Vitaminol. (Tokyo)* 34: 11, 1988.

58. Leedle, R. A., and Aust, D. S. The effect of glutathione on the vitamin E requirement for inhibition of liver microsomal lipid peroxidation. *Lipids* 25: 241, 1990.

59. Pascoe, G. A., Olafsdottir, K., Reed, D. J. Vitamin E protection against chemical-induced cell injury. I. Maintenance of cellular protein thiols as a cytoprotective mechanism. *Arch. Biochem. Biophys.* 256: 150, 1987.

60. Odeleye, O. E., Eskelson, C. D., Mufti, S. I., Watson, R. R., Vitamin E protection against chemically-induced esophageal tumor growth in mice immunocompromised by retroviral infection. *Carcinogenesis* 13: 1811, 1992.

61. Corash, L. M., Sheetz, M., Bieri, J. G. Chronic hemolytic anemia due to glucose-6-phosphate dehydrogenase deficiency or glutathione synthetase deficiency: the role of vitamin E in its treatment. *Ann. NY. Acad. Sci.* 393: 348, 1982.

62. Sundstrom, H., Korpela, H., Sajanti, E. Supplementation with selenium, vitamin E and their combination in gynecological cancer during cytotoxic chemotherapy. *Carcinogenesis* 10: 273, 1989.

63. Costagliola, C., and Menzione, M. Effect of vitamin E on the oxidative state of glutathione in plasma. *Clin. Physiol. Biochem.* 8: 140, 1990.

64. U.S. Department of Health and Human Services. *Cancer Rates and Risks*, U.S. DHHS, 1985.

65. American Cancer Society. *Cancer Facts and Figures*, ACS, 1991.

66. Gopalakrishna, R., and Jaken, S. Protein Kinase C signaling and oxidative stress. *Free Rad. Biol. Med.* 28(9): 1349–1361, 2000.

67. Suziki, Y. J., Forman, H. J., Sevanian, A. Oxidants as stimulators of signal transduction. *Free Radic. Biol. Med.* 22: 269–285, 1997.

68. Meyer, M., Schreck, R., Muller, J. M., Baeuerle, P. A. Redox control of gene expression by eukaryotic transcription factors NF-$_k$B, AP-1 and SRF/TCF, in Pasquier, C., Auclair, C., Olivier, R. Y., Packer, L., eds. *Oxidative stress, cell activation and viral infection.* Switzerland: Birkhauser Verlag; 1994: 217–235.

69. Burdon, R. H. Superoxide and hydrogen peroxide in relation to mammalian cell proliferation. *Free Radic. Biol. Med.* 18: 775–794, 1995.

70. Sundaresan, M., Yu, Z., Farran, V. J., Irani, K., Finkel, T. Requirement of generation of H_2O_2 for platelet-derived growth factor signal transduction. *Science* 270: 296–299, 1995.

71. Bae, Y. S., Kang, S. W., Seo, M. S., Baines, I. C., Tekle, E., Chock, P. B., Rhee, S. G. Epidermal growth factor (EGF)-induced generation of hydrogen peroxide. *J. Biol. Chem.* 272: 217–221; 1997.

72. Borek, C., Ong, A., Mason, H., Donahue, L., Biaglow, J. E. Selenium and vitamin E inhibit radiogenic and chemically induced transformation *in vitro* via different mechanisms. *Proc. Natl. Acad. Sci.* 83: 1490, 1986.

73. Prasad, K. N., and Edwards-Prasad, J. Effects of tocopherol (vitamin E) acid succinate on morphological alterations and growth inhibition in melanoma cells in culture. *Cancer Res.* 42: 550, 1982.

74. Horvath, P. M., and Ip, C. Synergistic effect of vitamin E and selenium in the chemoprevention of mammary carcinogenesis in rats. *Cancer Res.* 43: 5335, 1983.

75. Cook, M. G., and McNamara, P. Effect of dietary vitamin E on dimethylhydrazine induced colonic tumors in mice. *Cancer Res.* 40: 1329, 1980.

76. Odeleye, O. E., Eskelson, C. D., Mufti, S. I., Watson, R. R. Vitamin E inhibition of lipid per-

oxidation and ethanol mediated promotion of esophageal tumorigenesis. *Nutr. Cancer* 17: 223, 1992.

77. Odukoya, O., Hawach, F., Shklar, G. Retardation of experimental oral cancer by topical vitamin E. *Nutr. Cancer* 6: 98, 1984.

78. Trickler, D., and Shklar, G. Prevention by vitamin E of experimental oral carcinogenesis. *J. Natl. Cancer Inst.* 78: 165, 1987.

79. Shklar, G., Schwartz, J., Tricklar, D., Kiukian, K. Regression by vitamin E of experimental oral cancer. *J. Natl. Cancer Inst.* 78: 987, 1987.

80. Shklar, G., and Schwartz, J. Tumor necrosis factor in experimental cancer regression with alpha-tocopherol, beta-carotene, canthaxanthin and algae extract. *Eur. J. Cancer Clin. Oncol.* 24: 839, 1988.

81. Shklar, G., Schwartz, J., Trickler, D., Reid, S. Regression of experimental cancer by oral administration of combined alpha-tocopherol and beta-carotene. *Nutr. Cancer* 12: 321, 1989.

82. Perchellet, J. P., Abney, N. L., Thomas, R. M., Guislain, Y. L., Perchellet, E. M. Effects of combined treatments with selenium, glutathione and vitamin E on glutathione peroxidase activity, ornithine decarboxylase induction, and complete and multistage carcinogenesis in mouse skin. *Cancer Res.* 47: 477, 1987.

83. Gerrish, K. E., and Gensler, H. L. Prevention of photocarcinogenesis by dietary vitamin E. *Nutr. Cancer* 19: 125, 1993.

84. Berton, T. R., Conti, C. J., Mitchell, D. L., Aldaz, C. M. Lubet, R. A. Fischer, S. M. The effect of vitamin E acetate on ultraviolet-induced mouse skin carcinogenesis. *Molecular Carcinogenesis* 23 (3): 175–84, 1998 Nov.

85. Shklar, G., Schwartz, J., Trickler, D., Reid, S. Prevention of experimental cancer and immunostimulation by vitamin E (immunosurveillance). *J. Oral Pathol. Med.* 19: 60, 64, 1990.

86. Horwitt, M. K. Interpretations of requirements for thiamin, riboflavin, niacin-tryptophan, and vitamin E plus comments on balance studies and vitamin B_6. *Am. J. Clin. Nutr.* 44: 973, 1986.

87. Yang, C., Sun, Y., Yang, Q., et al. Vitamin A and other deficiencies in Linxian, a high esophageal cancer incidence area in Northern China. *J. Natl. Cancer Inst.* 73: 1449, 1984.

88. Lee, C. J., and Wan, J. M. Vitamin E supplementation improves cell-mediated immunity and oxidative stress of Asian men and women. *J. Nutr.* 130: 2932–2937, 2000.

89. Benzie, I. F. F., Janus, E. D., Strain, J. J. Plasma ascorbate and vitamin E in Hong Kong Chinese. *Eur. J. Clin. Nutr.* 52: 447–451.

90. Wald, N., Thompson, S., Densem, J., et al. Serum vitamin E and subsequent risk of cancer. *Br. J. Cancer* 56: 69, 1987.

91. Knekt, P., Aromaa, A., Maatela, J., Aaran, R., Nikkari, T., Hakama, M., Hakulinen, T., Peto, R., Saxen, E., Teppo, L. Serum vitamin E and risk of cancer among Finnish men during a ten-year follow-up. *Am. J. Epidemiol.* 127: 28, 1988.

92. Knekt, P. Serum vitamin E level and risk of female cancers. *Int. J. Epidemiol.* 17: 281, 1988.

93. Menkes, M., Comstock, G., Vuilleumier, J., et al. Serum beta-carotene, vitamins A and E, selenium, and the risk of lung cancer. *N. Engl. J. Med.* 315: 1250, 1986.

94. Miyamoto, H., Araya, Y., Ito, M., et al. Serum selenium and vitamin E concentrations in families of lung cancer patients. *Cancer* 60: 1159, 1987.

95. Schwartz, J., and Shklar, G. The selective cytotoxic effect of carotenoids and alpha-tocopherol on human cancer cell lines *in vitro*. *J. Oral . Maxillofac. Surg.* 50: 367–373, 1992.

96. Malafa, M. P., and Neitzel, L. T. Vitamin E succinate promotes breast cancer tumor dormancy. *J. Surg. Res.* 93(1): 163–70, 2000.

97. Wang, Y. M., Purewal, M., Nixon, B., Li, D. H., Soltysiak-Pawluczuk, D. Vitamin E and Cancer prevention in an Animal Model. *Ann. NY. Acad. Science* 571: 383–390, 1989.

98. London, R., Sundaram, G., Schultz, M., et al. Endocrine parameters and alpha-tocopherol therapy of patients with mammary dysplasia. *Cancer Res.* 41: 3811, 1981.

99. Wald, N., Boreham, J., Hayward, J., Bulbrook, R. Plasma retinal, beta-carotene and vitamin E levels in relation to the future risk of breast cancer. *Br. J. Cancer* 49: 321, 1984.

100. Bohlke, K., Spiegelman, D., Trichopoulou, A., Katsouyanni, K., Trichopoulos, D. Vitamin A, C, and E and the risk of breast cancer: results from a case-control study in Greece. *British J. of Cancer* 79(1): 23–9, 1999.

101. Michels, K. B., Holmberg, L., Bergkvist, L., Ljung, H., Bruce, A., Wolk, A. Dietary antioxidant vitamins, retinol, and breast cancer incidence in a cohort of Swedish women. *Inter. J. of Cancer* 91(4): 563–7, 2001.

102. Kok, F. J., Van Duigin, C. M., Hofman, A., Vermeeren, R., De Bruinj, A. M., Valkenburg, H. A. Micronutrients and the risk of lung cancer. *N. Engl. J. Med.* 316: 1416, 1987.

103. Le Gardeur, B. Y., Lopez, S. A., Johnson, W. D. A case-control study of serum vitamins A, E and C in lung cancer patients. *Nutr. Cancer* 14: 133, 1990.

104. Mayne, S. T., Janerick, D. T., Greenwald, P., et al. Dietary beta-carotene and lung cancer risk in US nonsmokers. *J. Natl. Cancer Inst.* 1994; 86: 33–38.

105. The Alpha-tocopherol Beta-Carotene Cancer Prevention Study Group. The effect of vitamin E and beta-carotene on the incidence of lung cancer and other cancers in male smokers. *N. Engl. J. Med.* 1994; 330: 1029–35.

106. Palan, P. R., Mikhail, M. S., Basu, J., Romney, S. L. Plasma levels of antioxidant beta-carotene and alpha-tocopherol in uterine cervic dysplasias and cancer. *Nutr. Cancer* 15: 13, 1991.

107. Verreault, R., Chu, J., Mandelson, M., Shy, K. A case-control study of diet and invasive cervical cancer. *Int. J. Cancer* 43: 1050, 1989.

108. Gridley, G., McLaughlin, J. K., Block, G., Blot, W. J., Gluch, M., Fraumeni, J. F. Vitamin supplement use and reduced risk of oral and pharyngeal cancer. *Am. J. Epidemiol.* 135: 1083, 1992.

109. Buiatti, E., Palli, D., Decarli, A., Amadori, D., Avellini, C., Bianchi, S., Bonaguri, C., et al. A case-control study of gastric cancer and diet in Italy. II. Association with nutrients. *Int. J. Cancer* 45: 896, 1990.

110. Bendich, A., and Machlin, L. J. Safety of oral intake of vitamin E. *Am. J. Clin. Nutr.* 8: 612, 1988.

111. Machlin, L. J. Vitamin E, in *Handbook of Vitamins: Nutritional, Biochemical, and Clinical Aspects*, Machlin, L. J., Ed. Marcel Dekker. New York, 1988, 100.

112. Federation of American Societies for Experimental Biology (FASEB), Evaluation of the health aspects of tocopherols and alpha-tocopherol acetate as food ingredients. *FASEB*, Washington, DC, 1975.

113. Committee on Dietary Allowances, Food and Nutrition Board, National Research Council, *Recommended Dietary Allowances,* 10th ed. National Academy Press, Washington, DC, 1989.

114. Shoulson, I. Deprenyl and tocopherol antioxidative therapy of Parkinsonism (DATATOP) Parkinson Study Group. *Acta. Neurol. Scand. Suppl.* 126, 171, 1989.

115. The Parkinson Study Group. Effect of deprenyl on the progression of disability in early Parkinson's disease. *N. Engl. J. Med.* 321: 1364, 1989.

116. Miller, E. R., and Hayes, K. E. Vitamin excess and toxicity, in *Nutritional Toxicology*, Hathcock, J., Ed. Academic Press, New York, 1982, 81.

117. Meydani, S. N., Meydani, M., Blumberg, J. B., et al. Vitamin E supplementation enhances in vivo immune response in healthy elderly: a dose-responsive study. *JAMA* 1997; 277(17): 1380–6.

118. Weber, P., Bendich, A., Machlin, L. J. Vitamin E and human health: Rational for determining Recommended intake levels. *Nutrition* 13(5): 450–460, 1997.

119. Meydani, M., and Meisler, J. G. A closer look at vitamin E: can this antioxidant prevent chronic diseases? *Postgraduate Medicine* 102(2): 199–207, 1997.

120. Blot, W. J., Li, J. Y., Taylor, P. R., et al. Nutrition intervention trials in Linxian, China, supplementation with specific vitamin/mineral combinations, cancer incidence, and disease specific mortality in the general population. *J. Natl. Cancer Inst.* 1993; 85(18):1483–92.

121. Benner, S. E., Winn, R. W., Lippman, S. M., et al. Regression of oral leukoplakia with alpha-tocopherol: a community clinical oncology program chemoprevention study. *J. Natl. Cancer Inst.* 1993; 85:44.

122. Losonczy, K. G., Harris, T. B., Havlik, R. J. Vitamin E and vitamin C supplement use and risk of all-cause and coronary heart disease mortality in older persons: the established populations for epidemiologic studies of the elderly. *Am. J. Clin. Nutr.* 1996; 64(2): 190–6.

123. Polyp Prevention Study Group. A clinical trial of antioxidant vitamins to prevent colorectal adenoma. *N. Engl. J. Med.* 1994; 331(3):141–7.

124. Hennekens, C. H., Stampfer, M. J., Willet, W. Micronutrients and cancer chemoprevention. *Cancer Detect. Prev.* 7: 147, 1984.

125. Bailar, J. C., and Smith, E. M. Progress against cancer? *N. Engl. J. Med.* 314: 1226, 1986.

126. Greenwald, P., Nixon, D. W., Malone, W. F., Kelloff, G. J., Stern, H. R., Witkin, K. M. Concepts in cancer chemoprevention research. *Cancer* 65: 1483, 1990.

4

Chemical Versus Food Forms of Selenium in Cancer Prevention

Cindy D. Davis and
John W. Finley

INTRODUCTION

Selenium (Se) was discovered in 1817 by Berzelius who named it after Selene, the Greek goddess of the moon. The history of biomedical research on Se is intriguing. Initially, Se was considered only as a highly toxic element causing such signs in farm animals as loss of hooves and hair, emaciation, stiffness, and even death. However, the pioneering work of Schwartz and Foltz (1999) demonstrated the nutritional essentiality of Se when a component containing Se was found to prevent hepatic necrosis in vitamin E-deficient rats. Conclusive evidence for a metabolic role of Se came after the discovery that the element is an essential constituent of glutathione peroxidase (GSH-Px), an enzyme that protects against oxidative injury (Rotruck et al. 1973). Selenium was first associated with cancer risk over 30 years ago when Shamberger and Frost (1969) observed an inverse association between the geographic distribution of Se in forage crops and cancer mortality rates in the United States.

Selenium is in the same group of the periodic table as sulfur, and the two elements are metabolized similarly resulting in the substitution of Se for sulfur in the sulfur-amino acids to form the Se analogues selenomethionine (SeMet) and selenocysteine (SeCys) (Lockitch 1989). These amino acids, particularly SeMet, comprise the predominant forms of Se in food (Levander 1983), although most foods are a mixture of multiple Se species. Inorganic Se salts such as selenite and selenate generally only enter the diet through supplements.

Most of the known metabolic functions of Se are associated with specific selenoproteins. In mammals, Se is covalently bound in all selenoproteins as the amino acid SeCys (Hatfield et al. 1999). The synthesis of selenoproteins is accomplished by an elaborate mechanism that involves activation of inorganic selenide to a selenophosphate (Glass et al. 1993) followed by transfer of the Se to a three-carbon intermediate at the level of transfer RNA to form SeCys (Stadtman 1996). Hydrogen selenide (H_2Se) is the obligate precursor for selenoprotein synthesis and this metabolite can be produced from several different food forms of Se.

SE IN DIET AND FOOD

For most individuals, diet is the primary source of Se; however, drinking water, and occupational and environmental pollution may be additional sources of exposure. Average Se intake in most countries ranges from about 30 to 200 µg/day, although lower and higher values may also occur (Vinceti et al. 2000).

Because of the unique metabolic routes of different forms of Se (see next section), specific information on the form of Se in a food would be useful in predicting the biopotency of Se-enriched foods. Characterization of the chemical form of Se in foods is hampered by methodological problems. The primary method currently in use is reverse phase liquid chromatography coupled to an inductively coupled plasma argon mass spectrometer (Ip et al. 2000a, Zheng et al. 2000). A major limitation to this method is a lack of sufficient standards.

Wheat and meat are the primary sources of dietary Se. Se in wheat is commonly considered to be almost completely SeMet, but there have been comparatively few attempts to completely speciate all forms of Se (Olson et al. 1970). Also the reports cited most often are old and used relatively crude analytical methods.

The form of Se in edible muscle meats depends on the form of Se supplied to the animal (Beilstein and Whanger 1986, van Ryssen et al. 1989, Whanger and Butler 1988) and, therefore, is affected by feedstuffs supplied to the animal as well as production practices. Meat from animals supplied only salts of Se (i.e., selenite and selenate) will contain primarily SeCys with minimal or no SeMet because there are no enzymes capable of converting selenide to SeMet. However, meat from animals fed SeMet will contain mixtures of both SeCys and SeMet.

Other food forms of Se have been used in cancer chemoprevention studies. Selenium-enriched yeast has been used in intervention studies (Clark et al. 1996). This so-called "selenized" yeast is often erroneously labeled as SeMet, but actual analyses have demonstrated that a substantial portion (about 15%) of it occurs in other forms such as selenite, selenolanthionine, SeCys, selenocystathionine, SeMSC, gamma-glutamyl-SeMSC, and Se-adenosyl selenohomocysteine (Ip et al. 2000a). Garlic that can accumulate very high concentrations (more than 1300 mg/g of Se) using fertilization contains mainly Se-methyl-selenocysteine (SeMSC) with minor amounts of SeCys and SeMet (Cai et al. 1995). In contrast, garlic that accumulates moderately high concentrations of Se (< 300 mg Se/g) contains 73% of total Se as gamma-glutamyl SeMSC and 13% of Se as SeMet (Ip et al. 2000a). High-Se broccoli produced with selenate-fertilization has SeMSC as the major Se-component of that broccoli with substantial amounts of selenite and selenate (Finley et al., unpublished observations).

SE METABOLISM

The chemical form of Se can be a determinant of its metabolism and its ultimate in vivo function. A generalized scheme of Se metabolism is shown in Figure 4.1. The metabolism of Se comprises four major pathways: (1) metabolism analogous to the sulfur amino acids, (2) reduction to hydrogen selenide (H_2Se) that utilizes glutathione, (3) formation of

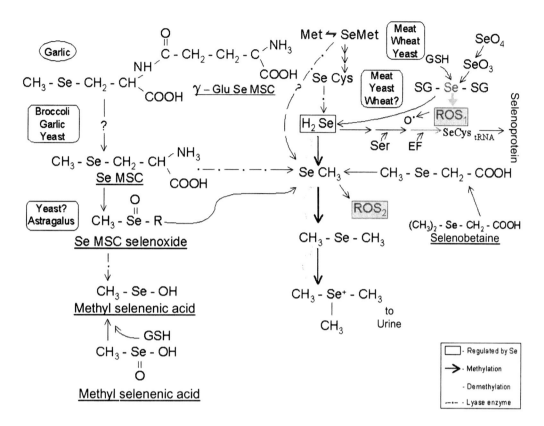

Figure 4.1.   Metabolism of different chemical forms of selenium. SeMet is incorporated into proteins or converted to SeCys. SeCys is metabolized to H$_2$Se. Selenate and selenite combine with GSH to form H$_2$Se. Hydrogen selenide can either be utilized as a precursor for the synthesis of selenoproteins or undergo a series of methylation steps to form methyl selenol (HSeCH$_3$, which has been associated with cancer suppression), dimethyl selenide (expired in the breath), or tri-methyl selenonium ion (which is excreted in the urine). SeMSC is a direct precursor of HSeCH$_3$. Selenobetaine may be metabolized to dimethyl selenide.

selenoproteins, and (4) methylation that produces tri-methyl selenonium ion for urinary excretion.

Selenomethionine (SeMet) may substitute for methionine (Met) in general body proteins because eukaryotic cells are not able to discriminate between Met and SeMet. When protein turns over, SeMet is released and a certain portion may continue this cycle. An alternative fate is for SeMet to move into the trans-sulfuration pathway and form selenocysteine (SeCys). Although SeCys is found at the active site of selenoproteins, preformed SeCys cannot be incorporated into selenoproteins. However, it is currently unknown whether SeCys may substitute for Cys in general body proteins. Preformed SeCys also may be metabolized by a specific lyase to H$_2$Se.

Oxygen anions of Se follow a reductive pathway to H$_2$Se. Selenate is first non-enzymatically converted to selenite using reducing equivalents from glutathione (GSH). Selenite then undergoes a sequence of reactions that require reduced GSH and reduced nicotinamide adenine dinucleotide phosphate (NADPH) to form selenodiglutathione. The selenodiglutathione is further metabolized by glutathione reductase and NADPH to form H_2Se. Once H_2Se is formed, it may enter either the pathway that results in selenoprotein biosynthesis or the methylation pathway in preparation for respiratory and/or urinary excretion.

Selenoprotein biosynthesis has been extensively reviewed (Burk and Hill 1993, Gladyshev and Hatfield 1999, Sunde 1990) and only a short overview is presented here. The formation of selenoproteins is a rigorously controlled process with a unique biological pathway that requires several unique protein and RNA factors. Hydrogen selenide reacts with the beta carbon of a serine already attached to a unique transfer RNA (tRNA[Sec]) that is capable of being joined to L-serine and possesses an anticodon complementary to UGA. This reaction is thought to proceed via a selenophosphate intermediate, and it results in the formation of tRNA-bound SeCys. This tRNA incorporates the SeCys into the growing polypeptide chain by using UGA as the insertion codon. The latter step requires the presence of a specific elongation factor; otherwise, UGA functions as a stop codon. In the presence of Se, the elongation factor binds to a stem-loop structure and facilitates the positioning of the tRNA over the UGA codon, thus forcing the polypeptide to accept SeCys. In the absence of Se, the elongation factor does not bind and the ribosome reads the UGA as a termination signal.

Over a dozen selenoproteins have been characterized and several families of them have been identified. Mammalian selenoproteins include glutathione peroxidases, thyroid hormone deiodinases, thioredoxin reductases, selenophosphate synthetase, selenoprotein P, selenoprotein W, and a 15-kd selenoprotein. A common feature among mammalian selenoproteins is that each appears to regulate and/or be regulated by intra- and/or extracellular redox processes (Gladyshev and Hatfield 1999). Nature may have taken advantage of utilizing SeCys at critical sites in certain enzymes because of the unique redox properties of Se (Boyington et al. 1997). Selenocysteine is capable of oxidation to the seleninic acid and then being reduced to the selenol by reduced glutathione. Although SeCys is structurally similar to cysteine, the Se in that molecule is a better nucleophile than the analagous sulfur and SeCys is ionized at physiological pH, while cysteines typically are protonated (Hatfield et al. 1999, Stadtman 1996).

The amount of H_2Se that does not enter the selenoprotein synthetic pathway enters a methylation pathway and ultimately results in excretion of Se in the urine. A specific methyl transferase catalyzes the formation of methylselenol from H_2Se; formation of methylselenol is necessary for the chemopreventive effects of Se (Ip 1998). Sequential methylation reactions produce dimethyl selenide (volatilized through the breath at very high intakes of Se) and ultimately the tri-methyl selenonium ion, which is excreted in urine.

Some seleno-compounds enter the methylation pathway without first forming H_2Se. A specific lyase may cleave SeMSC to directly form methylselenol. Selenobetaine may be metabolized directly to dimethylselenide. Tri-phenolic synthetic Se-compounds are probably metabolized directly to the tri-methylselenonium ion.

Specific lyases are needed to cleave terminal Se groups in many Se metabolic pathways (Soda et al. 1999). Beta-lyases cleave between the beta-carbon and Se, thus removing

H_2Se from SeCys. Ip et al. (2000a) demonstrated that methylselenic acid, a putative metabolite of SeMSC, was much more effective for inhibiting cell growth and stimulating apoptosis in TM12 and TM2H mouse mammary hyperplastic epithelial cells than SeMSC. Because these cells have very low beta-lyase activities, these findings indicated that beta-lyase activity is essential for the anticarcinogenic effect of SeMSC. A gamma-methionine lyase has been found in bacteria that catalyzes removal of methylselenol from SeMet (Soda et al. 1999). Although there is no indication that this enzyme occurs in mammals, the finding raises the possibility that undigested SeMet in the colon may be acted on by gut bacteria resulting in methylselenol production. This finding may explain the observation that a high-Se whole wheat product containing primarily SeMet was as protective against carcinogen-induced aberrant crypts, a preneoplastic lesion for colon cancer, as high-Se broccoli containing primarily SeMSC (Finley and Davis 2001). There also is an early report that an enzyme in cabbage leaf is able to cleave selenomethionine (Lewis et al. 1971), leaving open the possibility that mastication may begin metabolism of the compound.

EVIDENCE FOR ANTICARCINOGENIC EFFECTS OF SE—HUMAN STUDIES

Evidence for cancer-protective effects of Se in humans was initially obtained by means of ecological and correlational studies. Geographic correlation data in different regions worldwide and in the United States have noted an inverse association between Se levels in forage crops or diet and cancer mortality in the same area (Clark et al. 1991, Schrauzer et al. 1977, Shamberger et al. 1976, Yu et al. 1985). Furthermore, statistically significant inverse associations were obtained when cancer mortalities were correlated with the blood Se levels of healthy donors in different U.S. cities (Shamberger and Willis 1971), as well as with the apparent dietary Se intakes in different countries (Schrauzer et al. 1977). In China, the mean Se concentrations in blood samples drawn from healthy adults in 24 regions were compared to the corresponding cancer mortality rates. Strong and significant inverse correlations were observed for overall cancer mortality ($r = -0.62$), particularly for stomach and esophagus (Yu et al. 1985). These and subsequent studies (Burguera et al. 1990, Chen et al. 1992, Chu et al. 1984, Clark et al. 1991, Cogwill 1983, Schrauzer and White 1978, Yu et al. 1985) suggested significant protective effects of Se against major forms of cancer. However, other dietary and nondietary factors that differ among these regions might account for the association with Se.

Subsequently, a number of case-control studies were performed to investigate the correlation between Se status and cancer susceptibility. In these studies, Se levels in blood, serum, hair, or toenails were compared between healthy subjects and those of cancer patients. In most cases, a lower Se status in patients compared with controls was reported (Broghamer et al. 1976, Calautti et al. 1980, Fex et al. 1987, Gerhardsson et al. 1985, Glattre et al. 1989, Hardell et al. 1993, Hojo 1981, Itoh and Kikuchi 1997, Krishnaswamy et al. 1993, McConnell et al. 1975, McConnell et al. 1980, McConnell et al. 1987, Persson-Moschos et al. 2000, Psathakis et al. 1998, Russo et al. 1997, Schrauzer et al. 1985, Shamberger et al. 1973, Subramaniam et al. 1993, Sundstrom et al. 1986, Toma et al. 1991, van der Brandt et al. 1993a, van der Brandt et al. 1993b, Willett et al. 1983, Yoshizawa et al. 1998, Zachara et al. 1997). However, a few case-control studies detected either no difference between the two groups (Broghamer et al. 1978, Mannisto et al. 2000, Nelson et al. 1985, Robinson et al. 1979, Rogers et al. 1991, Shultz and Leklem 1983, Vernie et al. 1983) or even higher tissue Se in cancer patients (Glattre et al. 1989).

The inverse associations between short-term biomarkers of Se exposure, such as serum or plasma Se levels, and cancer stage and progression observed in some case-control studies have suggested that Se status can be utilized in the diagnosis and the prognosis of cancer (Avanzini et al. 1995, Deffuant et al. 1994). Some cohort studies have indicated that subjects with preclinical disease may also have lower serum Se concentrations because these studies have shown that subjects had lower serum Se concentrations 4 to 7 years prior to the appearance of lung (Knekt et al. 1998) or thyroid tumors (Glattre et al. 1989). However, other studies have found no association between serum Se concentrations and preclinical disease (Batieha et al. 1993, Breslow et al. 1995, Burney et al. 1989, Coates et al. 1988, Helzlsouer et al. 1989, Schober et al. 1987, van der Brandt et al. 1993a, and van der Brandt et al. 1993b).

Although these studies demonstrate low Se levels in certain cancer patients, it does not necessarily mean that low Se levels are a risk factor for cancer. Because Se levels were determined after the diagnosis of cancer, the lower Se levels may be a reflection of Se sequestration by the tumor, other metabolic consequences of the tumor, or poor dietary Se intake. Thus, low Se status may be a consequence of the illness, rather than a cause of cancer. Selenium can become concentrated in certain tumors, depriving the host tissues and perhaps thereby reducing circulating levels. This effect has been observed in animal models (Baumgartner et al. 1978) and in human tumors (Rizk and Sky-Peck 1984, Zachara et al. 1997).

Prospective studies, in which the tissue samples are collected before the onset of the disease, avoid many of the potential problems described above for case-control studies. However, the major disadvantage of prospective studies is that, even over a moderately extended period of time, the risk of any given individual developing cancer is generally quite low. Thus, samples must be taken from a large number of individuals who must then be followed over several years for onset of the disease to allow for an adequate sample size.

In prospective studies, low Se status has been associated with significant increased risks of cancer incidence and mortality. Risk has been from twofold to sixfold higher in the lowest tertile or quintile of serum Se concentration (Clark et al. 1993, Kok et al. 1987, Salonen et al. 1984, Virtami et al. 1987). Salonen et al. (1985) indicated that the adjusted risk of death was 5.8-fold in the lowest tertile of serum Se concentration compared with those with higher values. Clark et al. (1993) found in a cohort of 1738 Americans that initial plasma Se concentration was inversely related to subsequent risk of both non-melanoma skin cancer and colonic adenomatous polyps. Patients with plasma Se levels less than the population median (128 ng/mL) were four times more likely to have one or more adenomatous polyps and had more than three times the number of polyps per patient. A prospective study on the association between Se intake and prostate cancer involved 34,000 men from the Health Professionals' Cohort Study (Yoshizawa et al. 1998). Those in the lowest quintile of Se status, as measured by toenail Se, were found to have three times the likelihood of developing advanced prostate cancer as those in the highest quintile (P for trend = 0.03). Only cases diagnosed more than two years after collection of the samples were counted. In contrast, a study by Coates et al. (1988) failed to detect significant associations between serum Se concentration and subsequent risk of cancer and Hunter et al. (1990) did not find a relationship between toenail Se concentrations and risk of breast cancer in the Nurses' Health Study Cohort.

There have been few intervention trials looking at Se supplementation without supplementing other nutrients. In an intervention trial conducted in China, a community of about 21,000 was supplemented with selenite-fortified salt from 1985 through 1992, and residents of the community experienced a 35% drop in the incidence of primary liver cancer (Yu et al. 1997). In a study in which 226 hepatitis B antigen carriers were randomized to either 200 µg of Se-enriched yeast or a placebo, no cases of hepatocellular carcinoma occurred in the supplemented group after 4 years of supplementation, while seven cases of hepatocellular carcinoma occurred in the placebo group (Yu et al. 1997).

The Nutritional Prevention of Cancer Trial, carried out by Clark and coworkers (1996) in the United States, was the first double-blind, placebo-controlled intervention trial in a western population, designed to test the hypothesis that Se supplementation would reduce the risk of cancer. This study involved 1312 patients who were recruited because of a recent history of basal cell and/or squamous cell carcinoma of the skin. Supplementation of 200 µg Se/day did not significantly affect the incidence of basal cell or squamous cell skin cancer; however, Se supplementation significantly reduced total cancer mortality, and incidences of lung, colorectal, and prostate cancers.

Another clinical trial is being conducted to assess the role of Se in chemoprevention of prostate cancer. The SELECT (Se, vitamin E Chemoprevention Trial) is a 2×2 factorial double-blind randomized study to assess the efficacy of vitamin E and Se in preventing prostate cancer.

EVIDENCE FOR ANTICARCINOGENIC EFFECTS OF SE—ANIMAL STUDIES

Laboratory animal model studies support the epidemiologic evidence and demonstrate that Se supplementation in the diet or drinking water inhibits initiation and/or postinitiation stages of liver, esophageal, pancreatic, colon, and mammary carcinogenesis (Baines et al. 2000, Birt et al. 1986, Chen et al. 2000b, Dias et al. 2000, Griffin and Jacobs 1977, Ip and Ganther 1996, Ip and Lisk 1994a, Jacobs et al. 1981, Thirunavukkarasu and Sakthisekaran 2001) (Table 4.1). Perinatal Se exposure has been shown to decrease spontaneous liver tumorigenesis in CBA mice (Popova 2002).

The chemopreventive effect of Se depends on its chemical form. For example, it was recently observed that 3,2'-dimethyl-4-aminobiphenyl (DMABP)-induced aberrant crypt formation (a preneoplastic lesion for colon cancer) decreased significantly in rats supplemented with 0.1 or 2.0 mg Se/kg diet as selenite or selenate, but not as SeMet, compared

Table 4.1.   Examples of the Protective Effect of Supplemental Selenium on Carcinogenesis in Animal Models

Form of selenium[1]	Carcinogen[2]	Organ	Reference
BSC	AOM	Colon	Fiala et al. 1991; Kawamori et al. 1998; Reddy et al. 1996
Diallyl selenide	DMBA	Mammary	El-Bayoumy et al. 1996
Se-allylselenocysteine	MNU	Mammary	Ip et al. 1999
Selenobetaine	DMBA	Mammary	Ip and Ganther 1990
SeCys	DMBA	Mammary	Ip et al. 1991
Selenate	DMABP	Colon	Feng et al. 1999
Selenite	AOM	Colon	Reddy et al. 1996
Selenite	BOP	Pancreas	Birt et al. 1986
Selenite	DEN	Liver	Thirunavukkarasu and Sakthisekaran 2001
Selenite	DMABP	Colon	Feng et al. 1999
Selenite	DMBA	Mammary	Chidambaram and Baradarajan 1994; Dias et al. 2000; Ip et al. 1991
Selenite	DMH	Colon	Jacobs et al. 1981; Jao et al. 1996
Selenite	MNU	Mammary	Ip et al. 1999
Selenite	MeDAB	Liver	Griffin and Jacobs 1977
Selenite	Spontaneous	Liver	Popova 2002
Selenoxide	DMBA	Mammary	Ip et al. 1991
SeMet	AOM	Colon	Baines et al. 2000
SeMSC	DMBA	Mammary	Ip et al. 1991
SeMSC	MNU	Mammary	Ip et al. 1999
Se-propylselenocysteine	MNU	Mammary	Ip et al. 1999
Triphenylselenonium	DMBA	Mammary	Ip et al. 1994
Triphenylselenonium	NMU	Mammary	Ip et al. 1994
p-XSC	AOM	Colon	Rao et al. 2001; Reddy et al. 1996
p-XSC	Benzo[a]pyrene	Forestomach	El-Bayoumy 1985
p-XSC	DMBA	Mammary	El-Bayoumy et al. 1993, 1995; Ip et al. 1994
P-XSC	NNK	Lung	El-Bayoumy et al. 1995; Prokopczyk et al. 1997
p-XSC	NQO	Oral	Tanaka et al. 1997
p-XSe-SG	AOM	Colon	Rao et al. 2001

[1] p-XSC = 1,4-phenylenebis(methylene)selenocyanate; p-XSe-SG = glutathione conjugate of p-XSC.
[2] Carcinogens are abbreviated as follows: AOM = azoxymethane; BOP = n-nitrosobis(2-oxopropyl)amine; DEN = N-nitrosodiethylamine; BSC = benzylselenocyanate; DMABP = 3,2′-dimethyl-4-aminobiphenyl; DMBA = 7,12-dimethylbenzanthracene; DMH = dimethylhydrazine; MEDAB = 3′-methyl-4-dimethylaminoazobenzene; MNU = methylnitrosurea; NNK = 4-(methylnitrosamino)-1-(3-pyridyl)-1-butanone; NQO = 4-nitroquinoline-1-oxide.

to animals fed a Se deficient diet (Feng et al. 1999). The lack of an effect of SeMet on aberrant crypt formation may be related to the fact that SeMet can readily acylate met-tRNA and be incorporated into proteins in place of Met, thus being diverted from the direct formation of the putative anticarcinogenic metabolite methylselenol. In the study by Feng et al. (1999), colonic Se concentrations of rats fed SeMet were more than twofold higher than those of rats fed comparable levels of Se as selenite or selenate, a finding consistent with the incorporations of SeMet into the general protein pool. Ip (1988) observed that 3.0 mg Se/kg diet but not 2.0 mg Se/kg diet as SeMet was protective against mammary cancer and that low dietary Met decreased the biological activities (both glutathione peroxidase activity and anticarcinogenic efficacy) of SeMet but not those of selenite. Thus, when Met is limiting, a greater percentage of SeMet is sequestered into general body proteins and not available for the formation of selenoproteins or metabolism to anticarcinogenic metabolites (Ip 1988). It is believed that long-term feeding of SeMet, even when Met is limiting, should allow the establishment of an equilibrium between protein anabolism and catabolism so that SeMet would be available for selenoproteins or for further metabolism to anticarcinogenic metabolites. Future studies are needed to test this hypothesis. However, Reddy et al. (2000) found that 55 weeks of feeding a diet containing 3.6 and 5.4 mg Se/kg diet as SeMet did not affect AOM-induced colon carcinogenesis. This might also suggest that SeMet is more protective against mammary than colon cancer in experimental animals. SeMet was also more effective than selenite or SeCys in prolonging survival of Dalton's lymphoma-bearing mice (Mukhopadhyay-Sardar et al. 2000).

Ip and coworkers (1991) conducted a series of studies focused on finding less-toxic forms of Se that would retain chemopreventive activity. They observed that SeMSC > selenite > SeCys > selenoxide for the inhibition of mammary tumors. From that work, monomethylated forms of Se have emerged as a critical class of Se metabolites having powerful effects on carcinogenesis, while lacking some of the toxic effects produced by other forms such as inorganic selenite (Ip 1998, Ganther and Lawrence 1997).

Some investigators have also focused on the development of new organoselenium compounds that have a high efficacy as cancer chemopreventive agents, yet are much better tolerated than the traditional Se compounds, such as selenite or SeMet. Ideally, such agents would be employed to inhibit tumor development in different organs caused by a variety of chemical carcinogens, particularly those present in the human environment (El-Bayoumy et al. 1996). Bioassays using various animal tumor models have demonstrated that benzyl selenocyanate (BSC), 1,4-phenylenebis(methylene)selenocyanate (p-XSC), and related organoselenium compounds are effective in protecting against chemically induced tumorigenesis, including azoxymethane-induced colon tumors (Fiala et al. 1991, Rao et al. 2001, Reddy et al. 1996, Nayini et al. 1991, Reddy et al. 1992) 7,12-dimethylbenz[a]anthracene (DMBA)-induced mammary tumors (Chae et al. 1997, El-Bayoumy et al. 1995, Ip et al. 1994, El-Bayoumy et al. 1992), benzo[a]pyrene-induced forestomach tumors (El-Bayoumy et al. 1985), 4-(methylnitrosoamino)-1-(3-pyridyl)-1-butanone (NNK)-induced lung tumors (El-Bayoumy et al. 1993, Prokopczyk et al. 1997), and 4-nitroquinoline-1-oxide-induced oral cancer (Tanaka et al. 1997). Besides inhibiting tumorigenesis, recent studies have suggested that p-XSC can inhibit pulmonary metastasis of B16BL6 melanoma cells and inhibit the growth of these metastatic tumors in the lung, in part by inducing apoptosis (Tanaka et al. 2000). It should be noted that the Se from p-XSC is not well utilized as a source of Se for GSH-Px (Ip et al. 1994) indicating that the antitumorigenicity of p-XSC is not coupled to the nutritional role of Se in supporting the expression of selenoproteins (Combs and Gray 1998).

MECHANISMS FOR THE CHEMOPREVENTIVE EFFECTS OF SE

Potential interactions between Se and the cancer process may affect the phases of initiation, promotion, and progression. Many potential mechanisms have been advanced and Figures 4.2 and 4.3 summarize these mechanisms. Although mechanistic studies are ongoing and are yielding valuable information, there is an increasing consensus that Se may exert its effects at multiple levels. Combs and Gray (1998) have proposed a three-stage model for the biological action of Se. During Se deficiency, addition of small amounts of Se to the diet increases the activity of selenoproteins, improves immune function, and may regulate Phase I and Phase II metabolic enzymes. Supra-nutritional amounts of Se probably exert their effects via completely different pathways, and the primary targets are probably control of the cell cycle, apoptosis, and angiogenesis. Finally, very high concentrations of Se can be directly cytotoxic.

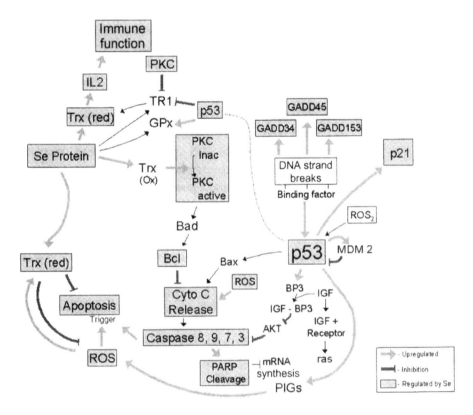

Figure 4.2.   Selenium as a regulator of apoptosis. Reactive oxygen species produced from the metabolism of selenium salts with GSH cause apoptosis by both p53 dependent and independent mechanisms. Induction of p53 will reduce TR but increase GSH-Px activity. ROS can down regulate PKC activity by oxidizing cysteine residues. Reduction of the cysteine residues on PKC is accomplished by reduced thioredoxin (Trx_{red}), which is accomplished by TR. Shaded areas might be influenced by Se.

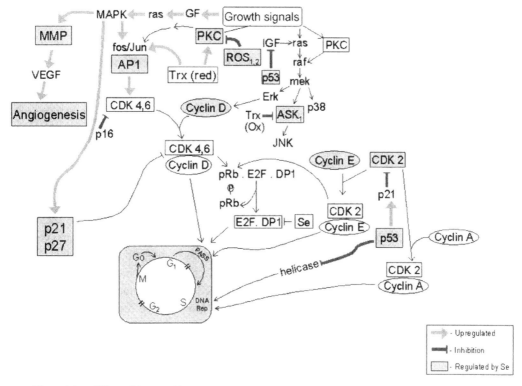

Figure 4.3.   Effect of Se on cell cycle regulation. Selenium may regulate expression of the cyclins p53, p21, p27, cdk2, and PKC to control cell cycle progression. Selenium may stimulate MAPK signaling pathways leading to suppression of angiogenesis.

Selenoprotein Production

It has been stated that the reduction in cancer by Se is not necessarily related to increases in the activity of selenoproteins (Ip et al. 1991) because the amounts of Se needed for chemoprevention are much larger than the amount of Se needed to maximize GSH-Px activity (Combs et al. 2001). Despite these data, there is increasing evidence that selenoproteins may indeed play a role in chemoprevention. First, while GSH-Px activity does plateau at a fairly low intake of Se, thioredoxin reductase (TR) activity can be influenced by chemopreventive levels of Se (Ganther 1999). For example, using rats fed a moderately high level (1 μg Se/g) of Se as selenite, TR activity increased approximately twofold in some tissues (lung, liver and kidney) but not in others, in comparison with rats fed a normal Se level (0.1 μg Se/g). In contrast to TR, GSH-Px activity was not increased by the high Se level in any tissue (Berggren et al. 1999). Also, there is increasing evidence that many of the putative effects of Se on cell cycle control and apoptosis are mediated via reactive oxygen species (ROS), and intracellular ROS are regulated by several selenoproteins including TR and the GSH-Px family of proteins. For example, Fu et al. (2001a and 2001b) demonstrated that diquat induced apoptosis in hepatocytes null for GSH-Px1 but not in wild type cells; however, GSH-Px status did not affect the cells susceptibility to reactive nitrogen species (Fu et al. 2001a, Fu et al. 2001b). Brigelius-Flohe et al. (2001) have proposed a major antioxidant role for gastrointestinal glutathione peroxidase in protection against food-borne hydroperoxides, redox-regulation of proliferation or apoptosis, and modulation of mucosal immunity. A previous report had suggested a similar role for phospholipid hydroperoxide glutathione peroxidase (Brigelius-Flohe et al. 2000), thus suggesting that selenoprotein production may play a role in the chemopreventive effects of Se.

The role of TR in carcinogenesis is perplexing because many of the biological effects of thioredoxin are growth stimulatory and may actually promote tumor development (Arner and Holmgren 2000, Becker et al. 2000, Powis et al. 1997). However, TR can also be protective against oxidative stress. Thioredoxin reductase has been reported to reduce methylated selenium compounds that may result in production of oxygen radicals (Gromer and Gross 2002). Furthermore, TR activity increases with increased Se status, which could benefit the cell by reducing oxidative stress (Ganther 1999). Thioredoxin reductase has been found to protect against oxidative stress in cultured human umbilical-vein endothelial cells (Anema et al. 1999) and this protection may be mediated by protein kinase C (PKC). Protein kinase C can also be influenced by selenoprotein status because its activity depends on reduction of sulfhydryls of surface cysteine residues by reduced thioredoxin, and TR is the only known mechanism of reducing thioredoxin (Gopalakrishna and Gundimeda 2001)

Carcinogen Metabolism and DNA Adduct Formation

Because Se has been shown to be protective against chemical carcinogenesis in animal models, many studies have investigated the effect of Se on carcinogen metabolism and DNA adduct formation. A number of studies have suggested that most of the chemical carcinogens in the environment are not active themselves in interacting with intracellular DNA but induce tumors only after metabolic activation by a variety of drug-metabolizing enzymes including cytochrome P-450 and phase II enzymes (Nelson et al. 1996, Pelkonen and Nebert 1982). Several studies suggest that dietary Se may affect activity of these enzymes and alter carcinogen metabolism (Arciszewska et al. 1982, Marshall et al. 1979) perhaps by altering cytochrome P-450 metabolism (Burk and Masters 1975, Shimada et al. 1997, Wrighton and Elswick 1989).

Activated carcinogens are able to covalently bind to DNA. The formation of carcinogen-induced DNA adducts is believed to be necessary for initiation of chemical carcinogenesis. Carcinogen-DNA adducts may distort the shape of the DNA molecule, potentially causing mistranslations or, when the DNA replicates, an adducted base can be misread, which causes a mutation in the new strand. Furthermore, repair of bulky adducts can result in DNA strand breaks that may result in mutations or deletions of genetic material.

Selenite, p-XSC, Se-enriched mushrooms, and Se-enriched garlic inhibit the formation of DMBA-DNA adducts in the mammary gland (Ejadi et al. 1989, El-Bayoumy et al. 1992, Ip and Lisk 1997, Liu et al. 1991, Spolar et al. 1999, Upadhyaya and El-Bayoumy 1998). Ip and Lisk (1997) observed that Se-enriched garlic did not significantly alter P-

450 1A1 (responsible for DMBA activation), 1A2, 2B1, 2E1 and 3A4; however, the phase II enzymes, glutathione S-transferase and uridine 5′-diphosphate-glucuronyltransferase activities were significantly elevated in liver and kidney. Consequently, an increased detoxification of carcinogens via the phase II conjugating enzymes might represent a mechanism of tumor suppression by Se-enriched garlic (Ip and Lisk 1997).

Selenite and p-XSC have been shown to inhibit NNK-induced DNA adducts in lungs and livers of female A/J mice and male Fischer-344 rats (Prokopczyk et al. 1996). Wortzman et al. (1980) demonstrated that selenite inhibited DNA adduct formation with 2-acetylaminofluorene, a liver carcinogen, in rat liver. Similar findings were observed with aflatoxin, another liver carcinogen in rats (Chen et al. 1982a). Se supplementation did not affect cytochrome P-450 content but did cause increased glucoronyl transferase activity, and adduct formation was more consistently related to transferase activity than to mixed function oxidase activities (Chen et al. 1982a). In humans, plasma Se concentrations were found to be significantly associated with an increased level of aflatoxin-albumin adducts in men in Southeastern China (Chen et al. 2000a). However, in contrast, selenite enhanced aflatoxin-induced DNA adduct formation in chicken liver (Chen et al. 1982b).

Supplementation with either 0.1 or 2.0 mg Se/kg diet as either selenite or selenate but not as SeMet resulted in significantly fewer (53–70%, $p < 0.05$) 3,2′-dimethyl-4-amino-biphenyl (DMABP)-DNA adducts in the colon, but not in the liver, than in rats fed a Se-deficient diet (Davis et al. 1999). This reduction in DMABP-DNA adduct formation in the colon correlated with a reduction in DMABP-induced aberrant crypt foci. The protective effect of selenite and selenate against DMABP-DNA adduct formation apparently is not a result of alterations in plasma or liver Se concentrations, GSH-Px, or glutathione transferase activities, but may be related to differences in the metabolism of the different forms of Se (Davis et al. 1999).

Fiala et al. (1991) observed that benzylselenocyanate (BSC) reduced DNA methylation in the colon but not in the liver of rats treated with the colon carcinogen azoxymethane. This is in good agreement with the inhibitory action of BSC on azoxymethane-induced colon carcinogenesis (Reddy et al. 1987). Thus, the observed inhibitory effects of Se compounds on DNA adduct formation are consistent with their ability to inhibit carcinogenesis in laboratory animals (El-Bayoumy 2001).

Selenium as a Regulator of Apoptosis and Cell Cycle Arrest

Selenium appears to have important roles in regulating the cell cycle and induction of programmed cell death, or apoptosis. Studies investigating the mechanism for the effect of Se on apoptosis are limited by a paucity of studies focusing on a specific mechanism. Also, the studies have been conducted in many diverse models with equally diverse techniques. Despite these limitations, the literature suggests that there appears to be separate pathways that result in either apoptosis or cell cycle arrest, and these pathways appear to be connected to specific chemical forms of Se. Other reviews have covered much of this topic and this review is not intended to be exhaustive, rather it is intended to concentrate on differences related to the chemical form of Se.

There appear to be four possible cell cycle/apoptotic regulatory mechanisms of Se: (1) Selenium in the reductive pathway to selenide, especially seleno-diglutathione and H_2Se, induces irreversible apoptosis with DNA strand breaks (Fig. 4.2). (2) Selenium in the methylation pathway appears to induce cell cycle arrest and/or apoptosis independent of DNA strand breaks. Mechanisms 1 and 2 may be either p53-dependent or p53-independent. (3) Selenium may induce global changes in the mitogen activated cell signaling pathway (Fig. 4.3). (4) Some forms of Se may be directly cytotoxic. The mechanism that initiates the above regulatory changes is still unknown, but activation of PKC and control of ROS are favored theories.

1. Selenium in the reductive pathway to selenide, especially diglutathione selenide, induces irreversible apoptosis with DNA strand breaks.

Selenite enters a reductive metabolic pathway that results in the formation of a complex with GSH and conversion to selenide. Selenium species in this pathway are known to be highly reactive and result in the formation of ROS. Because ROS are very damaging to DNA, it has been suggested that ROS produced by reactions of Se compounds in this pathway (i.e., selenite, selenium dioxide, and diselenides) with GSH, mediate Se-responsive cell cycle regulation (Davis et al. 1998, Spallholz 1994, Spallholz 1997, Spallholz et al. 2001, Stewart et al. 1999). This regulation may be mediated by DNA strand breaks and result in an irreversible decision for apoptosis rather than cell cycle arrest (Lu et al. 1995). Selenium in the reductive pathway has also been associated with the induction of p53 (Ghose et al. 2001a and 2001b). Antioxidants have been reported to protect against selenite-induced apoptosis (Shen et al. 2001).

This mechanism is supported by observations that in human mammary cells, selenite and selenocysteine, but not SeMet or selenate, decreased GSH concentrations or cell viability (Yan et al. 1991). However, both selenate and SeMet decreased cell growth. This may be because free radicals, such as superoxide and hydrogen peroxide, are produced from the reaction of selenite and selenocysteine with glutathione (Yan and Spallholz 1993), whereas almost no superoxide anions are generated by the reaction of selenate and SeMet with thiols. The induction of DNA strand breaks and apoptosis by forms of Se in the reductive pathway have also been reported in human leukemia cells (Cho et al. 1999), mouse leukemia cells (Wilson et al. 1992), mouse keratinocytes (Stewart et al. 1999), primary cultures of oral carcinomas (Ghose et al. 2001a and 2001b), human hepatic carcinoma cells (Shen et al. 2000), human oral squamous carcinoma cells (Lanfear et al. 1994), human colon carcinoma cells (Stewart et al. 1997), and human prostate cancer cells (Zhong and Oberley 2001).

A novel hypothesis proposed by Gopalakrishna and Gundimeda (2001) is that cell-cycle regulation by Se is mediated through control of PKC activity. Similar to Se in the reductive pathway, methyl selenol also may generate ROS (Spallholz et al. 2001). Protein kinase C activity is dependent on the presence of reduced cysteine residues on the protein, and methyl selenol is capable of oxidizing these residues (Gopalakrishna and Jaken 2000) thus down-regulating PKC activity. Interestingly, reduction of the cysteine residues on

PKC is accomplished by reduced thioredoxin, and thioredoxin reduction is reduced by the selenoprotein TR (Gopalakrishna and Gundimeda 2001).

2. Se in the methylation pathway appears to induce cell cycle arrest and/or apoptosis independent of DNA strand breaks.

In contrast to Se metabolized through the reductive pathway, Se in the methylation pathway induces reversible cell cycle arrest in the absence of DNA strand breaks (Lu et al. 1995, Wilson et al. 1992). Methylated forms of Se may exert their activity by activating key enzymes in the caspase pathway. Human prostate cancer cells exposed to methyl seleninic acid exhibited activation of multiple caspases (caspase-3, -7, -8, and -9), mitochondrial release of cytochrome c, poly(ADP-ribose) polymerase (PARP) cleavage, and DNA fragmentation whereas selenite induced apoptosis by activation of the c-Jun and mitogen/stress-activated pathways (Jiang et al. 2001). Similar activation of the caspase apoptotic pathway by methylated forms of Se also has been reported in human umbilical endothelial cells (Wang et al. 2001), human leukemia cells (Jung et al. 2001, Kim et al. 2001), and human prostate cancer cells (Jiang et al. 2001).

Methylated forms of Se also may induce cell cycle arrest independent of caspase induction. Sinha and Medina (1997) reported that SeMSC prolonged S-phase cell cycle arrest in mouse mammary epithelial cells. S-phase arrest was accompanied by decreased cdk2 kinase activity and induction of gadd 34, 45, and 153 (Sinha et al. 1999). The authors suggested that the primary upstream regulatory target may be PKC as total PKC activity was reduced in both the cytosolic and membrane fractions within 30 minutes of exposure to 50 μM SeMSC (Sinha et al. 1999). In contrast, SeMet and sulfurmethyl-L-cysteine (the sulfur analogue of SeMSC) did not affect PKC activity. Dong et al. (2002) utilized cDNA microarrays to characterize the effects of SeMSC on premalignant human breast cells. They found that cells exposed to SeMSC exhibited G0-G1 cell cycle arrest accompanied by alterations in the mRNA expression of cdcs, cdks, E2F family proteins, serine/threonine kinases, and the apoptotic regulatory genes Apo-3, c-jun, and cdk5/cyclin D1.

Whether methylated forms of Se exert their effects through p53 is not presently clear. Se-allylselenocysteine (ASC), a compound with many similarities to SeMSC, inhibits mammary epithelial cell growth in vitro and mammary carcinogenesis in the rat (Ip et al. 1999, Zhu et al. 2000). Mammary epithelial cells exposed to ASC had upregulated p53, Cip1/p21, and Kip1/p27 and decreased cyclin D1 and E; however, SeMSC has been shown to induce apoptosis in mouse mammary epithelial cells with nonfunctional p53, suggesting that p53 regulation is not essential for cell cycle regulation by this pathway (Ip et al. 2000b).

3. Selenium may induce global changes in the mitogen activated cell signaling pathway.

Ghose et al. (2001a) theorized that Se regulation of carcinogenesis may be by regulation of cell signaling pathways such as mitogen activated cell signaling pathways independent of p53. Oral carcinoma cells exposed to selenodiglutathione and *p*-XSC had enhanced sensitivity to apoptosis coupled with induction of the stress pathway kinases c-Jun N-terminal kinase (JNK) and p38 kinase (Ghose et al. 2001a). In contrast, Park et al. (2000) observed that selenite suppresses both the c-Jun N-terminal kinase/stress-activated protein kinase (JNK/SAPK) and the p38 mitogen-activated protein kinase pathway in 293T cells. Using cDNA micro-arrays, Dong et al. (2002) also demonstrated that methylseleninic altered multiple signaling molecules in the MAPK, extracellular signal-regulated protein kinase (ERK), and phosphatidylinositol 3'-kinase (PI3k) pathways.

4. Some forms of Se may be directly cytotoxic.

Some synthetic forms of Se such as BSC and *p*-XSC may exert their chemopreventive effects by direct cytotoxicity. However, these forms of Se are not found in nature and the amounts needed are well beyond physiological intakes (El-Bayoumy et al. 1992, El-Bayoumy et al. 1993, El-Bayoumy et al. 1995).

5. Other Mechanisms

That the effects of SeMet on apoptosis and cell cycle arrest do not appear consistent with the above mechanisms suggests that this form of Se may exert its anticarcinogenic effects by other mechanisms. As discussed previously, SeMet may enter the transulfuration pathway and be converted to SeCys, which can then be converted to hydrogen selenide by a beta lyase, thus suggesting that many of the effects of SeMet could be through the reductive pathway. However, because SeMet can substitute for Met, the Met status of the cell may regulate this pathway. It is also possible that through the action of bacteria in the lower gut SeMet may directly liberate methyl selenol.

The metabolism of SeMet, and thus its biological action, can be affected by Met status; however, the interpretation of SeMet effects in animal tumor models has been complicated by the fact that many investigators have not reported the dietary Met levels used in their studies. Chigbrow and Nelson (2001) reported that SeMet induced apoptosis and altered the cell cycle of HCT 116 colon cancer cells through cyclin expression and cdc2 kinase activity. Redman et al. (1997) reported that SeMet causes a depletion of polyamines leading to an induction of apoptosis and pertubations in the cell cycle of HT-29 cells. Menter et al. (2000) reported that LNCaP prostate cancer cells were less growth inhibited by SeMet than selenite, and that SeMet caused cell cycle arrest in the G2-M phase of the cell cycle. Moreover, SeMet induced apoptosis in cancerous, but not primary prostate cells (Menter et al. 2000). In contrast, SeMet did not cause apoptosis in keratinocytes (Stewart et al. 1999).

Selenium as an Effector of Angiogenesis and Metastasis

In addition to affecting the initiation and promotion stages of carcinogenesis, Se may affect tumor promotion by inhibiting angiogenesis and metastasis. When administered at very low levels, Se has been reported to stimulate angiogenesis (McAuslan and Reilly 1986). In contrast, several reports suggest that at higher concentrations Se may inhibit angiogenesis, thus slowing tumor growth (Lu and Jiang 2001). Jiang et al. (2000) reported that methylseleninic acid (MSeA) and methylselenocyanate inhibited matrix metalloproteinase-2 activity in human umbilical vein endothelial cells in a concentration-dependent manner. Likewise, MSeA but not selenite decreased cellular and secreted VEGF (vascular endothelial growth factor) protein levels in human prostate cancer and breast cancer cells (Jiang et al. 2000). The same group also reported that Se consumed as high-Se garlic reduced VEGF and intratumoral microvessel density in NMU-induced rat mammary carcinomas (Jiang et al. 1999). Dietary supplementation of SeMet also has been reported to reduce metastasis of melanoma cells in mice (Yan et al. 1999).

SE-ENRICHED FOODS FOR CANCER PREVENTION

Whenever possible, the American Dietetic Association recommends that the best nutritional strategy for promoting optimal health and reducing the risk of chronic disease is to obtain adequate nutrients from a wide variety of foods. Consuming foods enriched in Se is a much better way to obtain Se than supplements because food often contains multiple chemical forms of Se, the Se is supplied in a matrix with other health-promoting chemicals, and there is little chance of consuming a toxic dose of Se from food. Because there are multiple forms of Se in food, and because each form is metabolized uniquely, food provides multiple potential chemopreventive effects of Se (Table 4.2).

Various plant species have been designated as Se accumulators (seleniferous) in that they have the ability to accumulate large amounts of Se from the soil (Rosenfield and Beath 1964). Plants absorb Se preferentially as selenate via permease, which has a high

Table 4.2.   Protective Effect of Selenium-enriched Foods on Carcinogenesis in Animal Models

Selenium-enriched food	Carcinogen[1]	Organ	Reference
Brazil nut	DMBA	Mammary	Ip and Lisk 1994c
Broccoli	DMH	Colon	Finley et al. 2000, 2001
Broccoli	MNU	Mammary	Finley et al. 2001
Broccoli	Spontaneous	Intestinal	Davis et al. 2002
Garlic	DMBA	Mammary	Ip et al. 1996
			Ip and Lisk 1994a, 1994b, 1995
			Liu et al. 1991
Garlic	MNU	Mammary	Ip et al. 1996, 2000a
Ramps	MNU	Mammary	Whanger et al. 2000
Yeast	MNU	Mammary	Ip et al. 2000a

[1] DMBA = 7,12-dimethylbenzanthracene; DMH = dimethylhydrazine; MNU = methylnitrosurea.

affinity for sulfate. Plants are known to convert inorganic Se in soil to organic Se compounds following the sulfur assimilatory pathway (Shrift 1973). Organic Se compounds may be required for some species of Se accumulator plants, as plant growth is stunted in the absence of soil Se (Shrift 1973). They are thus useful as indicators of the presence of Se in the soils. Se accumulator plants such as *Astragalus*, store Se primarily as methylated species (Shibata et al. 1992, Spallholz 1994). Methylation is catalyzed by a SeCys specific methyl transferase (Neuhierl and Bock 2000) and insertion of this gene allows a nonaccumulating plant species to become a Se accumulator (Wang et al. 1999). Nonaccumulator plants such as grains contain Se predominantly as seleno amino acids such as SeMet.

Garlic was the first food plant that was demonstrated to accumulate large amounts of Se (Ip et al. 1994). Garlic was chosen as the experimental crop under special production conditions because the allyl sulfides present in garlic are known to have anticarcinogenic activity. A number of studies have shown that Se-enriched garlic is an effective anticarcinogen and that the anticarcinogenic activity of the Se-enriched garlic is superior to that of natural garlic or other chemically defined sources of Se such as selenite or SeMet (Ip and Lisk 1994a, 1994b). A major form of Se in Se-enriched garlic is SeMSC, which has also been shown to inhibit tumorigenesis (Lu et al. 1995). In addition, in Se-enriched garlic, most of the diallyl sulfide is replaced by diallyl selenide. Garlic containing diallyl selenide has been shown to be at least three hundred times more active than diallyl sulfide in the DMBA-induced mammary tumor model (El-Bayoumy et al. 1996). Furthermore, it has been reported that the chemopreventive activity of Se enriched garlic is likely to be accounted for by the effect of Se rather than the effect of garlic per se (Ip and Lisk 1995). Analytical studies of the chemical Se species have shown that the bulk of the Se in Se-enriched garlic and Se-enriched yeast is in the form of SeMSC or gamma-glutamyl-Se-methylselenocysteine (73%) and SeMet (85%), respectively (Ip et al. 2000a). The ratio of SeMSC to gamma-glutamyl-Se-methylselenocysteine is dependent on the selenium concentration. In rat feeding studies, supplementation of Se-enriched garlic in the diet at different levels consistently caused lower tissue Se levels when compared to Se-enriched yeast. On the other hand, Se-enriched garlic was significantly more effective in suppressing the development of premalignant lesions and the formation of adenocarcinomas in the mammary gland of carcinogen-treated rats (Ip et al. 2000a).

The forms of Se in garlic and broccoli are virtually identical and the broccoli can accumulate as much Se as garlic (Cai et al. 1995). Se-methylselenocysteine, which is the primary form of Se found in high-Se garlic, is also the primary form of Se found in broccoli. Garlic consumption may be limited by personal preferences and social concerns, therefore broccoli may be a much better food to provide supplemental Se.

Finley et al. (2000) demonstrated that Se from high-Se broccoli is more effective than selenate or selenite for the prevention of precancerous lesions in the colon of rats. Furthermore, the anticarcinogenic activity of Se in broccoli is caused by the chemical forms of Se in broccoli. A lesser amount of the Se in broccoli may be used to form selenoproteins, thus allowing more to enter a pool that is protective against colon carcinogenesis. In follow-up studies, Finley et al. (2001) observed that the cancer protective effect of

Se in high-Se broccoli extends to mammary cancer and that the protective forms of broccoli against colon cancer include high-Se broccoli sprouts.

Multiple intestinal neoplasia (Min) mice are a good model for the investigation of the effects of dietary alterations in a genetic model for intestinal cancer. These mice have a mutation in the *APC* gene and develop spontaneous tumors in both the small and large intestine. Min mice fed Se-enriched broccoli had fewer small intestinal and large intestinal tumors than those fed an equivalent amount of unenriched broccoli (Davis et al. 2002). Thus, Se-enriched broccoli is protective against both chemically induced colon tumor development in rats and spontaneous tumorigenesis in Min mice. Furthermore, Finley (1999) observed that healthy men fed stable isotopes of Se as selenate or Se that had been hydroponically incorporated into broccoli did not accumulate the Se from broccoli in the plasma as well as selenate, and Se-deficient rats repleted with broccoli did not accumulate as much Se in most tissues and organs as rats repleted with selenate, selenite, or SeMet (Finley 1998, Finley and Davis 2001).

Another vegetable that has been explored for uptake of Se and anticarcinogenic activity is Se-enriched ramps (*Allium tricoccum*) (Whanger et al. 2000). Although some minor differences exist, the organosulfur compounds in ramps and garlic have been shown to be generally similar (Calvey et al. 1997, Calvey et al. 1998), and thus ramps would be expected to take up Se like garlic (Whanger et al. 2000). Similar to Se-enriched garlic, broccoli, and onions, the predominant form of Se in the ramp bulbs at all concentrations of Se was SeMSC (Whanger et al. 2000). There was a 43% reduction in chemically induced mammary tumors when rats were fed a diet with Se-enriched ramps (Whanger et al. 2000).

The protective effect of Se-enriched foods on cancer susceptibility in humans has been demonstrated in Finland. Since 1984, Se supplementation through fertilizers has been employed in Finland, which has led to an increase in the Se content of grains (Varo et al. 1988). This, in turn, increased the average daily Se intake from 20–30 µg/d to 80–90 µg/d, and the concentration of Se in the blood of 108 healthy adults changed from 83 to 126 ng Se/mL blood (Makela et al. 1993). Improved Se status has been associated with a reduction in lung cancer (Knekt et al. 1998).

CONCLUSIONS

The trace element Se has been shown to have chemopreventive potential by a converging body of evidence from epidemiologic, clinical, and experimental studies. In particular, the results of recent clinical intervention trials have shown strong protective effects of Se-enriched yeast for cancers of the lung, colon, and prostate. Yet, it is clear that the cancer-protective activities of Se, like other biological activities of Se, depend on the Se compounds present and not on the element per se. Different chemical forms of Se are metabolized differently and exert different biochemical effects. Selenium appears to exert its chemopreventive effects via changes in selenoprotein production, carcinogen metabolism and DNA adduct formation, regulation of apoptosis and cell cycle arrest, and/or inhibition of angiogenesis. Selenium-enriched foods often contain mixtures of different Se compounds and thus can affect multiple carcinogenic pathways to inhibit carcinogenesis.

Furthermore, Se-enriched foods have been shown to have equal or higher chemopreventive activity in animal models than purified compounds suggesting that Se-enriched foods are feasible anticarcinogenic agents.

REFERENCES

Anema, S. M., Walker, S. W., Howie, A. F., Arthur, J. R., Nicol, F., and Beckett, G. J. 1999. Thioredoxin reductase is the major selenoprotein expressed in human umbilical-vein endothelial cells and is regulated by protein kinase C. *Biochem. J.* 342: 111–117.

Arciszewska, L. K., Martin, S. E., and Milner, J. A. 1982. The antimutagenic effect of selenium on 7,12-dimethylbenz(a) anthracene and metabolites in the Ames Salmonella/microsome system. *Bio. Trace Elem. Res.* 4: 259–267.

Arner, E. S., and Holmgren, A. 2000. Physiological functions of thioredoxin and thioredoxin reductase. *Eur. J. Biochem.* 267: 6102–6109.

Avanzini, P., Vinceti, M., Ilariucci, F., Masini, L., D'Inca, M., and Vivoli, G. 1995. Serum selenium concentrations in patients with newly diagnosed lymphoid malignancies. *Haematologica* 80: 505–511.

Baines, A. T., Holubec, H., Basye, J. L., Thorne, P., Bhattacharyya, A. K., Spallholz, J., Shriver, B., Cui, H., Roe, D., Clark, L. C., Earnest, D. L. and Nelson, M. A. 2000. The effects of dietary selenomethionine on polyamines and azoxymethane-induced aberrant cryps. *Cancer Lett.* 160: 193–198.

Batieha, A. M., Armenian, H. K., Norkus, E. P., Morris, J. S., Spate, V. E., and Comstock, G. W. 1993. Serum micronutrients and the subsequent risk of cervical cancer in a population-based nested case-control study. *Cancer Epidemiol. Biomarkers. Prev.* 2: 335–339.

Baumgartner, W. A., Hill, V. A., and Wright, E. T. 1978. Antioxidant effects in the development of Ehrlich ascites carcinoma. *Am. J. Clin. Nutr.* 31: 457–465.

Becker, K., Gromer, S., Schirmer, R. H., and Muller, S. 2000. Thioredoxin reductase as a pathophysiological factor and drug target. *Eur. J. Biochem.* 267: 6118–6125.

Beilstein, M., and Whanger, P. 1986. Chemical forms of selenium in rat tissues after administration of selenite or selenomethionine. *J. Nutr.* 116:1711–1719.

Berggren, M. M., Mangin, J. F., Gasdaska, J. R., and Powis, G. 1999. Effect of selenium on rat thioredoxin reductase activity. Increase by supranutritional selenium and decrease by selenium deficiency. *Biochem. Pharmacol.* 57: 187–193.

Birt, D. F., Julius, A. D, Runice, C. E., and Salmasi, S. 1986. Effects of dietary selenium on bis-(2-oxypropyl)-nitrosamine-induced carcinogenesis in Syrian hamsters. *J. Natl. Cancer Inst.* 77: 1281–86.

Boyington, J. C., Gladyshev, V. N., Khangulov, S. V., Stadtman, T. C., and Sun P. D. 1997. Crystal structure of formate dehydrogenase H: Catalysis involving M., molybdopterin, selenocysteine, and an Fe_4S_4 cluster. *Science* 275: 1305–1308.

Breslow, R. A., Alberg, A. J., Helzlsouer, K. J., Bush, T. L., Norkus, E. P., Morris, J. S., Spate, V. E., and Comstock, G. W. 1995. Serological precursors of cancer: malignat melanoma, basal and squamous cell skin cancer, and prediagnostic levels of retinal, beta-carotene, lycopene, alpha-tocopherol, and selenium *Cancer Epidemiol. Biomarkers Prev.* 4: 837–842.

Brigelius-Flohe, R., Maurer, S., Lotzer, K., Bol, G., Kallionpaa, H., Lehtolainen, P., Viita, H. and YlaHerttuala, S. 2000. Overexpression of PHGPx inhibits hydroperoxide-induced oxidation, NF kappaB activation and apoptosis and affects oxLDL-mediated proliferation of rabbit aortic smooth muscle cells. *Atherosclerosis.* 152: 307–316.

Brigelius-Flohe, R., Muller, C., Menard, J., Florian, S., Schmehl, K., and Wingler, K. 2001. Functions of GI-GPx: lessons from selenium-dependent expression and intracellular localization. *Biofactors.* 14: 101–106.

Broghamer, W. L., McConnell, K. P., and Blotcky, J. L. 1976. Relationship between serum selenium levels and patients with carcinoma. *Cancer* 37: 1384–1388.

Broghamer, W. L., McConnell, K. P., Grimaldi, M., and Blotcky, J. L. 1978. Serum selenium and reticuloendothelial tumors. *Cancer* 41: 1462–1466.

Burguera, M., Gallignani, M., Alarcon, O. M., and Burguera, J. 1990. Blood serum selenium in the province of Merida, Venezuela, related to sex, cancer incidence and soil selenium. *Trace Elem. Electrol. Health Dis.* 4: 73–77.

Burk, R., and Hill, K. 1993. Regulation of selenoproteins. In: Olson R, Bier D, McCormick D, eds. *Annual Review of Nutrition.* Palo Alto, CA: Annual Reviews, Inc., pp. 65–81.

Burk, R. F., and Masters, B. S. 1975. Some effects of selenium deficiency on the hepatic microsomal cytochrome P-450 system in the rat. *Arch. Biochem. Biophy.* 170: 124–131.

Burney, P. G., Comstock, G. W., and Morris, J. S. 1989. Serological precursors of cancer: serum micronutrients and the subsequent risk of pancreatic cancer. *Am. J. Clin. Nutr.* 49: 895–900.

Cai, X. J., Block, E., Uden, P. C., Zhang, Z., Quimby, B. D., and Sullivan, J. J. 1995. Allium chemistry: identification of selenoamino acids in ordinary and selenium-enriched garlic, onion, and broccoli using gas chromatography equipped with atomic emission detection. *J. Agric. Food Chem.* 43: 1754–1757.

Calautti, P., Moschini, G., Stievano, B. M., Tomio, L., Calzavara, E., and Perona, G. 1980. Serum selenium levels in malignant lymphoproliferative diseases. *Scand. J. Haematol.* 23: 63–66.

Calvey, E. M., Matuski, J. E., White, K. D., DeOrazio, R., Sha, D., and Block, E. 1997. Allium chemistry: supercritical fluid extraction and LC-APCIMS of thiosulfinates and related compounds from homogenates of garlic, onion and ramp. Identification in garlic and ramp and synthesis of 1-propane-sulfinothioic acid S-allyl ester. *J. Agric. Food Chem.* 45: 4406–4413.

Calvey, E. M., White, K. D., Matuski, J. E., Sha, D., and Block, E. 1998. Allium chemistry: identification of organosulfur compounds in ramp (*Allium trioccum*) homogenates. *Phytochemistry* 49: 359–364.

Chae, Y.-H., Upadhyaya, P., and El-Bayoumy, K. 1997. Structure-activity relationships among the ortho-, meta-, and para-isomers of phenylenebis(methylene)selenocyanate (XSC) as inhibitors of 7,12-dimethylbenz[*a*]anthracene-DNA binding in mammary glands of female CD rats. *Oncol. Rep.* 4: 1067–1071.

Chen, J., Geissler, C., Parpia, B., Li, J., and Campbell, T. C. 1992. Antioxidant status and cancer mortality in China. *Int. J. Epidemiol.* 21: 625–635.

Chen, J., Goetchius, M. P., Campbell, T. C., and Combs, G. F., Jr. 1982a. Effects of dietary selenium and vitamin E on hepatic mixed-function oxidase activities and in vivo covalent binding of aflatoxin B1 in rats. *J. Nutr.* 112: 324–331.

Chen, J., Goetchius, M. P., Combs, G. F., Jr., Campbell, T. C. 1982b. Effects of dietary selenium and vitamin E on covalent binding of aflatoxin to chick liver cell macromolecules. *J. Nutr.* 112: 350–355.

Chen, S. Y., Chen, C. J., Tsai, W. Y., Ahsan, H., Liu, T. Y., Lin, T. J., and Santella, R. M. 2000a. Associations of plasma aflatoxin B1-adduct level with plasma selenium level and genetic polymorphisms of glutathione S-transferase M1 and T1. *Nutr. Cancer.* 38: 179–185.

Chen, X., Mikhail, S. S., Ding, Y. W., Yand, G.-Y., Bondoc, F., and Yang, C. S. 2000b. Effects of vitamin E and selenium supplementation on esophageal adenocarcinogenesis in a surgical model with rats. *Carcinogenesis.* 21: 1531–1536.

Chidambaram, N., and Baradarajan, A. 1994. Effect of selenium on lipids and some lipid metabolising enzymes in DMBA induced mammary tumors. *Cancer Biochem. Biophys.* 15: 41–47.

Chigbrow, M., and Nelson, M. 2001. Inhibition of mitotic cyclin B and cdc2 kinase activity by selenomethionine in synchronized colon cancer Cells. *Anticancer Drugs* 12: 43–50.

Cho, D. Y., Jung, U., and Chung, A. S. 1999. Induction of apoptosis by selenite and selenodiglutathione in HL-60 cells: correlation with cytotoxicity. *Biochem. Mol. Biol. Int.* 47: 781–793.

Chu, Y.-J, Liu, Q.-Y., Hou, C., and Yu, S.-Y. 1984. Blood selenium concentration in residents of areas in China having a high incidence of lung cancer. *Biol. Trace Elem. Res.* 6: 133–137.

Clark, L., Hixon, L., Combs, G. F., Jr., Reid, M., Turnbull, B. W., and Sampliner, R. 1993. Plasma selenium concentration predicts the prevalence of colorectal adenomatous polyps. *Cancer Epidemiol. Biomarkers Prev.* 2: 41–46.

Clark, L. C., Cantor, K. P., and Allaway, W. H. 1991. Selenium in forage crops and cancer mortality in U. S. counties. *Arch. Environ. Health* 46: 37–42.

Clark, L. C., Combs, G. F., Turnbull, B. W., Slate, E. H., Chalker, D. K., Chow, J., Davis, L. S., Glover, R. A., Graham, G. F., Gross, E. G., Krongrad, A., Lesher, J. L., Park, H. K., Sanders, B. B., Smith, C. L., and Taylor, J. R. 1996. Effects of selenium supplementation for cancer prevention in patients with carcinoma of the skin. A randomized controlled trial. *JAMA* 276: 1957–1963.

Coates, R. J., Weiss, N. S., Daling, J. R., Morris, J. S., and Labbe, R. F. 1988. Serum levels of selenium and retinol and the subsequent risk of cancer. *Am. J. Epidemiol.* 128: 515–523.

Cogwill, U. 1983. the distribution of selenium and cancer mortality in the continental United States. *Biol. Trace Elem. Res.* 5: 336–345.

Combs, G. F., and Gray, W. P. 1998. Chemopreventive agents: Selenium. *Pharmacol. Ther.* 79: 179–192.

Combs, G. F., Jr., Clark, L. C., and Turnbull, B. W. 2001. An analysis of cancer prevention by selenium. *BioFactors* 14:153–9.

Davis, C. D., Feng, Y., Hein, D. W., and Finley, J. W. 1999. The chemical form of selenium influences 3,2'-dimethyl-4-aminobiphenyl-DNA adduct formation in rat colon. *J. Nutr.* 129: 63–69.

Davis, C. D, Zeng, H., and Finley, J. W. 2002. Selenium-enriched broccoli decreases intestinal tumorigenesis in multiple intestinal neoplasia mice. *J. Nutr.* 132: 307–309.

Davis, R. L., Spallholz, J. E., and Pence, B. C. 1998. Inhibition of selenite-induced cytotoxicity and apoptosis in human colonic carcinoma (HT-29) cells by copper. *Nutr. Cancer* 32:181–189.

Deffuant, C., Celerier, P., Boiteau, H. L., Litoux, P., and Dreno, B. 1994. Serum selenium in melanoma and epidermotropic cutaneous T-cell lymphoma. *Acta Derm venerol.* 74: 90–92.

Dias, M. F., Sousa, E., Cabrita, S., Patricio, J., and Oliveira, C. F. 2000. Chemoprevention of DMBA-induced mammary tumors in rats by a combined regimen of alpha-tocopherol, selenium, and ascorbic acid. *Breast J.* 6: 14–19.

Dong, Y., Ganther, H. E., Stewart, C., and Ip, C. 2002. Identification of molecular targets associated with selenium-induced growth inhibition in human breast cells using cDNA microarrays. *Cancer Res.* 62:708–714.

Ejadi, S., Bhattacharya, I. D., Voss, K., Singletary, K., and Milner, J. A. 1989. In vitro and in vivo effects of sodium selenite on 7,12-dimethylbenz(*a*)anthracene (DMBA) -DNA adduct formation in isolated rat mammary epithelial cells. *Carcinogenesis.* 10: 823–826.

El-Bayoumy, K. 1985. Effects of organoselenium compounds on induction of mouse forestomach tumors by benzo[*a*]pyrene. *Cancer Res.,* 45: 3631–3635.

El-Bayoumy. K. 2001. The protective role of selenium on genetic damage and on cancer. *Mutat. Res.* 475: 123–139.

El-Bayoumy, K., Chae, Y.-H., Upadhyaya, P., and Ip, C. 1996. Chemoprevention of mammary cancer by diallyl selenide, a novel organoselenium compound. *Anticancer Res.* 16: 2911–2916.

El-Bayoumy, K., Chae, Y.-H., Upadhyaya, P., Meschter, C., Cohen, L. A., and Reddy, B. S. 1992. Inhibition of 7,12-dimethylbenz[a]anthracene-induced tumors and DNA adduct formation in the mammary glands of female Sprague-Dawley rats by 7,12-dimethylbenz[a]anthracene-induced tumors and DNA adduct formation in the mammary glands of female Sprague-Dawley rats by the synthetic organoselenium compound 1,4-phenylenebis(methylene)selenocyanate. *Cancer Res.* 45: 2402–2407.

El-Bayoumy, K., Upadhyaya, P., Chae, Y.-H., Shon, O. S., Rao, C. V., Fiala, E. S., and Reddy, B. S. 1995. Chemoprevention of cancer by organoselenium compounds. *J. Cell. Biochem.* 22: 92–100.

El-Bayoumy, K., Upadhyaya, P., Desai, D., Amin, S., and Hecht, S. S. 1993. Inhibition of 4-(methyl-nitrosamin)-1-(3-pyridyl)-1-butanone tumorigenicity in mouse lung by the synthetic organoselenium compound 1,4-phenylenebis(methylene)selenocyanate. *Carcinogenesis.* 14:1111–1113.

Feng, Y., Finley, J. W., Davis, C. D., Becker, W. K., Fretland, A. J., and Hein, D. W. 1999. Dietary selenium reduces the formation of aberrant crypts in rats administered 3,2'-dimethyl-4-amino-biphenyl. *Toxicol. Appl. Pharmacol.* 157, 36–42.

Fex, G., Petterson, B., and Akesson, B. 1987. Low plasma selenium as a risk ractor for cancer in middle aged men. *Nutr. Cancer* 10: 221–229.

Fiala, E. S., Joseph, C., Sohn, O.-S., E.-Bayoumy, K., and Reddy, B. S. 1991. Mechanism of benzylselenocyanate inhibition of azoxymethane-induced colon carcinogenesis in F344 rats. *Cancer Res.* 51: 2826–2830.

Finley, J. 1998. Selenium from broccoli is metabolized differently than selenium from selenite, selenate or selenomethionine. *J. Agric. Food Chem.* 46: 3702–3707.

Finley, J. 1999. The retention and distribution by healthy young men of stable isotopes of selenium consumed as selenite, selenate or hydroponically grown broccoli are dependent on the chemical form. *J. Nutr.* 129: 865–871.

Finley, J. W., and Davis, C. D. 2001. Selenium (Se) from high-selenium broccoli is utilized differently than selenite, selenate and selenomethionine but is more effective in inhibiting colon carcinogenesis. *Biofactors* 14: 191–196.

Finley, J. W., Davis, C. D., and Feng, Y. 2000. Selenium from high-selenium broccoli protects rats from colon cancer. *J. Nutr.* 130: 2384–2389.

Finley, J. W., Ip, C., Lisk, D. J., Davis, C. D., Hintze, K. J., and Whanger, P. D. 2001. Cancer-protective properties of high-selenium broccoli. *J. Agric. Food Chem.* 49: 2679–2683.

Fleming, J., Ghose, A., and Harrison, P. R. 2001. Molecular mechanisms of cancer prevention by selenium compounds. *Nutr. Cancer.* 40: 42–49.

Fu, Y., Porres, J. M., Porres, J. M., and Lei, X. G. 2001a. Comparative impacts of glutathione peroxidase-1 gene knockout on oxidative stress induced by reactive oxygen and mitrogen species in mouse hepatocytes. *Biochem. J.* 359: 687–695.

Fu, Y., Sies, H., and Lei, X. G. 2001b. Opposite roles of selenium-dependent glutathione peroxidase-1 in superoxide generator diquat- and peroxynitrite-induced apoptosis and signaling. *J. Biol. Chem.* 276: 43004–43009.

Ganther, H. E. 1999. Selenium metabolism, selenoproteins and mechanisms of cancer prevention: complexities with thioredoxin reductase. *Carcinogenesis.* 20:1657–66.

Ganther, H. E., and Lawrence, J. R. 1997. Chemical transformations of selenium in living organisms. Improved forms of selenium for cancer prevention. *Tetrahedron.* 53: 12229–12310.

Ghose, A., Fleming, J., El Bayoumy, K., and Harrison, P. R. 2001a. Enhanced sensitivity of human oral carcinomas to induction of apoptosis by selenium compounds: involvement of mitogen-activated protein kinase and Fas pathways. *Cancer Res.* 61:7479–7487.

Ghose, A., Fleming, J., and Harrison, P. R. 2001b. Selenium and signal transduction: roads to cell death and anti-tumour activity. *BioFactors*. 14:127–133.

Gladyshev, V. N., and Hatfield, D. L. 1999. Selenocysteine-containing proteins in mammals. *J. Biomed. Sci.* 6: 151–160.

Glass, R. S., Singh, W. P., Jung, W., Veres, Z., Scholz, T. D., and Stadtam, T. C. 1993. Monoselenophosphate: synthesis, characterization, and identity with the prokaryotic biological selenium donor, compound SePX. *Biochemistry* 32: 12555–12559.

Glattre, E. M., Thomassen, Y., Thorensen, S. Q., Haldorsen, T., Lund-Lasen, P. G., Theodorsen, L., and Aaseth, J. 1989. Prediognostic serum selenium in a case-control study of thyroid cancer. *Int. J. Epidemiol.* 18: 45–49.

Gopalakrishna, R., and Gundimeda, U. 2001. Protein kinase C as a molecular target for cancer prevention by selenocompounds. *Nutr.Cancer.* 40:55–63.

Gopalakrishna, R., and Jaken, S. 2000. Protein kinase C signaling and oxidative stress. *Free Radic. Biol. Med.* 28:1349–1361.

Griffin, A. C., and Jacobs, M. M. 1977. Effects of selenium on azo dye hepatocarcinogenesis. *Canc. Lett.* 3: 177–181.

Gromer, S., and Gross, J. H. 2002. Methylseleninate is a substrate rather than an inhibitor of mammalian thioredoxin reductase. Implications for the antitumor effects of selenium. *J. Biol. Chem.* 277: 9701–9706.

Hardell, L., Danell, M., Angqvist, C.-A., Marklund, S. L., Fredriksson, M., Zakari, A.-L., and Kjellgren, A. 1993. Levels of selenium in plasma and glutathione peroxidase in erythrocytes and risk of breast cancer. A case-control study. *Biol. Trace Elem. Res.* 36: 99–108.

Hatfield, D. L., Gladyshev, V. N., Park, J., Park, S. I., Chittum, H. S., Baek, H. J., Carlson, B. A., Yang, E. S., Moustafa, M. E., and Lee, B. J. 1999. Biosynthesis of selenocysteine and its incorporation into protein as the 21st amino acid. *Comp. Nat. Prod. Chem.* 4: 353–380.

Helzlsouer, K. J., Comstock, G. W., and Morris, J. S. 1989. Selenium, lycopene, alpha-tocopherol, beta-carotene, retinol, and subsequent bladder cancer. *Cancer Res.* 49: 6144–6148.

Hojo, Y. 1981. Subject groups high and low in urinary selenium levels: workers exposed to heavy metals and patients with cancer and epilepsy. *Bull. Environ. Contam. Toxicol.* 26: 466–471.

Hunter, D. J., Morris, J. S., Stampfer, M. J., Colditz, G. Z., Speizer, F. E., and Willett, W. C. 1990. A prospective study of selenium status and breast cancer risk. *JAMA* 264: 1128–1131.

Ip, C. 1988. Differential effect of dietary methionine on the biopotency of selenomethionine and selenite in cancer chemoprevention. *J. Natl. Cancer Inst.* 80: 258–262.

Ip, C. 1998. Lessons from basic research in selenium and cancer prevention. *J. Nutr.* 128: 1845–1854.

Ip, C., and Ganther, H. E. 1990. Activity of methylated forms of selenium in cancer prevention. *Cancer Res.* 50, 1206–1211.

Ip, C., and Lisk, D. J. 1994a. Characterization of tissue selenium profiles and anticarcinogenic responses in rats fed natural sources of selenium-rich products. *Carcinogenesis* 15: 573–576.

Ip, C., and Lisk, D. J. 1994b. Enrichment of selenium in allium vegetables for cancer prevention. *Carcinogenesis.* 15: 1881–1885.

Ip, C., and Lisk, D. J. 1994c. Bioactivity of selenium from brazil nut for cancer prevention and selenoenzyme maintenance. *Nutr. Cancer.* 21: 203–212.

Ip, C., and Lisk, D. J. 1995. Efficacy of cancer prevention by high selenium-garlic is primarily dependent on the action of selenium. *Carcinogenesis* 16: 2649–2652.

Ip, C., and Lisk, D. J. 1997. Modulation of phase I and phase II xenobiotic-metabolizing enzymes by selenium-enriched garlic in rats. *Nutr. Cancer* 28: 184–188.

Ip, C., Birringer, M., Block, E., Kotrebai, M., Tyson, J. F., Uden, P. C., and Lisk, D. J. 2000a. Chemical speciation influences comparative activity of selenium-enriched garlic and yeast in mammary cancer prevention. *J. Agric. Food Chem.* 48: 2062–2070.

Ip, C., El-Bayoumy, K., Upadhyaya, P., Ganther, H., Vadhanavikit, S., and Thompsom, H. 1994. Comparative effect of inorganic and organic selenocyanate derivatives in mammary cancer chemoprevention. *Carcinogenesis.* 15: 187–192.

Ip, C., Hayes, C., Budnick, R. M., and Ganther, H. E. 1991. Chemical forms of selenium, critical metabolites and cancer prevention. *Cancer Res.* 51: 595–600.

Ip, C., Lisk, D., and Thompson, H. J. 1996. Selenium-enriched garlic inhibits the early stage but not the late stage of mammary carcinogenesis. *Carcinogenesis.* 17: 1979–1982.

Ip, C., Thompson, H., and Ganther, H. 1994. Activity of triphenylselenonium chloride in mammary cancer prevention. *Carcinogenesis.* 15: 2879–2882.

Ip, C., Thompson, H. J., Zhu, Z., and Gangehr, H. E. 2000b. In vitro and in vivo studies of methylseleninic acid: evidence that a monomethylated selenium metabolite is critical for cancer chemoprevention. *Cancer Res.* 60: 2882–2886.

Ip, C., Zhu, Z., Thompson, H. J., Lisk, D., and Ganther, H. E. 1999. Chemoprevention of mammary cancer with Se-allylselenocysteine and other selenoamino acids in the rat. *Anticancer Res.* 19:2875–2880.

Itoh, Y., and Kikuchi, H. 1997. Serum selenium contents and the risk of cancer. *Biomed. Res. Trace Elem.* 8: 75–76.

Jacobs, M., Frost, C. F., and Beams, F. A. 1981. Biochemical and clinical effects of selenium on dimethylhydrazine-induced colon cancer in rats. *Cancer Res.* 44: 4458–4465.

Jao, S.-W., Shen, K.-L., Lee, W., and Ho, W.-S. 1996. Effect of selenium on 1,2-dimethylhydrazine-induced intestinal cancer in rats. *Dis. Colon Rectum.* 39: 628–631.

Jiang, C., Ganther, H., and Lu, J. 2000. Monomethyl selenium-specific inhibition of MMP-2 and VEGF expression: implications for angiogenic switch regulation. *Mol. Carcinog.* 29: 236–250.

Jiang, C., Jiang, W., Ip, C., Ganther, H., and Lu, J. 1999. Selenium-induced inhibition of angiogenesis in mammary cancer at chemopreventive levels of intake. *Molec. Carcinogenesis* 26: 213–225.

Jiang, C., Wang, Z., Ganther, H., and Lu, J. 2001. Caspases as key executors of methyl selenium-induced apoptosis (anoikis) of DU-145 prostate cancer cells. *Cancer Res.* 61:3062–3070.

Jung, U., Zheng, X., Yoon, S. O., and Chung, A. S. 2001. Se-methylselenocysteine induces apoptosis mediated by reactive oxygen species in HL-60 cells. *Free Radic. Biol. Med.* 31:479–489.

Kawamori, T., El-Bayoumy, K., Ji, B.-Y., Rodriguez, J. G. R., Rao, C. V., and Reddy, B. S. 1998. Evaluation of benzyl selenocyanate glutathione conjugate for potential chemopreventive properties in colon carcinogenesis. *Int. J. Oncol.* 13: 29–34.

Kim, T., Jung, U., Cho, D.-Y., and Chung, A.-S. 2001. Se-Methylselenocysteine induces apoptosis through caspase activation in HL-60 cells. *Carcinogenesis.* 22: 559–565.

Knekt, P., Marniemi, J., Teppo, L., Heliovaara, M., and Aromaa, A. 1998. Is low selenium status a risk factor for lung cancer? *Am. J. Epidemiol.* 148: 975–982.

Kok, F. J., de Bruijn, A. M., Hoffman, A., Verneeren, R., and Valkenberg, H. A. 1987. Is serum selenium a risk factor for cancer in men only? *Am. J. Epidemiol.* 125: 12–16.

Krishnaswamy, K., Trasad, M. P. R., Krishna, T. P., and Pasricha, S. 1993. A case control study of selenium and cancer. *Ind. J. Med. Res [B]* 98: 124–128.

Lanfear, J., Fleming, J., Wu, L., Webster, G., and Harrison, P. R. 1994. The selenium metabolite selenodiglutathione induces p53 and apoptosis: relevance to the chemopreventive effects of selenium? *Carcinogenesis.* 15: 1387–1392.

Levander, O. A. 1983 Considerations in the design of selenium bioavailability studies. *Fed. Proc.* 42: 1721–1725.

Lewis, B. G., Johnson, C. M., Broyer, T. C. 1971. Cleavage of Se-methylselenomethionine selenomium salt by a cabbage leaf enzyme fraction. *Biochim. Biophys. Acta* 237:603–5.

Liu, J., Gilbert, K., Parker, H. M., Haschek, W. M., and Milner, J. A. 1991. Inhibition of 7,12-dimethylbenz(*a*)anthracene-induced mammary tumors and DNA adducts by dietary selenite. *Cancer Res.* 51: 4613–4617.

Lockitch, G. 1989. Selenium: clinical significance and analytical concepts. *Crit. Rev. Clin. Lab. Sci.* 27: 483–541.

Lu, J., and Jiang, C.2001. Antiangiogenic activity of selenium in cancer chemoprevention: metabolite-specific effects. *Nutr. Cancer* 40: 64–73.

Lu, J., Jiang, C., Kaeck, M., Ganther, H., Vadhanavikit, S., Ip, C., and Thompson, H. 1995. Dissociation of the genotoxic and growth inhibitory effects of selenium. *Biochem. Pharmacol.* 50: 213–219.

Makela, A., Nanto, V., Makela, P., and Wang, W. 1993. The effect of nationwide selenium enrichment of fertilizers on selenium status of healthy Finnish medical students living in South Western Finland. *Biol. Trace Elem. Res.* 36: 151–157.

Mannisto, S., Alfthan, G., Virtanen, M., Kataja, V., Uusitupa, M., and Pietinen, P. 2000. Toenail selenium and breast cancer- a case-control study in Finland. *Eur. J. Clin. Nutr.* 54: 98–103.

Marshall, M. V., Arnott, M. S., and Jacobs, M. M. 1979. Selenium effects on the carcinogenicity and metabolism of 2-acetylaminofluorene. *Cancer Lett.* 7: 331–338.

McAuslan, B. R., and Reilly, W. 1986. Selenium-induced cell migration and proliferation: relevance to angiogenesis and microangiopathy. *Microvasc. Res.* 32: 112–120.

McConnell, K. P., Broghamer, W. L., and Blotcky, A. J. 1975. Selenium levels in human blood and tissue in health and disease. *J. Nutr.* 105: 1026–1031.

McConnell, K. P., Jager, R. M., Bland, K. I., and Blotcky, A. J. 1980. The relationship of dietary selenium and breast cancer. *J. Surg. Oncol.* 15: 67–70.

McConnell, K. P., Jager, R. M., Bland, K. I., and Blotcky, A. J. 1987. The relationship of dietary selenium and breast cancer. *J. Surg. Oncol.* 15: 67–70.

Menter, D. G., Sabichi, A. L., and Lippman, S. M. 2000. Selenium effects on prostate cell growth.*Cancer Epidemiol. Biomarkers Prev.* 9: 1171–1182.

Mukhopadhyay-Sardar, S., Rana, M. P., and Chatterjee, M. 2000. Antioxidant associated chemprevention by selenomethionine in murine tumor mode. *Mol. Cell Biochem.* 206: 17–25.

Nayini, J. R., Sugie, S., El-Bayoumy, K., Rao, C. V., Rigotty, J., Sohn, O.-S., and Reddy, B. S. 1991. Effect of dietary benzylselenocyanate on azoxymethane-induced colon carcinogenesis in male F344 rats. *Nutr. Cancer* 15: 129–139.

Nelson, D. R., Koymans, L., Kamataki, T., Stegeman, J. J., Feyereisen, R., Wazman, D. J., Waterman, M. R., Gotoh, O., Coon, M. J., Estabrook, R. W., Gunsalus, I. C., and Nebert, D. W. 1996. P450: superfamily: update on new sequences, gene mapping, accession numbers and nomenclature. *Pharmocogenetics.* 6: 1–42.

Nelson, R. L., Davis, F. G., Sutter, E., Kikendall, J. W., Sobin, L. H., Milner, J. A., and Bowen, P. E. 1985. Serum selenium and colonic neoplastic risk. *Dis. Colon Rectum.* 38: 1306–1310.

Neuhierl, B., and Bock, A. 2000 On the mechanism of selenium tolerance in selenium-accumulating plants: Purification and characterization of a specific selenocysteine methyltransferase from cultured cells of *Astragalus bisculatus*. *Eur J Biochem* 239: 235–238

Olson, O. E., Novacek, E., Whitehead, E., and Palmer, I. 1970. Investigations on selenium in wheat. *J.Trace Elem.Electrolytes Health Dis* 7:107–8.

Park, H.-S., Park, E., Kim, M.-S., Ahn, K., Kim, I. Y., and Choi, E.-J. 2000. Selenite inhibits the c-Jun N-terminal kinase/stress-activated protein kinase (JNK/SAPK) through a thiol redox mechanism. *J. Biol. Chem.* 275: 2527–2531.

Pelkonen, O., and Nebert, D. W. 1982. Metabolism of polycyclic aromatic hydrocarbons: etiologic role in carcinogenesis. *Pharmacol. Rev.* 34: 189–222.

Persson-Moschos, M. E. K., Stavenow. L., Akesson, B., and Lindgarde, F. 2000. Selenoprotein P in plasma in relation to cancer morbidity in middle-aged Swedish men. *Nutr. Cancer* 36: 19–26.

Popova, N. V. 2002. Perinatal selenium exposure decreases spontaneous liver tumorigenesis in CBA mice. *Cancer Lett.* 179: 39–42.

Powis, G., Gasdaska, J. R., Gasdaska, P. Y., Berggren, M., Kirkpatrick, D. L., Engman, L., Cotgreave, I. A., Angulo, M., and Baker, A. 1997. Selenium and the thioredoxin redox system: effects on cell growth and death. *Oncol Res.* 9: 303–312.

Prokopczyk, B., Amin, S., Desai, D. H., Kurtzke, C., Upadhyaya, P., and El-Bayoumy, K. 1997. Effects of 1,4-phenylenebis(methylene)selenocyanate and selenomethionine on 4-(methylnitrosamino)-1-(3-pyridyl)-1-butanone-induced tumorigenesis in A/J mouse lung. *Carcinogenesis* 18: 1855–1857.

Prokopczyk, B., Cox, J. E., Upadhyaya, P., Amin, S., Desai, D., Hoffman, D., and El-Bayoumy, K. 1996. Effects of dietary 1,4-phenylenebis(methylene)selenocyanate on 4-(methylnitrosamino)-1-(3-pyridyl)-1-butanone-induced DNA adduct formation in lung and liver of A/J mice and F344 rats. *Carcinogenesis.* 17: 749–753.

Psathakis, D., Wedemeyer, N., Oevermann, E., Krug, F., Siegers, C.-P., and Bruch, H.-P. 1998. Blood selenium and glutathione peroxidase status in patients with colorectal cancer. *Dis. Colon Rectum* 41: 328–335.

Rao, C. V., Wang, C.-Q., Simi, B., Rodriquez, F. G., Cooma, I., El-Bayoumy, K., and Reddy, B. S. 2001. Chemoprevention of colon cancer by a glutathione conjugate of 1,4- phenylenebis(methylene)selenocyanate, a novel organoselenium compound with low toxicity. *Cancer Res.* 61: 3647–3652.

Reddy, B. S., Hirose, Y., Lubet, R. A., Steele, V. E., Kelloff, G. C., and Rao, C. V. 2000. Lack of chemopreventive efficacy of DL-selenomethionine in colon carcinogenesis. *Int. J. Mol. Med.* 5: 327–330.

Reddy, B. S., Rivenson, A., Kulkarni, N., Upadhyaya, P., and El-Bayoumy, K. 1992. Chemoprevention of colon carcinogenesis by synthetic organoselenium compound 1,4-phenylenebis(methylene)selenocyanate. *Cancer Res.* 52: 5635–5640.

Reddy, B. S., Sugie, S., Maruyama, H., El-Bayoumy, K., and Marra, P. 1987. Chemoprevention of colon carcinogenesis by dietary organoselenium, benzylselenocyanate, in F344 rats. *Cancer Res.* 47: 5901–5904.

Reddy, B. S., Wynn, T. T., El-Bayoumy, K., Upadhyaya, P., Fiala, E. S., and Rao, C. V. 1996. Evaluation of organoselenium compounds for potential chemopreventive properties in colon cancer. *Anticancer Res.* 16: 1123–1128.

Redman, C., Xu, M. J., Peng, Y. M., Scott, J. A., Payne, C., Clark, L. C., and Nelson, M. A. 1997. Involvement of polyamines in selenomethionine induced apoptosis and mitotic alterations in human tumor cells. *Carcinogenesis.* 18: 1195–1202.

Rizk, S. L., and Sky-Peck, H. H. 1984. Comparison between concentrations of trace elements in normal and neoplastic human breast tissue. *Cancer Res.* 44: 5390–5394.

Robinson, M. F., Godfrey, P. J., Thomson, C. D., Rea, H. M., and van Rij, A. M. 1979. Blood selenium and glutathione peroxidase activity in normal subjects and in surgical patients with and without cancer in New Zealand. *Am. J. Clin. Nutr.* 32: 1477–1485.

Rogers, M. A. M., Thomas, D. B., Davis, S., Weiss, N. S., Vaughan, T. L., and Nevissi, A. L. 1991 A case-control study of oral cancer and pre-diagnostic concentrations of selenium and zinc in nail tissue. *Int. J. Cancer Res.* 48: 182–188,

Rosenfield, I., and Beath, O. A. 1964. *Selenium, geobotany, toxicity and nutrition.* New York: Academy Press.

Rotruck, J. T., Pope, A. L., Ganther, H. E., Swanson, A. B., Hafeman, D. G., and Hoekstra, W. G. 1973. Selenium: biochemical role as a component of glutathione peroxidase. *Science 179: 588–590.*

Russo, M. W., Murray, S. C., Wurzelmann, J. I., Woosley, J. T., and Sandler, R. S. 1997. Plasma selenium and the risk of colorectal adenomas. *Nutr. Cancer* 28: 125–129.

Salonen, J. T., Alfthan, G., Huttunen, J. K., and Puska, P. 1984. Association between serum selenium and the risk of cancer. *Am. J. Epidemiol.* 120: 339–342.

Salonen, J. T., Salonen, R. Lappetelainen, R., Maenpaa, P. H., Alfthan, G., and Puska, P. 1985. Risk of cancer in relation to serum concentration of selenium and vitamins A and E: matched case-control analysis of prospective data. *Br. Med. J.* 290: 417–420.

Schober, S. E., Comstock, G. W., Helsing, K. J., Salkeld, R. M., Morris, J. S., Rider, A. A., and Brookmeyer, R. 1987. Serologic precursors of cancer. I. Prediagnostic serum nutrients and colon cancer risk. *Am. J. Epidemiol.* 126: 1033–1041.

Schrauzer, G. N., and White, D. A. 1978. Selenium in human nutrition: dietary intakes and effects of supplementation. *Bioinorg. Chem.* 8: 303–318.

Schrauzer, G. N., Molenaar, T., Mead, S., and Kuehn, K. 1985. Selenium in the blood of Japanese and American women with and without breast cancer and fibrocystic disease. *Jpn. J. Cancer Res.* 76: 374–377.

Schrauzer, G. N., White, D. A., and Schneider, C. J. 1977. Cancer mortality correlation studies. III. Statistical association with dietary selenium intakes. *Bioinorg. Chem.* 7:23–34.

Schwartz, K., and Foltz, M. 1999. Selenium as an integral part of factor 3 against dietary necrotic liver degeneration 1951. *Nutrition* 3: 255.

Shamberger, R. J., and Frost, D. V. 1969. Possible inhibitory effect of selenium on human cancer. *CMAJ.* 100:682.

Shamberger, R. J., and Willis, C. E. 1971. Selenium distribution and human cancer mortality. *Crit. Rev. Clin. Lab. Sci.* 2: 211–221.

Shamberger, R. J., Rukovena, E., Longfield, A. K., Tytko, S. A., Deodhar, S., and Willis, C. E. 1973. Antioxidants and cancer. I. Selenium in the blood of normal and cancer patients. *J. Natl. Cancer. Inst.* 50: 867–870.

Shamberger, R. J., Tytko, S. A., and Willis, C. E. 1976. Antioxicants and cancer. Part VI. Selenium and age-adjusted human cancer mortality. *Arch. Environ. Health* 31: 231–235.

Shen, C. L., Song, W., and Pence, B. C. 2001. Interactions of selenium compounds with other antioxidants in DNA damage and apoptosis in human normal keratinocytes. *Cancer Epidemiol. Biomarkers Prev.* 10:385–390.

Shen, H., Yang, C., Liu, J., and Ong, C. 2000. Dual role of glutathione in selenite-induced oxidative stress and apoptosis in human hepatoma cells. *Free Radic. Biol. Med.* 28: 1115–1124.

Shibata, Y., Masatoshi, M., and Fuwa, K. 1992. Selenium and arsenic in biology: the chemical forms and biological functions. *Adv. Biophys.* 28: 31–80.

Shimada, T., El-Bayoumy, K., Upadhaya, P., Sutter, T. R., Guengrich, P., and Yamazaki, H. 1997. Inhibition of human cytochrome P450-catalyzed oxidations of xenobiotics and procarcinogens by synthetic organoselenium compounds. *Cancer Res.* 57(21): 4757–4768.

Shrift, A. 1973. Metabolism of selenium by plants and microorganisms. In *Organic selenium compounds: Their chemistry and biology,* edited by Klayman, D. K., and Gunter, W. H., pp. 763–814. New York: Wiley-Interscience.

Shultz, T. D., and Leklem, J. E. 1983. Selenium status of vegetarians, nonvegetarians, and hormone-dependent cancer subjects. *Am. J. Clin. Nutr.* 37: 114–118.

Sinha, R., and Medina, D. 1997. Inhibition of cdk2 kinase activity by methylselenocysteine in synchronized mouse mammary epithelial tumor cells. *Carcinogenesis.* 18:1541–1547.

Sinha, R., Kiley, S. C., Lu, J. X., Thompson, H. J., Moraes, R., Jaken, S., and Medina, D. 1999. Effects of methylselenocysteine on PKC activity, cdk2 phosphorylation, and *gadd* gene expression in synchronized mouse mammary epithelial cells. *Cancer Lett.* 146: 135–145.

Soda, K., Oikawa, T., Esaki, N. 1999. Vitamin B6 enzymes participating in selenium amino acid metabolism. *BioFactors* 10:257–62

Spallholz, J. E. 1994. On the nature of selenium toxicity and carcinostatic activity. *Free Radical Biol. Med.* 17: 45–64.

Spallholz, J. E. 1997. Free radical generation by selenium compounds and their prooxidant toxicity. *Biomed. Environ. Sci.* 10: 260–270.

Spallholz, J. E., Shriver, B. J., and Reid T. W. 2001. Dimethyldiselenide and methylseleninic acid generate superoxide in an in vitro chemiluminescence assay in the presence of glutathione: implications for the anticarcinogenic activity of L-selenomethionine and L-Se-methylselenocysteine. *Nutr. Canc.* 40: 34–41.

Spolar, M. R., Schaffer, E. M., Beelman, R. B., and Milner, J. A. 1999. Selenium-enriched Agaricus bisporus mushrooms suppress 7, 12-dimethylbenz[a]anthracene bioactivation in mammary tissue. *Cancer Lett.* 138: 145–150.

Stadtman, T. C. 1996. Selenocysteine. *Ann. Rev. Biochem.* 65: 83–100.

Stewart, M. J., Spallholz, J. E., Neldner, K. H., and Pence, B. C. 1999. Selenium compounds have disparate abilities to impose oxidative stress and induce apoptosis. *Free Rad. Biol. Med.* 26: 42–48.

Stewart, M. S., Davis, R. L., Walsh, L. P., and Pence, B. C. 1997. Induction of differentiation and apoptosis by sodium selenite in human colonic carcinoma cells (HT29). *Cancer Lett.* 117: 35–40.

Subramaniam, S., Shyama, S., Jagadeesan, M., and Dhyamala-Devi, C. S. 1993. Oxidant and antioxidant levels in the erythrocytes of breast cancer patients treated with CMF. *Med. Res. Sci.* 21:79–80.

Sunde R. 1990. Molecular biology of selenoproteins. In *Annual review of nutrition,* edited by Olson, R., Bier, D., and McCormick, D., pp 451–474. Palo Alto, CA: Annual reviews Inc.

Sundstrom, H., Ylikorkala, O., and Kauppila, A. 1986. Serum selenium and thromboxane in patients with gynaecological cancer. *Carcinogenesis* 7: 1051–1052.

Tanaka, T., Kohno, H., Murakami, M., Kagami, S., and El-Bayoumy, K. 2000. Suppression effects of dietary supplementation of the organoselenium 1,4-phenylenebis(methylene)selenocyanate and the citrus antioxidant auraptene on lung metastasis of melanoma cells in mice. *Cancer Res.* 60: 3713–3716.

Tanaka, T., Makita, H., Kawabata, K., Mori, H., and El-Bayoumy, K. 1997. 1,4-Phenylenebis(methylene)selenocyanate exerts exceptional chemopreventive activity in rat tongue carcinogenesis. *Cancer Res.* 57: 3644–3648.

Thirunavukkarasu, C., and Sakthisekaran, D. 2001. Effect of selenium on N-nitrosodiethylamine-induced multistage hepatocarcinogenesis with reference to lipid peroxidation and enzymic antioxidants. *Cell. Biochem. Function* 19: 27–35.

Toma, S., Micheletti, A., Giacchero, A., Coialbu, T., Collecchi, P. , Esposito, M., Rotundi, M., Ablanese, E., and Cantoni, E. 1991. Selenium therapy in patients with precancerous and malignant oral cavity lesions: preliminary results. *Cancer Detect. Prevention* 15: 491–494.

Upadhyaya, P., and El-Bayoumy. 1998. Effect of dietary soy protein isolate, genistein, and 1,4-phenylenebis(methylene)-selenocyanate on DNA binding of 7,12-dimethylbenz(*a*)anthracene in mammary glands of CD rats. *Oncol. Rep.* 5: 1541–1545.

van der Brandt, P. A., Goldbohm R. A., van't Veer P., Bode, P., Dorant, E., Hermus, R. J., and Sturmans, F. 1993a. A prospective cohort study on selenium status and the risk of lung cancer. *Cancer Res.* 53: 4860–4865.

van der Brandt, P. A., Goldbohm R. A., van't Veer P., Bode, P., Dorant, E., Hermus, R. J., and Sturmans, F. 1993b. A prospective study on toenail selenium levels and risk of gastrointestinal cancer. *J. Natl. Cancer Inst.* 85: 224–229.

van Ryssen, J. B., Deagen, J. T., Beilstein, M., and Whanger, P. 1989. Comparative metabolism of organic and inorganic selenium by sheep. *J.Ag.and Food Chem.* 37:1358–63.

Varo, P., Alfthan, G., Ekholm, P., Aro, A., and Koivistoienen, P. 1988. Selenium intake and serum selenium in Finland: effects of soil fertilization with selenium. *Am. J. Clin. Nutr.* 48: 324–329.

Vernie, L. N., De Vries, M., Benckhuijsen, C., De Goeij, J. J. M., and Zegers, C. 1983. Selenium levels in blood and plasma and glutathione peroxidase activity in blood of breast cancer patients during adjuvant treatment with cyclophosphamide, methotrexate and 5-fluorouracil. *Cancer Lett.* 18: 283–289.

Vinceti, M., Rovesti, S., Bergomi, M., and Vivoli, G. 2000. The epidemiology of selenium and human cancer. *Tumori* 86: 105–118.

Virtami, J., Valkeila, E., Alfthan, G., Punsar, S., Huttunen, J. K., and Karvonen, M. J. 1987. Serum selenium and risk of cancer: a prospective follow up of nine years. *Cancer* 60: 145–148.

Wang, Y., Block, A., and Neuhierl, B. 1999, Acquisition of selenium tolerance by a selenium non-accumulating Astragalus species via selection. *Biofactors* 9:3–10.

Wang, Z., Jiang, C., Ganther, H., and Lu, J. 2001. Antimitogenic and proapoptotic activities of methylseleninic acid in vascular endothelial cells and associated effects on PI3K-AKT, ERK, JNK and p38 MAPK signaling. *Cancer Res.* 61: 7171–7178.

Whanger, P., and Butler, J. 1988. Effects of various dietary levels of selenium as selenite or selenomethionine on tissue selenium levels and glutathione peroxidase activity in rats. *J.Nutr.* 118:846–52.

Whanger, P. D., Ip, C., Polan, C. E., Uden, P. C., Welbaum, G. 2000. Tumorigenesis, metabolism, speciation, bioavailability and tissue deposition of selenium in selenium-enriched ramps (*Allium tricoccum*). *J. Agric. Food Chem.* 48: 5723–5730.

Willett, W., Polk, B., Morris, S., Stampfer, M., Preissel, S., Rosner, B., Taylor, J., Schneider, K., and Hames, C. 1983. Prediagnostic serum selenium and risk of cancer. *Lancet* ii:130–133.

Wilson, A. C., Thompson, H. J., Schedin, P. J., Gibson, N. W., and Ganther, H. E. 1992. Effect of methylated forms of selenium on cell viability and the induction of DNA strand breakage. *Biochem. Pharmacol.* 43: 1137–1141.

Wortzman, M. S., Besbris, H. J., and Cohen, A. M. 1980. Effect of dietary selenium on the interaction between 2-acetylaminofluorene and rat liver DNA in vivo. *Cancer Res.* 40: 2670–2676.

Wrighton, S. A., and Elswick, B. 1989. Modulation of the induction of rat hepatic cytochromes P-450 by selenium deficiency. *Biochemical Pharmacol.* 38: 3767–3771.

Yan, L., and Spallholz, E. 1993. Generation of reactive oxygen species from the reaction of selenium compounds with thiols and mammary tumor cells. *Biochemical Pharmacol.* 45: 429–437.

Yan, L., Yee, J. A., Boylan, L. M., and Spallholz, J. E. 1991. Effect of selenium compounds and thiols on human mammary tumor cells. *Biol. Trace Elem. Res.* 30: 145–162.

Yan, L., Yee, J. A., Li, D., McGuire, M. H., and Graef, G. L. 1999. Dietary supplementation of selenomethionine reduces metastasis of melanoma cells in mice. *Anticancer Res.* 19: 1337–1342.

Yoshizawa, K., Willet, W. C., Morris, S. J., Stampfer, M. J., Spiegelman, D., Rimm, E. B., and Giovanucci, E. 1998. Study of prediagnostic selenium level in toenails and the risk of advanced prostate cancer. *J. Natl. Cancer Inst.* 90: 1219–1224.

Yu, M.-W., Zhu, Y. J., and Li, W. G. 1997. Protective role of selenium against hepatitis B virus and primary liver cancer in Qidong. *Biol. Trace Elem. Res.* 56: 117–124.

Yu, S.-Y., Chu, Y.-J., Gong, X.-G., and Hou, C. 1985. Regional variation of cancer mortality incidence and its relation to selenium levels in China. *Biol. Trace Elem. Res.* 67: 21–29.

Zachara, B. A., Marchaluk-Wisniewska, E., Maciag, A., Peplinski, J., Skokowski, J., and Lambrecht, W. 1997. Decreased selenium concentration and glutathione peroxidase activity in blood and increase of these parameters in malignant tissue of lung cancer patients. *Lung* 175: 321–332.

Zheng, J., Ohata, M., Furuta, N., and Kosmus, W. 2000. Speciation of selenium compounds with ion-pair reversed-phase liquid chromatography using inductively coupled plasma mass spectrometry as element-specific detection. *J. Chromatogr.* 874: 55–64.

Zhong, W., and Oberley, T. D. 2001. Redox-mediated effects of selenium on apoptosis and cell cycle in the LNCaP human prostate cancer cell line. *Cancer Res.* 61: 7071–7078.

Zhu, Z., Jiang, W., Ganther, H. E., Ip, C., and Thompson, H. J. 2000. Activity of Se-allylselenocysteine in the presence of methionine γ-lyase on cell growth, DNA integrity, apoptosis, and cell-cycle regulatory molecules. *Molec. Carcin.* 29: 191–197.

5

Nutrients to Stimulate Cellular Immunity: Role in Cancer Prevention and Therapy

Satoru Moriguchi,
Satoe Yamashita,
and Eiji Shimizu

INTRODUCTION

Nutrition plays an important role in two respects: one is the inhibitory factor for carcinogenesis via its immunoenhancing effects and the other is the determinant for prognosis of cancer patients. In this chapter, the relationship between the malnourished status of cancer patients and immune responses, and the beneficial effect of nutritional support using enteral and parenteral feeding are described first. The rest of this chapter discusses the immunomodulating action of each nutrient, such as fat, protein (amino acid), vitamins, and minerals, in cancer patients or animals with tumors. Finally, some foods that promote health are described in regard to their action on host immunity.

NUTRITIONAL STATUS IN CANCER PATIENTS AND IMMUNITY

Not only cancer itself but also conventional approaches to therapy for cancer such as chemotherapy, operative therapy, and radiation therapy are known to produce profound changes in host immunity. The effects of chemotherapy upon immune responses are related both to the dosage and duration of therapy and are readily reversible. Operative therapy likewise suppresses both humoral and cell-mediated immunity for 2 to 3 weeks, as manifested by in vitro and in vivo tests of these functions. And radiation therapy induces the decrease of host immune responses for more prolonged periods of time over 10 years. One of the factors inducing the decrease of host immunity following cancer and its therapies is malnutrition. Nutritional status affects both limbs of the immune system. Enteral and parenteral (intravenous hyperalimentation) nutrition are safe and effective methods for correcting deficits in cancer patients. In the malnourished gastric cancer patient, one week of pre- or postoperative parenteral nutrition significantly increased natural killer cell (NK) activity, T-helper proportion, T-helper/T-suppressor ratio, and total T lymphocyte count (Yan 1990). This evidence suggests that perioperative nutrition support can improve the immunocompetence of gastric cancer patients. The other study has shown that a marked depression of NK activity of peripheral blood mononuclear cells (PBMC) was observed in malnourished cancer patients with moderate protein-calories malnutrition, but not in well-nourished cancer patients nor in the healthy controls (Villa et al. 1991). Although the decreased NK activity in this study was restored to normal by rIL-2, but not by α-rIFN, the ability to produce IL-2 in vitro in each cancer patient did not correlate with NK activity. This evidence suggests that malnutrition, rather than malignancy, plays a major role in the immune dysfunction of cancer patients. When compared with immune functions after operation in patients with esophageal or gastric cancer, ConA- and PHA-stimulated lymphocyte proliferation decreased significantly 7 days after esophagectomy, but was unchanged in the patients receiving gastrectomy (Tashiro et al. 1999). Since serum cortisol level was significantly increased in patients after surgery, stress response may induce in part the suppression of immune functions. In patients with hepatocellular carcinoma, the phagocytic and bactericidal activities of neutrophils and the percentage of NK cells were significantly reduced (Iida et al. 1999). In particular, the phagocytic and bactericidal activities of neutrophils were low in patients with poor nutritional status compared to those with a good nutritional status. Taken together, nutritional supplementation such as enteral and parenteral nutrition for malnourished cancer patients appears to be useful for preventing further decrease of host immune functions.

It is a well-known fact that food restriction results in longer longevity than ad libitum feeding (Sheldon et al. 1995). Some previous animal studies have found that food restriction has a beneficial effect on the incidence of cancer. Using mice treated with 3-methylcholanthrene (MC), 40% dietary restriction caused a great inhibition of tumor incidence at 114 days after treatment(Konno et al. 1991). Since the optimum duration and degree of dietary restriction cause the enhancements of both splenic lymphocyte proliferation and phagocytic activity of alveolar macrophages in rats (Fig. 5.1), the decreased incidence of cancer may be related to the changes of host immune functions following dietary restriction. In fact, the above study has shown that dietary restriction causes a marked increase of the proportion of Thy1.2+, L3T4+T cells, and increased T cell responses against ConA and IL-2 in MC-treated diet-restricted mice. The increase of host immune functions might be one of the major causes for the reduction of tumor occurrence by dietary restriction. In conclusion, caution should be employed in the nutritional manipulation of malnourished cancer patients.

ROLE OF LIPIDS IN CANCER PREVENTION AND IMMUNITY

There is in vitro and in vivo evidence to suggest that dietary lipids play an important role in modulating immune functions. It is known that diets high in polyunsaturated fat, relative to diets high in saturated fat, are more immunosuppressive and are better promoters of tumorigenesis (Vitale and Broitman 1981). It has been also shown that rats fed diets high in lipid and cholesterol develop more 1,2-dimethylhydrazine (DMH)-induced bowel tumors than those fed diets low in lipid or without cholesterol. When rats were fed diets containing 20% safflower or coconut oil, with or without cholesterol (1%) and cholic acid (0.3%), for 35 weeks and concomitantly given DMH, the suppression of PHA response was observed in the polyunsaturated fat (safflower oil) diet group compared with the saturated fat (coconut oil) diet group (Kraus et al. 1987). And the addition of cholesterol to

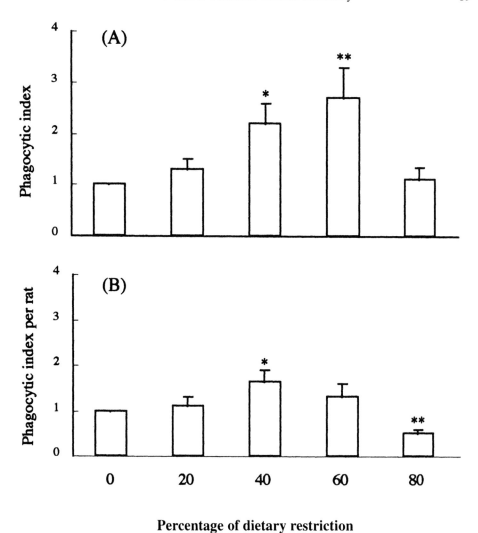

Percentage of dietary restriction

Figure 5.1.   Phagocytic activity of alveolar macrophages (AM) (2×105) in rats (**A**) or AM per rat (**B**) fed mildly or moderately restricted diets (20 to 80% restriction to control) for 2 weeks. Phagocytic index was calculated by assigning 1 to phagocytic activity of control group and comparing this to phagocytic activity of other groups. Values are means ± SD of triplicate cultures; significantly different from controls (*$P < 0.05$, **$P < 0.001$). (Reproduced from J. Nutr. Sci. Vitaminol., 35; Moriguchi, S., Toba, M. and Kishino, Y., Effects of dietary restriction on cellular immunity in rats, 49–59. Copyright 1989, with permission from the Center for Academic Publications Japan)

either the polyunsaturated or saturated fat diet diminished PHA response, to a lesser degree, of T lymphocytes from rats fed these diets. However, natural killer (NK) cell activity was unaffected by either the difference of dietary fat or cholesterol. The other study has shown that the splenic lymphocyte transformation response induced by ConA, PHA, or pokeweed mitogen is significantly depressed in the rats fed 24% corn oil (vehicle-treated) and in the DMH-treated rats fed 5% fat compared with the vehicle-treated rats fed 5% fat (Locniskar et al. 1986). This study has also found that splenic NK cell cytotoxic activity was not significantly affected by dietary fat, DMH treatment, or tumor development. On the other hand, it has been found that corn oil administered by oral gavage retards mononuclear cell leukemia proliferation, which is mediated at least in part by enhancing immune competence (Hursting et al. 1994).

As described previously in this chapter, the beneficial effect of early postoperative enteral nutrition enriched with not only arginine and RNA but also omega-3 fatty acids was found in 78 patients undergoing curative operations for gastric or pancreatic cancer (Braga et al. 1996). Since prealbumin concentration, retinol-binding protein (RBP) concentration, delayed hypersensitivity responses, phagocytic ability of monocytes, and concentration of interleukin-2 (IL-2) receptors had recovered more in the patients receiving the enriched enteral solution, early enteral feeding is likely to induce the recovery of both their nutritional and immunological status quicker than those supported with standard enteral diet or total parenteral nutrition (TPN). The recent study has also shown that the supplementation of eicosapentaenoic acid (EPA) with soybean oil emulsion significantly improved the lymphocyte proliferation and natural killer cell activity compared with the group receiving only soybean oil emulsion (Furukawa et al. 1999). Furthermore, the other study was conducted to investigate the effect of immunological effects of three TPN regimens such as calories derived solely from glucose and a half of total calories derived from lipid emulsion (one as long-chain triglycerides and the other containing half the fat as long-chain triglycerides and a half as medium-chain triglycerides) in patients undergoing preoperative parenteral nutrition. This study has shown that NK activity and lymphokine-activated killer (LAK) activity were significantly higher after TPN with long-chain and middle-chain triglyceride solutions and a significant fall in LAK activity occurred after TPN with long-chain triglyceride solution (Fig. 5.2) (Sedman et al. 1991).The design of TPN regimens is also an important factor for cancer patients to improve or maintain their immune functions.

ROLE OF PROTEIN OR AMINO ACIDS IN CANCER PATIENTS AND IMMUNITY

As described above, nutritional status is the most important determinant in the prognosis for cancer patients. It is well accepted that protein-calorie malnutrition impairs host immunity with particular detrimental effects on the T-cell system, resulting in increased opportunistic infection and increased morbidity and mortality in hospitalized patients including cancer patients (Daly et al. 1990). Levels of vitamins A and E, having a potent enhancing effect on host immune functions and being low in tumor bearing animals, decreased further when maintained in the restricted diet without soybean, but were raised to normal following addition of soybean in the diet (Mukhopadhyay et al. 1994). As soybean protein has high arginine content, the enhancing effect of soybean on immune functions in animals fed the restricted diet may be in part due to arginine. In fact, there are many reports showing that arginine has an immunoenhancing effects and an inhibitory

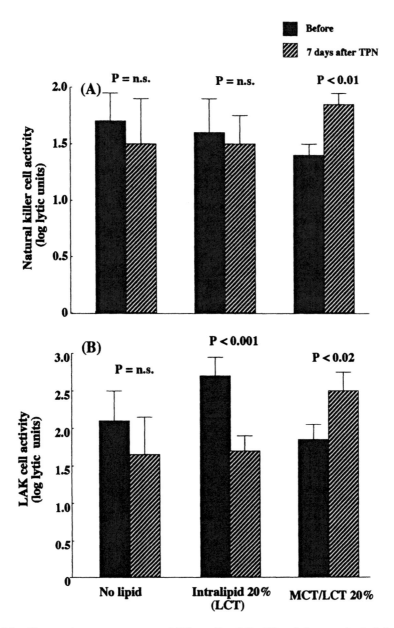

Figure 5.2. Changes in spontaneous natural killer cell activity (A) and the capacity to induce lymphokine-activated killer (LAK) cells in response to interleukin-2 (B) before and 7 days after total parenteral nutrition (TPN) with each of the three TPN regimens. Histograms denote means ± SEM of logtransformed data. MCT/LCT , medium-chain triglycerides/long-chain triglycerides. (Reproduced from Br. J. Sur, 78; Sedman, P. C., Somers, S. S., Ramsden, C. W., Brennan, T. G., and Guillou, P. J., Effects of different lipid emulsions on lymphocyte functions during total parenteral nutrition, 1396–1399. Copyright 1991, with permission from Butterworth-Heinemann Ltd.)

effect on tumor growth and metastasis. In vitro incubation with arginine induced threefold increase of NK cell activity of human PBL and 1.5-fold increase of human monocyte-mediated cytotoxicity (Fig. 5.3) (Moriguchi et al. 1987). Production of tumor cytotoxic factor from human monocytes also significantly increased after in vitro incubation with arginine. This evidence suggests that arginine action against tumor cells is due to not only the enhancement of host immune functions such as NK activity and human monocyte cytotoxicity but also to increased production of cytokines having the direct effect on tumor cells. Using arginine-enriched amino acids solution, growth and metastases of Yoshida sarcoma were suppressed (Tachibana et al. 1985). Since arginine supplementation enhanced the phagocytic activity of rat alveolar macrophages, the authors concluded that

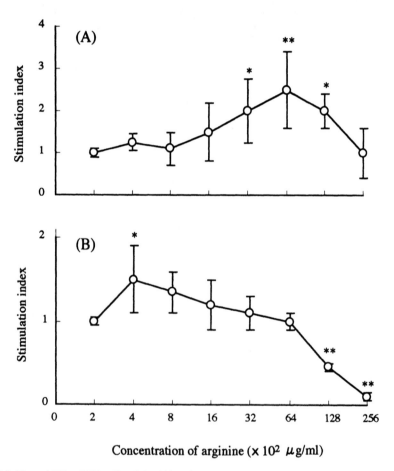

Concentration of arginine ($\times 10^2$ μg/ml)

Figure 5.3. Natural killer (NK) cell activity (**A**) and monocyte cytotoxicity (**B**) after incubation with various concentrations of arginine for 48 hours. Bars are means ± SD of triplicate cultures and compared with that of control culture (2×10^2 µg/ml of arginine). NK activity and percent cytotoxicity of monocytes in control culture are 22.0 ± 1.6% and 11.0 ± 0.8 %, respectively; significantly different from control culture (*P < 0.05, **P < 0.01). (Reproduced from Nutr. Res., 7; Moriguchi, S., Mukai, K., Hiraoka, I., and Kishino, Y., Functional changes in human lymphocytes and monocytes after in vitro incubation with arginine, 719–729. Copyright 1987, with permission from Elsevier Science)

the suppressive effect of arginine-enriched solution on tumor growth and metastases may be due to its activation of the immunologic system. Some of the clinical studies and animal studies were designed to evaluate the effect of arginine plus other nutrients such as glutamine, RNA, omega-3 fatty acid, and ornithine 2-oxoglutarate on host immune response (Gianotti et al. 1999, Chuntrasakul et al. 1998, Kemen et al. 1995).

Supplemented diet or enteral diet has a beneficial effect on host immune functions. Recently, it has been found that arginine is a substrate for nitric oxide showing various physiological activities such as the regulation of arterial smooth muscle, blood pressure, and immune functions (Palmer et al. 1987, Haynes et al. 1993, Ding et al. 1988). On the other hand, it has been reported that the expression of adhesion molecule CD44 is closely associated with the degree of metastasis of tumors (Sikorska et al. 2002, Lakshmi et al. 1997). In fact, the higher metastatic B16 melanoma cells showed the higher expression of CD44 as shown in Figure 5.4 (Moriguchi et al. 2002). In addition, the expression of CD44 was significantly suppressed following in vitro incubation with SIN-1, spontaneously generating NO (Fig. 5.5), which resulted in the decreased lung metastases of B16 melanoma in mice fed the high arginine diet. These results suggest that arginine has an inhibitory effect on tumor growth and metastases via two different mechanisms, such as immunoenhancement and depressed expression of adhesion molecule CD44.

The prolonged use of total parenteral nutrition provokes mucosal atrophy of the small intestine (Grant and Snyder 1988), which is related to the lack of glutamine in standard currently available parenteral solutions. Because glutamine is poorly soluble and instable, it has been not generally used as one of the amino acids in parenteral nutrition. However, glutamine is a nutrient necessary for the intestinal mucosal metabolism as a major oxidative fuel. Alanylglutamine, glutamine-containing dipeptide, was found as a source of free glutamine in parenteral nutrition (Furst et al. 1989). On the other hand, although free glutamine is highly consumed by rapidly proliferating tumor cells, it was not clearly known whether tumor growth rate was increased by intravenous supplementation of alanylglutamine. In addition, it is known that glutamine is preferentially used for the provision of fuels in proliferating lymphocytes (Ardawi and Newsgolme 1982) and macrophages (Newsholme and Newsholme 1989). A study was undertaken and evaluated the changes of tumor volume and weight, and cellular immune response following the administration of an alanylglutamine-enriched solution. As a result, in vivo administration of alanylglutamine did not accelerate the growth of transplanted Yoshida sarcoma cells as measured by changes in the weight and volume (Kweon et al. 1991). And the addition of alanylglutamine to culture medium showed a significant increase in phagocytic activity of alveolar macrophages and in blastogenic response of splenocytes. These results suggest that alanylglutamine infusion does not stimulate tumor growth due to maintenance of some immunoenhancing effects by glutamine liberated from alanylglutamine in tumor-bearing hosts.

ROLE OF VITAMINS IN CANCER PREVENTION AND IMMUNITY

Vitamin A is a nutrient having the most impact on both tumor incidence and growth and host immune system. Continuous administration of vitamin A and its derivatives (retinoids) has been shown to prevent cancer of the skin (Verma et al. 1982), lung (Saffiotti et al. 1967), bladder (Moon et al. 1982), and breast (Moon et al. 1983) in experimental animals exposed to carcinogens. Epidemiological results also suggest that dietary retinoids may be chemopreventive to some forms of cancer in humans as well (Wald et al.

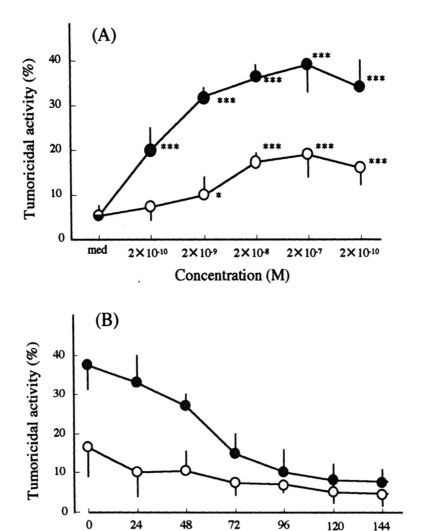

Figure 5.4. Tumoricidal activity of human monocytes treated in vitro with various concentrations (2×10^{-10} to 2×10^{-6} M) of beta-carotene or beta-carotene encapsulated in liposomes for 24 hours (**A**) and maintenance of the tumoricidal state of human monocytes after in vitro incubation with 2×10^{-7} M of beta-carotene or beta-carotene encapsulated in liposomes (**B**). Values are means ± SD for triplicate cultures; significantly different from cultures with medium containing 0.2% ethanol (*P < 0.05, ***P < 0.001). (Reproduced from Nutr. Res., 10; Moriguchi, S., and Kishino, Y ., In vitro activation of tumoricidal properties of human monocytes by beta-carotene encapsulated in liposomes, 837–846. Copyright 1990, with permission from Elsevier Science)

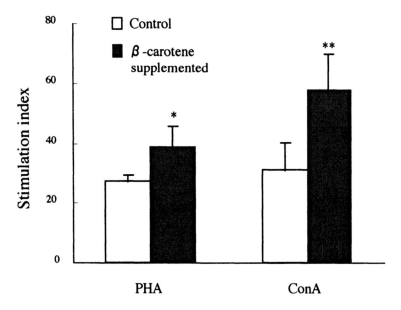

Figure 5.5. Proliferation of peripheral blood lymphocytes with PHA or ConA in control and beta-carotene supplemented subjects. Values are means ± SD; significantly different from control subjects (*P < 0.05, **P < 0.01). (Reproduced from Nutr. Res., 16; Moriguchi, S., Okishima, N., Sumida, S., Okamura, K., Doi, T., and Kishino, Y., Beta-carotene supplementation enhances lymphocyte proliferation with mitogens in human peripheral blood lymphocytes, 211–218. Copyright 1996, with permission from Elsevier Science)

1980, Kark et al. 1981). However, the toxicity of vitamin A precludes its use as a form of cancer prevention. The development of new vitamin A derivatives having low toxicity and high chemopreventive activity is required. The effect of selected doses of dietary retinyl palmitate and 13-*cis*-retinoic acid has been measured by using mouse skin papilloma promotion by 12-*O*-tetradecanoylphorbol-13-acetate (TPA). Dietary retinyl palmitate yields a dose-dependent inhibition of the number and weight of tumors, whereas dietary 13-*cis*-retinoic acid resulted in a decrease of weight but not in number of tumors (Gensler et al. 1987). This result suggests that retinyl palmitate inhibits both incidence and growth of tumors, whereas 13-*cis*-retinoid acid inhibits not the incidence of tumors but tumor growth. Using the same dietary regimens, the high retinyl palmitate diets significantly increased phagocytic ability and tumoricidal activity of peritoneal macrophages and mitogenesis of splenocytes and thymocytes in mice (Moriguchi et al. 1985). This evidence suggests that high retinyl palmitate diets may cause activation of both peritoneal macrophages and lymphocytes. Furthermore, in nude mice, defecting thymus gland development and lacking functional mature T lymphocytes, retinyl palmitate diets significantly stimulated phagocytosis of peritoneal macrophages only at the highest level. T-cell-dependent mitogens did not also cause significant mitogenesis in any dietary group, while lipopolysaccharide (LPS), a B-cell mitogen, did (Watson and Moriguchi 1989). These results suggest that mature T cells may be needed for retinyl palmitate to produce normal activation of macrophages, except at very high retinyl palmitate levels. As the in vitro study showed that both retinoids and carotenoids at higher concentrations have inhibitory effects on human lymphocyte functions, the use of vitamin A or its derivatives for chemoprevention and therapeutic trials for cancer patients should be carefully considered in its design.

Beta-carotene is one of the carotenoids, which are pigments contributing to the yellow, orange, and/or red coloration in vegetables and fruits. Epidemiological studies have demonstrated that a high intake of food rich in beta-carotene is associated with reduced risk of certain types of cancers, especially lung cancer (Le Marchand et al. 1989). Since other carotenoids lacking provitamin A activity had the similar anticancer effect as that of beta-carotene, it has been suggested that the anticancer effects of beta-carotene is not due to its provitamin A activity. Thus, the anticancer and antibacterial effects of beta-carotene are considered to be due to not provitamin A functions but antioxidant and immunomodulatory functions (Bendich and Shapiro 1986). Proliferation of peripheral blood lymphocytes with PHA or ConA was 1.4- to 1.9-fold higher in the beta-carotene supplemented group compared to the control group, whereas there was no significant difference in NK cell activity between both groups (Fig. 5.6) (Moriguchi et al. 1996). In addition, the study on in vitro effect of beta-carotene (beta) and beta-carotene encapsulated in liposomes (L + beta) on tumoricidal activity of human monocytes has found that the use of liposomes with beta-carotene could induce higher tumoricidal activity of human monocytes following short-term incubation and incubation with lower concentration compared to those of beta-carotene (Fig. 5.7) (Moriguchi and Kishino 1990). Since many other reports support the action of beta-carotene against inhibition of tumorigenesis and tumor cell growth (Kune et al. 1989), and the enhancement of immune responses (Bendich 1989), it is believed that beta-carotene is a nutrient for improving cancer patients and aged people showing decreased cellular immunity. Other fat-soluble vitamins, D and E, are also known to have both inhibitory effects on tumor incidence and growth (Mehta and Mehta 2002, Yu et al. 2002) and enhancing effects on host immune response (Lemire 2000, Moriguchi and Muraga 2000).

Water-soluble vitamins B_6 and C are also known to have the immunoenhancing effects. In the experiment using athymic nude mice, vitamin B_6 supplementation caused increased response of B lymphocytes with lipopolysaccharide (LPS), but did not inhibit the development of human malignant melanoma (M21-HPB) xenografts (Gebhard et al. 1990). This evidence suggests that tumor inhibition by high dietary vitamin B_6 may be mediated by T-lymphocyte-dependent mechanisms. Vitamin C is also an essential nutrient playing a role in protecting against carcinogenesis. As one of the inhibitory actions of vitamin C against carcinogenesis, the enhancement of cellular immunity is involved (Glatthaar et al. 1986). However, when desiring stable immunoenhancement, a daily high-level intake of vitamin C (> 1000 mg/day) is needed (Anderson et al. 1980).

ROLE OF MINERALS IN CANCER PREVENTION AND IMMUNITY

Selenium (Se) is an essential nutritional factor with a chemopreventive potential. An inverse correlation between cancer incidence and dietary intake of Se has been well estab-

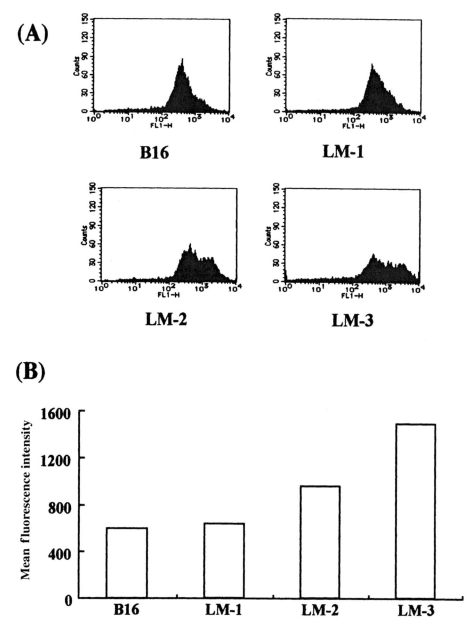

Figure 5.6. Expression of adhesion molecule, CD44 in B16 melanoma with various degrees of lung metastatic ability in male C57B1/6 mice. B16 melanoma cells with various degrees of lung metastatic ability were isolated from the lungs of mice. B16 melanoma cell lines in order of frequency of lung metastasis are LM-3, LM-2, LM-1, and B16. Distribution of melanoma cells with different fluorescence intensity (A) and mean fluorescence intensity in each melanoma cell line (B) are indicated. As shown in both figures, LM-3 cells having the high ability of lung metastasis showed the highest expression of CD44.

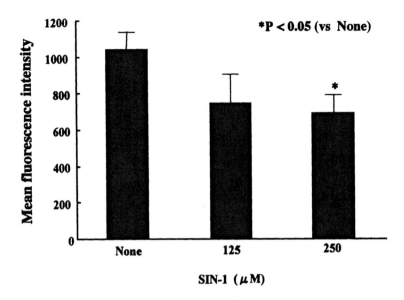

Figure 5.7.   In vitro effect of nitric oxide (NO) generated from SIN-1 on expression of adhesion molecule, CD44, in LM-2 melanoma cell line. After LM-2 melanoma cells were incubated with various concentrations of SIN-1, NO generator for 4 hours, they were washed and stained with anti-CD44 antibody conjugated with FITC. Then their fluorescence intensity was measured by using Flow cytometer. Values are means ± SD; significantly different from the culture with medium only (*P < 0.05).

lished in epidemiological and experimental studies. It is known that patients either with newly diagnosed cancers or with metastases or who are undergoing therapy have statistically significant less blood, urine, and hair Se than age- and sex-matched healthy controls. It seems that Se supplementation is important for cancer patients because Se has an ability to enhance various humoral and cellular immune responses.

The ability of C57BL/6J mice, maintained for 8 weeks on a Se-deficient (0.02 ppm Se), normal (0.20 ppm Se), or Se-supplemented (2.00 ppm Se) diet, to generate cytotoxic lymphocytes (CTL) and to destroy tumor cells was examined. Lymphocytes from mice fed the Se-supplemented diet had a greater ability to destroy tumor cells than those from mice fed the normal diet, whereas Se deficiency reduced the cytotoxicity (Roy et al. 1990). In addition, it is proposed that the enhancement of in vivo cytotoxicity of NK or CTL following Se supplementation is likely to act synergistically with tumor growth inhibition in the reduction of tumor incidence (Fig. 5.8) (Petrie et al. 1989). It seems that Se's direct effects on host defense cells to suppress or enhance their actions as well as effects on tumor cells occur in the promotion phase (Talcott et al. 1984).

Zinc is also an important nutrient for maintaining cellular immune functions. Zinc status was determined in patients with newly diagnosed squamous cell carcinoma of the oral cavity, oropharynx, larynx, and hypopharynx. In this case, patients with metastatic disease and with severe comorbidity were excluded. Results showed that approximately 50% of the subjects were zinc-deficient based on cellular zinc criteria and had decreased production of Th1 cytokines but not Th2 cytokines, decreased NK cell activity, and decreased

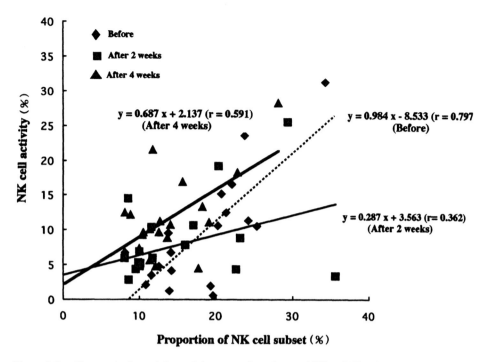

Figure 5.8.   Changes in the activity and the proportion of natural killer (NK) cells in peripheral blood lymphocytes (PBL) of subjects with Aojiru drinking for 4 weeks. Nineteen female university students were selected as subjects (aged 20 to 22) in this study. They daily drank 90 ml of Aojiru juice for 4 weeks. At 2 and 4 weeks, peripheral blood was taken and their PBL were isolated. NK activity in the vertical axis and proportion of NK cell subset in the horizontal axis were plotted. As shown in this figure, NK activity of subjects with lower proportion of NK cell subset was largely enhanced following Aojiru drinking.

proportion of CD4+CD45RA+ cells in the peripheral blood (Prasad et al. 1998). Zinc concentration in polymorphonuclear cells was also decreased in the hospitalized subjects (Goode et al. 1991).

ROLE OF SOME FOODS IN CANCER PREVENTION AND IMMUNITY

Both epidemiological and animal studies have found anticarcinogenic potential in garlic and its constituent compounds. A review on a historical perspective on garlic and cancer was recently published (Milner, 2001). This review shows that water- and lipid-soluble allyl sulfur compounds have an ability to block experimentally induced tumors in a variety of sites including skin, breast, and colon, which mechanism is related to changes in DNA repair and immunocompetence. In vitro effects of garlic derivative (alliin) on both peripheral blood mononuclear cell (PBMC) proliferation and cytokine production induced by the mitogen were examined and increases in pokeweed mitogen (PWM)-induced lymphocyte proliferation, and interleukin (IL)-1 beta and tumor necrosis factor (TNF)-a productions were found (Salman et al. 1999). Lamm and Riggs (2001) have also reviewed the antitumor effect of garlic and described that the immune stimulation of garlic is able to reduce the incidence of cancer. In addition, it has been also reported that aged garlic extract (AGE) significantly inhibits the growth of Sarcoma-180 (allogenic) and LL/2 lung carcinoma (syngenic) cells transplanted into mice and increases natural killer (NK) and killer activities of spleen cells in Sarcoma-180-bearing mice (Kyo et al. 2001).

In Japan, 40,000 households periodically purchase and drink Aojiru. Aojiru is named from its color and is a juice prepared from kale, which is a plant related to cabbage. The beneficial effect of Aojiru was investigated by measuring the activity of natural killer (NK) cells, which play an important role in protecting the body from bacteria and viral infections, and in excluding transformed cells and suppressing carcinogenesis (Cooley et al. 1999, Hirose and Kuroda 1999, and Baraz et al. 1999). NK activity of splenocytes from rats fed the freeze-dried Aojiru supplemented diet was about three times higher than that of control rats (Moriguchi and Muraga 2000).

To investigate its mechanism, the effect of Aojiru drinking on NK activity of peripheral blood lymphocytes of young female university students was examined. NK activity following Aojiru drinking for 4 weeks was significantly increased. As shown in Figure 5.8, the enhancement of NK activity is due not to increased proportion of NK cells but to increased activity of NK cell per se (Ogawa et al. 2001). Measuring cytokines in serum of these subjects, there was a significant increase of interleukin-2 (IL-2), inducing the activation of NK cells, after 4 weeks of Aojiru drinking (Fig. 5.9).

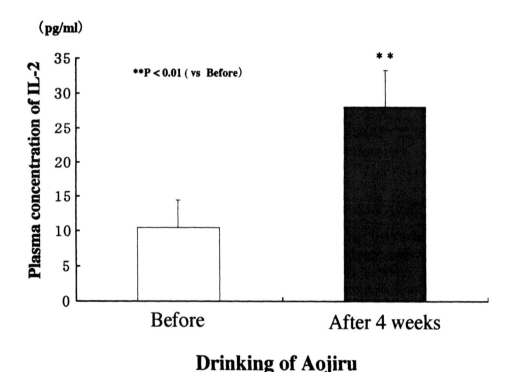

Figure 5.9.   Plasma concentration of IL-2 in female university students following Aojiru drinking for 4 weeks. Values are means ± SD (n = 19); significantly different from plasma concentration of IL-2 of subjects before Aojiru drinking (**P <0.01).

These results suggest that the intake of some foods having immunoenhancing effect is beneficial for preventing carcinogenesis and maintaining health.

CONCLUSION

Nutritional supplementation is important for both maintenance of host immune function for perioperative cancer patients and the suppression of cancer incidence and promotion.

As described in this chapter, there are many nutrients having immunoenhancing effects. Some of them act directly to inhibit tumorigenesis and tumor growth. Even if cancer patients fall into the immunodeficient status following malnutrition, enteral or parenteral nutrition for supplying adequate nutrition can improve their nutritional status and immune functions and result in prolonging their survival time. In addition, to protect tumorigenesis in our body simply and with certainty, we have two options: one is not eating foods with possible carcinogens and the other is eating foods with immunoenhancing effects described in this chapter.

REFERENCES

Anderson, R., Oosthuizen, R., Maritz, R., Theron, A., and Van Rensburg, A. J. 1980. The effects of increasing weekly doses of ascorbate on certain cellular and humoral immune functions in normal volunteers. Am. J. Clin. Nutr. 33(1): 71–76.

Ardawi, M. S., and Newsgolme, E. A. 1982. Maximum activities of some enzymes of glycolysis, the tricarboxylic acid cycle and ketone-body and glutamine utilization pathways in lymphocytes of the rat. Biochem. J. 208(3): 743–748.

Baraz, L., Khazanov, E., Condiotti, R., Kotler, M., and Nagler, A. 1999. Natural killer (NK) cells prevent virus production in cell culture. Bone Marrow Transplan. 24(2): 179–189.

Bendich, A. 1989. Carotenoids and the immune response. J. Nutr. 119(1): 112–115.

Bendich, A., and Shapiro, S. S. 1986. Effect of beta-carotene and canthaxanthin on the immune responses of rat. J. Nutr. 116(11): 2254–2262.

Braga, M., Vignali, A., Gianotti, L., Cestari, A., Profili, M., and Carlo, V. D. 1996. Immune and nutritional effects of early enteral nutrition after major abdominal operations. Eur. J. Surg. 162(2): 105–112.

Chuntrasakul, C., Siltham, S., Sarasombath, S., Sittapairochana, C., Leowattana, W., Chockvivatamavanit, S., and Bunnak, A. 1998. Metabolic and immune effects of dietary arginine, glutamine and omega-3 fatty acids supplementation in immunocompromized patients. J. Med. Assoc. Thai 81(5): 334– 343.

Cooley, S., Burns, L. J., Repka, T., and Miller, J. S. 1999. Natural killer cell cytotoxicity of breast cancer targets is enhanced by two distinct mechanisms of antibody-dependent cellular cytotoxicity against LFA-3 and HER2/neu. Exp. Hematol. 27: 1533–1541.

Daly, J. M., Reynolds, J., Sigal, R. K., Shou. J., and Liberman, M. D. 1990. Effect of dietary protein and amino acids on immune function. Crit. Care Med. 18(2 Suppl.): S86–S93.

Ding, A. H., Nathan, C., and Stuehr, D. J. 1988. Release of reactive nitrogen intermediates and reactive oxygen intermediates from mouse peritoneal macrophages. J. Immunol. 141(7): 2407–2412.

Furst, P., Albers, S., and Stehle, P. 1989. Availability of glutamine supplied intravenously as alanyl-glutamine. Metabolism 38(8 Suppl. 1): 67–72.

Furukawa, K., Tashiro, T., Yamamori, H., Takagi, K., Morishima, Y., Sugiura, T., Otsubo, Y.,

Hayashi, N., Tabashi, T., Sano, W., Toyoda, Y., Nitta, H., and Nakajima, N. 1999. Effects of soybean oil emulsion and eicosapentaenoic acid on stress response and immune function after a severely stressful operation. Ann. Surg. 229(2); 255–261.

Gebhard, K. J., Gridley, D. S., Stickney, D. R., and Shulz, T. D. 1990. Enhancement of immune status by high levels of dietary vitamin B-6 without growth inhibition of human malignant melanoma in athymic nude mice. Nutr. Cancer 14(1): 15–26.

Gensler, H. L., Watson, R. R., Moriguchi, S., and Bowden, G. T. 1987. Effects of dietary retinyl palmitate or 13-cis-retinoic acid on the promotion of tumors in mouse skin. Cancer Res. 47(2): 967–970.

Gianotti, L., Braga, M., Fortis, C., Soldini, L., Vignali, A., Colombo, S., Radaelli, G., and Di Carlo, V. 1999. A prospective, randomized clinical trial on perioperative feeding with an arginine-, omega-3 fatty acid-, and RNA- enriched enteral diet: effect on host response and nutritional status. J. Parenter. Enteral Nutr. 23(6): 314–320.

Glatthaar, B. E., Hornig, D. H., and Moser, U. 1986. The role of ascorbic acid in carcinogenesis. Adv. Exp. Med. Biol. 206: 357–377.

Goode, H. F., Penn, N. D., Kelleher, J., and Walker, B. E. 1991. Evidence of cellular zinc depletion in hospitalized but not in healthy elderly subjects. Age Ageing 20(5): 345–348.

Grant, J. P., and Snyder, P. J. 1988. Use of L-glutamine in total parenteral nutrition. J. Surg. Res. 44(5): 506–513.

Haynes, W. G., Noon, J. P., Walker, B. R., and Webb, D. J. 1993. L-NMMA increases blood pressure in man. Lancet 342: 931–932.

Hirose, M., and Kuroda, Y. 1999. Successful induction of natural killer/cytotoxic T-lymphocyte cells in the treatment of Langerhans' cell histiocytosis. Int. J. Hematol. 69(4): 272–273.

Hursting, S. D., Switzer, B. R., French, J. E., and Kari, F. W. 1994. Inhibition of rat mononuclear cell leukemia by corn oil gavage: in vivo, in situ and immune competence studies. Carcinogenesis 15(2): 193–199.

Iida, K., Kadota, J., Kawakami, K., Shirai, R., Abe, K., Yoshinaga, M., Iwashita, T., Matsubara, Y., Ishimatsu, Y., Ohmagari, K., and Kohno, S. 1999. Immunological function and nutritional status in patients with hepatocellular carcinoma. Hepatogastroenterology 46(28): 2476–2482.

Kark, J. D., Smith, A. H., Switzer, B. R., and Hames, C. G. 1981. Serum vitamin A (retinol) and cancer incidence in Evans Country, Georgia. J. Natl. Cancer Inst. 66: 7–16.

Kemen, M., Senkal, M., Homann, H. H., Mumme, A., Dauphin, A. K., Baier, J., Windeler, J., Newmann, H., and Zumtobel, V. 1995. Early postoperative enteral nutrition with arginine-, omega-3 fatty acids and ribonucleic acid-supplemented diet versus placebo in cancer patients: an immunologic evaluation of Impact. Crit. Care Med. 23(4): 652–659.

Konno, A., Hishinuma, K., Hashimoto, Y., Kimura, S., and Nishimura, T. 1991. Dietary restriction reduces the incidence of 3-methylcholanthrene-induced tumors in mice: close correlation with its potentiating effect on host T cell functions. Cancer Immunol. Immunother. 33(5): 293–298.

Kraus, L. J., Williams, R. N., Murphy. K., and Broitman, S. A. 1987. T-cell mitogenesis and natural killer cell activity in colonic tumor-bearing and nontumor-bearing rats fed diets high in lipid with and without cholesterol. Nutr. Cancer 9(2-3): 159–170.

Kune, G. A., Kune S., Watson, L. F., Pierce, R., Field, B., Vitetta, L., Merenstein, D., Hayes, A., and Irving, L. 1989. Serum levels of beta-carotene, vitamin A, and zinc in male lung cancer cases and controls. Nutr Cancer 12(2): 169–176.

Kweon, M. N., Moriguchi, S., Mukai, K., and Kishino, Y. 1991. Effect of alanylglutamine-enriched infusion on tumor growth and cellular immune function in rats. Amino Acids 1(1): 7–16.

Kyo, E., Uda, N., Kasuga, S., and Itakura, Y. 2001. Immunomodulatory effect of aged garlic extract. J. Nutr. 131(3S): 1075S–1079S.

Lakshmi, M. S., Parker, C., and Sherbet, G. V. 1997. Expression of the transmembrane glycoprotein CD44 and metastasis associated 18A2/MTS1 gene in B16 murine melanoma cells. Anticancer Res. 17(5A): 3451–3455.

Lamm, D. L., and Riggs, D. R. 2001. Enhanced immunocompetence by garlic: role in bladder cancer and other malignancies. J. Nutr. 131(3S): 1067S–1070S.

Le Marchand, L., Yoshizawa C. N., Kolonel, L. N., Hankin, J. H., and Goodman, M. T. 1989. Vegetable consumption and lung cancer risk: a population-based case-control study in Hawaii. J. Natl. Cancer Inst. 81(15): 1158–1164.

Lemire, J. 2000. 1,25-Dihydroxyvitamin D_3—a hormone with immunomodulatory properties. Rheumatol. 59 (Supple): 24–27.

Locniskar, M., Nauss, K. M., and Newberne, P. W. 1986. Effect of colon tumor development and dietary fat on the immune system of rats treated with DMH. Nutr. Cancer 8(2): 73–84.

Mehta, R. G., and Mehta, R. R. 2002. Vitamin D and cancer. J. Nutr. Biochem. 13(5): 252–264.

Milner, J. A. 2001. A historical perspective on garlic and cancer. J. Nutr. 131(3S): 1075S–1079S.

Moon, R. C., McCormik, D. L., and Mehta, R. G. 1983. Chemoprevention of animal tumors by retinoids. In: *Modulation and Mediation of Cancer by Vitamins*, Meyskens, F. L., and Prasad, K. N., pp. 47–57, Basel: Karger.

Moon, R. C., McCormik, D. L., Becci, P. J., Shealy, Y. F., Frickel, F., Paust, J., and Sporn, M. B. 1982. Influence of 15 retinoic acid amides on urinary bladder carcinogenesis in the mouse. Carcinogenesis (Lond.) 3: 1469–1472.

Moriguchi, S., and Kishino, Y. 1990. In vitro activation of tumoricidal properties of human monocytes by beta-carotene encapsulated in liposomes. Nutr. Res. 10: 837–846.

Moriguchi, S., and Muraga, M. 2000. Vitamin E and immunity. In *Vitamins and Hormones* 59, edited by Litwack, G., pp.305–336. Ames: Academic Press.

Moriguchi, S., Mukai, K., Hiraoka, I., and Kishino, Y. 1987. Functional changes in human lymphocytes and monocytes after in vitro incubation with arginine. Nutr. Res. 7: 719–729.

Moriguchi, S., Okishima, N., Sumida, S., Okamura, K., Doi, T., and Kishino, Y. 1996. Beta-carotene supplementation enhances lymphocyte proliferation with mitogens in human peripheral blood lymphocytes. Nutr. Res. 16(2): 211–218.

Moriguchi, S., Werner, L., and Watson, R. R. 1985. High dietary vitamin A (retinyl palmitate) and cellular immune functions in mice. Immunology 56: 169–177.

Moriguchi, S., Yamashita, S., and Kurihara, Y. 2002. Inhibitory effect of arginine on lung metastasis of B16 melanoma in C57 Bl/6 mice. Reports of the Research Committee of Essential Amino Acids 164: 6–11.

Mukhopadhyay, P., Gupta, J. D., Sanyal, U., Das, S., and Senyal, U. 1994. Influence of dietary restriction and soybean supplementation on the growth of a murine lymphoma and host immune function. Cancer Lett. 78(1-3): 151–157.

Newsholme, P., and Newsholme, E. A. 1989. Rates of utilization of glucose, glutamine and formation of endoproducts by mouse peritoneal macrophages in culture. Biochem. J. 261(1): 211–218.

Ogawa, K., Yamashita, S., Nakata, K., and Moriguchi, S. 2001. Effect of Aojiru drinking on cellular immunity and physiological functions in female university students 55th Annual Meeting in Japanese Society of Nutrition and Food Science, 6–8, May, at Kyoto International Conference Hall, Kyoto, Japan.

Palmer, R. M. J., Ferrige, A. G., and Moncada, S. 1987. Nitric oxide release accounts for the biological activity of endothelium-derived relaxing factor. Nature 327: 524–526.

Petrie, H. T., Klassen, L. W., Klassen, P. S., O'Dell, J. R., and Kay, H. D. 1989. Selenium and the immune response: 2. Enhancement of murine cytotoxic T-lymphocyte and natural killer cell cytotoxicity in vivo. J. Leukoc. Biol. 45(3): 215–220.

Prasad, A. S., Beck, F. W., Doerr, T. D., Shamsa, F. H., Penny, H. S., Marks, S. C., Kaplan, J., Kucuk, O., and Mathog, R. H. 1998. Nutritional and zinc status of head and neck cancer patients: an interpretive review. J. Am. Coll. Nutr. 17(5): 409–418.

Roy, M., Kiremidjian-Schumacher, L., Wishe, H. I., Cohen, M. W., and Stotzky, G. 1990. Selenium and immune cell functions. II. Effect on lymphocyte-mediated cytotoxicity. Proc. Soc. Exp. Biol. Med. 193(2): 143–148.

Saffiotti, U., Montesano, R., Sellakumar, A. R., and Bork, S. A. 1967. Experimental cancer of the lung. Inhibition by vitamin A of the induction of tracheobronchial squamous metaplasia and squamous cell tumors. Cancer (Phila.) 20: 857–864.

Salman, H., Bergman, M., Bessler, H., Punsky, I., and Djaldetti, M. 1999. Effect of a garlic derivative (alliin) on peripheral blood cell immune response. Int. J. Immunopharmacol. 21(9): 589–597.

Sedman, P. C., Somers, S. S., Ramsden, C. W., Brennan, T. G., and Guillou, P. J. 1991. Effects of different lipid emulsions on lymphocyte function during total parenteral nutrition. Br. J. Surg. 78(11): 1396–1399.

Sheldon, W. G., Bucci, T. J., Hart, R. W., and Turturro, A. 1995. Age-related neoplasia in a lifetime study of ad libitum-fed and food-restricted B6C3F1 mice. Toxicol. Pathol. 23(4): 458–476.

Sikorska, B., Danilewicz, M., and Wagrowska-Danilewicz, M. 2002. Prognostic significance of CD44v6 and nm 23 protein immunoexpression in laryngeal squamous cell carcinoma. Pol. J. Pathol. 53(1): 17–24.

Tachibana, K., Mukai, K., Hiraoka, I., Moriguchi, S., Takama, S., and Kishino, Y. 1985. Evaluation of the effect of arginine- enriched amino acid solution on tumor growth. J. Parenter. Enteral Nutr. 9(4): 428–434.

Talcott, P. A., Exon, J. H., and Koller, L. D. 1984. Alteration of natural killer cell-mediated cytotoxicity in rats treated with selenium, diethtylnitrosamine and ethylnitrosourea. Cancer Lett. 23(3): 313–322.

Tashiro, T., Yamamori, H., Takagi, K., Hayashi, N., Furukawa, K., Nitta, H., Toyoda, Y., Sano, W., Itabashi, T., Nishiya, K., Hirano, J., and Nakajima, N. 1999. Changes in immune function following surgery for esophageal carcinoma. Nutrition 15(10): 760–766.

Verma, A. K., Conrad, E. K., and Boutwell, R. K. 1982. The differential effects of retinoic acid and 7,8-benzoflavone on the induction of mouse skin tumors by the complete carcinogenesis process and by the initiation-promotion regimen. Cancer Res. 42: 3519–3525.

Villa, M. L., Ferrario, E., Bergamasco, E., Bozzetti, F., Cozzaglio, L., and Clerici, E. 1991. Reduced natural killer cell activity and IL-2 production in malnourished cancer patients. Br. J. Cancer 63(6): 1010–1014.

Vitale, J. J., and Broitman, S. A. 1981. Lipids and immune function. Cancer Res. 41(9 Pt. 2): 3706–3710.

Wald, N., Idles, M., Boreham, J., and Bailey, A. 1980. Low serum-vitamin A and subsequent risk of cancer. Lancet 2: 813–815.

Watson, R. R., and Moriguchi, S. 1989. Effect of retinyl palmitate and 13-cis retinoic acid on immune functions in immunodeficient, nude mice. Life Sci. 44(6): 387–395.

Yan, M. 1990. Effects of perioperative parenteral nutrition on immunocompetence in patients with gastric cancer. Zhonghua Wai Ke Za Zhi 28(12): 739–741.

Yu, A., Somasundar, P., Balsubramaniam, A., Rose, A. T., Vona-Davis, L., and McFadden, D. W. 2002. Vitamin E and the Y4 agonist BA-129 decrease prostate cancer growth and production of vascular endothelial growth factor. J. Surg. Res. 105(1): 65–68.

6

Nutrition and Skin Cancer Risk Prevention

Steven Pratt,
Hubert T. Greenway,
and Craig Naugle

INTRODUCTION

Skin cancer reached epidemic proportions during the last decade. Skin cancer comprises basal cell carcinoma (BCC), squamous cell carcinoma (SCC), and malignant melanoma. BCC is the most common cancer of white populations, with an estimated incidence of 900,000 cases per year occurring in the United States (Miller and Weinstock 1994). SCC develops in 200,000 persons per year in the United States and is more aggressive than BCC with a greater likelihood of metastases (Miller and Weinstock 1994). SCC has been shown to metastasize 7.4% of the time on the skin and 15.8% on the lip (Dinehart and Pollack 1989). Malignant melanoma has the highest metastatic potential and will affect 1 in 88 persons currently living in the United States with an estimated 41,600 persons developing melanoma in 1998 (Landis et al. 1998). This incidence is likely underestimated secondary to the frequent nonreporting of melanoma in situ lesions.

Over the past decade there has been a dramatic increase in all types of skin cancer resulting in the aforementioned skin cancer epidemic. The etiology is likely multifactorial, however, experts attribute the majority of the increase to ultraviolet light (UV). UV radiation is divided into UVA (320–399 nm), UVB (290–320 nm), and UVC (< 290 nm). For years the UVA spectrum was thought of as innocuous. However, literature over the past decade has clearly illustrated that this spectrum causes immediate and delayed tanning of the skin, photoaging, and immunosuppression (Fitzpatrick 1999). UVA results in the production of singlet oxygen and superoxide anion, which can induce damage to cell membranes and DNA, leading to DNA strand breaks and eventual mutations. Sunscreens have evolved in response to this research with UVA/UVB sunscreens containing UVA blockers such as avobenzone, micronized titanium oxide, and micronized zinc oxide entering the market. UVB is classically known as sunburn irradiation and is the primary cause of sunburn and skin cancer. UVB and UVC are absorbed by the stratospheric ozone layer. Chlorofluorocarbon is one of many chemicals that has been shown to reduce ozone and significantly affect the amount of UVB and UVC radiation that reaches our skin (Slaper et al. 1996).

Vitamin supplementation and micronutrients are emerging as a part of the armamentarium used in the defense against skin cancer. Vitamins A, C, and E, carotenoids, various polyphenols, and polyunsaturated fatty acids (omega-3) have been shown to be modestly photoprotective (Lee et al. 2001; Greenway et al. 2001a, pp. 109–116; Kune 1990). An increase in cell-mediated immunity via vitamin supplementation may enhance tumor surveillance (Wu et al. 1999). At least 30% of all cancers are considered to have a dietary component (Correa 1981, Block et al. 1992). The intake of cruciferous vegetables has been shown to be inversely related to the incidence of cancer (Verhoeven et al. 1996). As a group, as little as 10 g of cruciferous vegetables (broccoli, kale, cabbage, brussels sprouts, cauliflower, collards) per day can play an important role in the prevention of at least one type of cancer (colorectal) (Kohlmeir et al. 1997). Vegetables have been associated with a decreased incidence of photoaging (Purba et al. 2001), and crucifers have been inversely related to the incidence of skin cancer in at least one publication (Kune 1992). The phytochemical profile of cruciferous vegetables is well suited to play a role in cancer prevention. These vegetables are loaded with indoles, isothiocyanates, and sulforaphane (Zhang et al. 1994). These "anticancer" compounds appear to prevent cancer by such mechanisms as inactivating carcinogens, activating protective detoxification enzymes, and interfering with cancer cell replication (Jeffrey et al. 2001). Crucifers, especially broccoli, are also a rich source of vitamins (especially vitamin C), several carotenoids (lutein, beta-carotene), and polyphenols (Kurilich et al. 1999). Although we await specific studies looking at the relationship between skin cancer and intake of cruciferous vegetables (and the phytonutrients somewhat unique to this class of foods), it seems prudent to include these well-documented "cancer fighters" in any overall dietary strategy to decrease the incidence of skin cancer.

Finally, green tea polyphenols have been shown to reduce UV-light induced oxidative stress and immunosuppression (Katiyar et al. 2000b).

SKIN CANCER RISK FACTORS

The most significant risk factor for skin cancer is exposure to ultraviolet radiation. First and foremost, the cornerstone of a preventive plan for skin cancer begins with daily application of a UVA/UVB sunscreen. Studies have suggested that intermittent sun exposure as a child, especially resulting in sunburn, may be more important in determining BCC risk than cumulative exposure (Rossa et al. 1996). Other factors that increase risk for skin cancer include light skin, inability to tan, blue eyes, and living in latitudes near the equator.

Another possible risk factor for skin cancer is a high fat diet. Black et al. studied a low fat diet and found a potential benefit in reduction of actinic keratoses (Black et al. 1994). In addition, cigarettes increase the risk of squamous cell carcinoma (Thomas et al. 1974).

Over the past decade genetic influences have been elucidated. Mutations in the p53 tumor-suppressor gene via UV-induced mutations are thought to interfere with programmed cell death resulting in increased incidence of BCC and SCC (Kastan et al. 1998). More recently, malignant melanoma has been strongly associated with defects in the tumor suppressor gene CDKN2a (Serrano et al. 1993). Therefore, a family history of skin cancer puts one at increased risk.

Another major factor in the skin cancer epidemic is the perceived attractiveness of a tan population. Many attribute this belief to Coco Chanel, who was one of the central figures that glamorized the transition from a tan representing the "working class" to being a status symbol of the bourgeois. Clearly, environmental, genetic, and social factors intertwine, resulting in increased incidence of skin cancer worldwide.

Other populations at risk for skin cancer include those that are immunocompromised. SCC is greatly increased in those persons with chronic lymphocytic leukemia, post solid organ transplant, with HIV/AIDS, and those on chronic glucocorticoid therapy. Also, persons with a past history of skin cancer have a risk approaching 45% of developing a second skin cancer (Marghood et al. 1993). Persons in these groups are prime targets for any effective strategies to reduce skin cancer risk, such as through vitamin supplementation and ingestion of phytonutrients.

Patients with basal cell carcinoma and squamous cell carcinoma are at increased risk for cancers of the prostate, breast, larynx, lung, testicle, salivary gland, lip, and bladder (Riou et al. 1995). This is particularly true in those patients diagnosed with skin cancer before the age of 60. In addition, leukemia, melanoma, and non-Hodgkin's lymphoma are also more prevalent in patients with a history of nonmelanoma skin cancer (Riou et al. 1995). Finally, death rates from these cancers are 20–40% higher among patients who report a history of nonmelanoma skin cancer than in individuals who do not (Frisch et al. 1996).

PHOTOAGING

Cutaneous aging is the result of intrinsic aging (natural aging) and extrinsic aging. Intrinsic aging is due to such factors as oxidative stress and programmed cell death. Extrinsic aging is due to "unnatural" processes such as UV radiation and cigarette smoke. The exposure to excessive ultraviolet radiation results in benign extrinsic changes in the skin manifested as wrinkles, mottled hyperpigmentation, sagging, and textural changes. This aging process is associated with many skin changes that can be illustrated histologically. There are topical and oral treatments that one can use that have been proven to reverse some of the extrinsic signs of aging both clinically and histologically. Included in this class of cosmeceuticals is topical tretinoin (Retin-A or Renova), which when used with daily application of sunscreen can improve fine lines, mottled hyperpigmentation, and textural changes (Kligman et al. 1986). In addition, fruit acids such as glycolic acid are proven to modestly improve extrinsic aging. Evidence is mounting that in addition to these cosmeceuticals, specific fruits and vegetables or their components may reduce signs of extrinsic aging. A fascinating area of research includes benefits in slowing the natural progression of intrinsic aging through antioxidant properties of vitamins and micronutrients.

SKIN DEFENSES AGAINST OXIDATIVE STRESS FROM ULTRAVIOLET LIGHT

The skin has several intrinsic "lines of defense" against ultraviolet light and the subsequent oxidative stress. The stratum corneum acts to absorb and scatter light and melanin acts as a UV-absorbing filter and free radical scavenger. In addition, our skin uses antioxidant nutrients for protection from UV. These include vitamin C, vitamin E, carotenoids (beta-carotene, lycopene, lutein, beta cryptoxanthin, alpha-carotene), glutathione, coenzyme Q, vitamin A, polyphenolic flavonoids, and minerals such as zinc, selenium, and copper (Wu et al. 1999). Our antioxidant defense system helps minimize the damage to DNA caused by sunlight and is elaborated upon in the following sections. It is important to remember that many studies assess the efficacy of one or maybe two micronutrients and that there may be synergy between multiple vitamins and minerals. The synergistic benefits of vitamins A, C, E, glutathione, selenium, and polyphenols cannot be overemphasized (Jacob 1995).

PHOTOPROTECTION THROUGH VITAMIN C, VITAMIN E, CAROTENOIDS, AND POLYUNSATURATED FATTY ACIDS

The injured skin reacts to excessive UV irradiation with vasodilatation and a resultant cascade of inflammatory mediators resulting in sunburn. Scientists measure UV irradiation by the minimal erythema dose (MED). One MED is the amount of UV irradiation necessary to produce redness approximately 20 hours after exposure. Most studies of photoprotection utilize MED to assess blockage of UV absorption or inhibition of the inflammatory cascade. In addition, the MED is used to calculate sunscreen protection factor (SPF).

Chronic exposure to UV results in signs of extrinsic photoaging. The goal of photoprotection should be to first inhibit development of skin cancer and second prevent photoaging, reducing wrinkles, hyperpigmentation, sagging, and textural changes. Supplementation with carotenoids, vitamins C and E, and polyunsaturated fatty acids is an effective method of inhibiting photodamage.

Vitamin C

Vitamin C in its active form is called L-ascorbic acid. As discussed earlier, UV irradiation produces free radicals, which can damage DNA, cell enzymes, and cell membranes. Ascorbic acid acts as an antioxidant by scavenging free radicals (Beyer 1994). Vitamin C inhibits the damage caused by the superoxide anion (Scarpa et al. 1983), hydroxyl radicals (Cabelli et al. 1983), and singlet oxygen (Chou et al. 1983). In addition, vitamin C regenerates vitamin E from its radical form. Through vitamin C's interaction with vitamin E, it indirectly inhibits lipid peroxidation.

Vitamin C does not have the ability to absorb ultraviolet radiation and is most likely photoprotective secondary to its antioxidant and anti-inflammatory characteristics. There have been three clinical studies of topical vitamin C and two studies of oral vitamin C assessing photoprotection. Percutaneous absorption studies reveal that a 10% solution of L-ascorbic acid allows adequate pharmacologic levels of ascorbic acid to reach the skin. Absorption studies have shown that 12% ascorbic acid crosses the stratum corneum in 72 hours (Pinnell et al. 1988). Darr found decreased skin levels of vitamin C after UV exposure in pigs and was able to show elevated skin levels after topical application of vitamin C (Darr et al. 1992). Murray et al. applied 10% L-ascorbic acid to volar forearms of human subjects with controls treated with vehicle. Subjects then received UV irradiation and those sites treated with topical ascorbic acid showed decreased MED and less erythema than controls (Murray et al. 1991). Both studies assessing oral vitamin C and photoprotection have been done in coordination with vitamin E. Fuchs used very high doses of alpha-tocopherol (2 g/day) and ascorbate (3 g/day) on 40 volunteers for 50 days (Fuchs et al. 1998). Buccal mucosal keratinocyte analysis revealed adequate bioavailability in subjects tested. MED increased significantly in subjects treated with both vitamins, however, placebo treated subjects also had a modest increase in MED. The authors contributed this to seasonal influences. Vitamins C and E were clearly photoprotective, but diets would seldom produce levels approaching the doses studied. Eberlein-Konig et al. (1998) treated ten subjects with 671 mg vitamin E/day and 2 g vitamin C/day for a short period of 8 days. MED increased in 8 of 10 subjects. Clearly more studies are needed assessing the photoprotection gained by oral and topical supplementation with ascorbic acid. However, despite few double-blinded studies, many cosmetic companies are marketing topical vitamin C with claims ranging from improvement of fine lines to restoration of skin tone.

Vitamin E

Vitamin E encompasses tocotrienols and tocopherols and is present in a variety of foods. Studies evaluating the role of alpha-tocopherol both in the prevention of skin cancer, including melanoma, as well as evaluating plasma levels have produced conflicting results (Knekt 1992, and Wei et al. 1994). Therefore, evidence supporting Vitamin E supplementation for skin cancer needs further delineation. There have been four studies assessing the photoprotective potential of alpha-tocopherol. Studies by Fuchs et al. and Eberlein-Konig et al. were in combination with vitamin C and showed impressive increases in MED. These studies were outlined in the prior section. La Ruche and Cesarini (1991) studied 14 mg alpha-tocopherol in combination with 2700 micrograms retinol versus trace elements and placebo for 3 weeks. Those treated with the vitamins had decreased sunburn cells after exposure to UV irradiation versus controls, however, MED was not affected. Similar results were achieved in those receiving supplementation with the trace elements. Werninghaus et al. (1994) treated 12 healthy volunteers with 400 IU of alpha-tocopherol acetate/day or placebo for 6 months. MED was not significantly affected and there was no change in sunburn cells, in contrast to the study by La Ruche. Since the only clear increase in MED occurred in those subjects treated with ascorbic acid and vitamin E, it would seem likely that ascorbic acid is offering the bulk of the photoprotection. However, as aforementioned, other antioxidants such as vitamin C are likely necessary to enhance tocopherol's photoprotective effects by preventing its degradation in the skin. In addition, all studies are on few subjects at vastly different dosages and treatment durations making it difficult to compare outcomes.

Studies have suggested that vitamin E may have a role in the treatment of facial hyperpigmentation. A recent study by Funasaka et al. (1999) studied alpha-tocopherol ferulate solubilized in ethanol or in 0.5% lecithin on human melanoma cells in culture (Funasaka et al. 1999). They found a significant reduction of melanization secondary to inhibition of tyrosinase likely at the posttranslational level. Further studies are clearly needed.

In addition, up to 13% of the total vitamin E in the skin consists of tocotrienols. This percentage has been reported to be more than one order of magnitude higher than in other studied tissues (Podda et al. 1996). As a result for maximum protective effect from vitamin E one should probably consider both tocopherols and tocotrienols.

Carotenoids

There have been many studies assessing the photoprotective potential of carotenoids. Plasma carotenoid levels can be decreased markedly by UV exposure (White et al. 1988). The antitumor and photoprotective properties of carotenoids suggest that decreasing their plasma concentrations could lead to an increased possibility of photooxidative damage.

Dietary beta-carotene, alpha-carotene, and beta-cryptoxanthin are converted into vitamin A. Lutein and zeaxanthin, while related to beta-carotene, do not interconvert in the skin. Lycopene, another carotenoid, has been detected in the skin and is preferentially oxidized over beta-carotene during sunlight exposure (Ribaya-Mercado et al. 1995). Lycopenemia has been reported and is a harmless reddish discoloration of the skin from the excess ingestion of red-colored foods such as tomatoes. Beta-carotene is a precursor to vitamin A (retinol) and capable of scavenging reactive oxygen species generated under conditions of photooxidative stress. Beta-carotene is proven to be efficacious in patients with erythropoietic protoporphyria (EPP), a genetic disease resulting in blistering sun sensitivity in affected individuals. Matthews-Roth found that daily carotene in 133 patients with EPP experienced an 84% reduction in their tolerance to sunlight and had a much improved lifestyle with less skin burning and blistering upon UV exposure (Matthews-Roth et al. 1977).

There has only been one large randomized, controlled trial of beta-carotene in prevention of skin cancer (Greenberg et al. 1990). Eighteen hundred patients with a recent diagnosis of nonmelanoma skin cancer were studied for a 5 year period. Subjects received either 50 mg beta-carotene daily or placebo. Supplementation with beta-carotene did not result in a significant effect on prevention of subsequent nonmelanoma skin cancer. Interestingly, further evaluation of the data revealed that there was a greater relative risk of development of a new nonmelanoma skin cancer in those who smoked at study entry and received beta-carotene when compared to those that did not smoke and received beta-carotene. These findings, while not the reason for the study, suggest that there is a deleterious interaction between cigarette smoking, single nutrient beta-carotene supplements, and skin cancer. Heinonen et al. subsequently reported an increased risk of lung cancer in those smokers who received beta-carotene supplementation versus those that did not (Heinonen et al. 1994).

Lee et al. (2000) treated 22 subjects daily with 30 mg of a natural carotenoid mixture (29.4 mg beta-carotene, 0.36 mg alpha-carotene, 0.084 mg cryptoxanthin, 0.072 mg zeaxanthin, and 0.054 mg lutein). The patients were treated initially with 30 mg/day and increased every 8 weeks to a maximum dose of 90 mg/day. The two highest doses resulted in decreased serum lipid peroxidation. In addition, supplementation with 60 mg/day and 90 mg/day of carotenoids resulted in increased MEDs. Stahl treated 20 healthy subjects with 25 mg of a natural carotenoid mix daily, alone or in combination with 335 mg alpha-tocopherol (Stahl et al. 2000). After 12 weeks of daily supplementation, both groups showed elevated concentrations of beta-carotene in skin and serum and slight yellowing of the skin. Erythema post-UV exposure was lower 8 weeks after supplementation, and in those patients treated with carotenoids and vitamin E an even higher level of protection was obtained. Heinrich found similar results on 12 subjects treated with 50 mg of a natural carotenoid mix (Heinrich et al. 1998). The skin had a subtle yellow color and there was decreased erythema post-UV irradiation. Postaire et al. (1997) analyzed dosages of carotenoids and assessed chromametric changes in skin color. Subjects treated with 13 mg beta-carotene, 2 mg lycopene, 5 mg tocopherol, and 30 mg ascorbic acid daily for 8 weeks showed yellow discoloration of the skin and increase in melanin concentration. However, subjects treated with 3 mg beta-carotene and 3 mg lycopene showed no skin discoloration, but did have increases in melanin concentrations at 4 weeks of therapy. Photoprotection was not assessed in this study; however, the authors speculate that carotenoid supplementation stimulates melanogenesis. Gollnick et al. in another chromametric study showed that 30 mg/day of beta-carotene for 10 weeks increased the yellow color of the skin, however, it was not perceptible to the naked eye (Gollnick et al. 1996). They concluded that beta-carotene prior to UV exposure protects against sunburn and they found a synergistic effect when beta-carotene was combined with sunscreen. Garmyn studied much higher doses of beta-carotene (120 mg/day) and found no benefit in reduction of erythema after UV radiation (Garmyn et al. 1995). Wolf treated 23 healthy volunteers with 60 mg beta-carotene and 90 mg canthaxanthin daily for 4 weeks. They found the carotenoid mix not beneficial in reducing erythema post-UV irradiation (Wolf et al. 1988). Greenway and Pratt (Unpublished data) evaluated sun-damaged skin in patients with nonmelanoma skin cancer and found a sevenfold higher level of carotenoids, but not retinol, in the skin of the nose of one patient (six patients studied) with a similar distribution pattern in skin as in plasma, but with much lower values than expected in all six cases (Greenway et al. 2001b, unpublished data). Recently, lycopene was studied via dietary ingestion of tomato paste (approximately 16 mg/day of lycopene). Stahl et al. found a 40% reduction in erythema after UV irradiation at 10 weeks of daily ingestion. There was no difference in controls at 4 weeks of ingestion (Stahl et al. 2001).

Human cancer risks have been shown to be inversely associated with dietary beta-carotene (Peto et al. 1981). There have been few studies assessing beta-carotene and skin cancer. More double-blinded studies are needed to effectively assess the benefits of carotenoids in patients with a history of skin cancer. However, given the photoprotection offered by carotenoids, one can likely reduce skin cancer risk by daily mixed carotenoid supplementation and a frequent consumption of fruits and vegetables/tomato sauces high in a variety of carotenoids.

Polyunsaturated Fatty Acids

The importance of fatty acids and skin is clearly exhibited in essential fatty acid deficiencies. This group of diseases manifest with erythema, dryness, and scaling of the skin. In opposition, certain types of fat may function as immunosuppressants, possibly increasing the risk of melanoma and actinic keratoses (Wei et al. 1994). There have been four studies in the last twenty years assessing omega-3 polyunsaturated fatty acids and photoprotection.

Orengo found a small increase in MED in subjects treated with fish oil (2.8 g/day of eicosapentaenoic acid [EPA] and 1.2 g/day of docosahexaenoic acid) versus controls (Orengo et al. 1992). Rhodes et al. found that dietary supplementation with 10 g fish oil/day resulted in an increase in the MED after 6 months. However, they found that skin in subjects treated with fish oil was susceptible to lipid peroxidation because of the unstable nature of n-3 fatty acids (Rhodes et al. 1994). A second study by Rhodes found an increase in MED after 3 months of supplementation. They also performed suction blister fluid analysis and found decreased prostaglandin E2 levels in irradiated and nonirradiated skin treated with fish oil (Rhodes et al. 1995). Finally, a recent study assessed 28 healthy subjects treated with 4 g of EPA or 98% oleic acid daily for 3 months (Rhodes et al. 2002). A single dose of UVB irradiation was administered, and they found decreased UV-induced erythema and p53 induction. The oleic acid treated group had no significant changes.

GREEN TEA POLYPHENOLS AND SKIN CANCER

The tea plant *Camellia sinensis* was discovered in Southeast Asia. Many types of tea plant preparations are made from *C. sinensis*, with black and green tea the most common. Green tea is primarily consumed in Asian countries, but has gained popularity in Western cultures. The polyphenols in green tea are called catechins. The primary catechins in green tea are epicatechin, epicatechin-(3)-gallate, epigallocatechin, and epigallocatechin-(3)-gallate (EGCG) (Ahmad et al. 1999). EGCG is considered to be the most important for chemopreventive activity (Barthelman et al. 1998). Black tea also has several polyphenols that differ from green tea. Research over the past decade has focused on the polyphenols derived from green tea and their anti-inflammatory, antioxidant, and photoprotective properties.

Mukhtar and colleagues initially showed protection against polycyclic aromatic hydrocarbon-induced skin tumor initiation in mice by green tea polyphenols (Wang et al. 1989). Green tea polyphenols were found protective both topically and orally. A follow-up study found protection against UVB-induced photocarcinogenesis in mice given green tea (Wang et al. 1991). However, the mice treated topically did not do as well as the orally treated group. Early studies proved that green tea extract could cause partial regression of pre-existing skin papillomas in mice and when given chronically to mice resulted in protection against chemical and UVB-induced skin tumors (Mukhtar et al. 1994). Gensler and colleagues treated mice with purified topical EGCG at doses of 10 and 50 mg three times weekly prior to UV radiation. Skin cancer incidence was 96% at 28 weeks after the first UV treatment. EGCG at 10 and 50 mg reduced this incidence to 62% and 29%, respectively (Gensler et al. 1996). Notably, the mice treated with oral EGCG had no reduction in skin cancers.

Two studies analyzing oral administration of black and green teas assessed the effect of caffeine on inhibition of UV-light induced carcinogenesis (Huang et al. 1997 and Lou et al. 1999). The results indicated that decaffeinated teas were much less effective than their caffeinated counterpart. More studies are needed assessing the activity of oral green tea polyphenols and the effect of caffeine.

Katiyar and colleagues extended studies on mice to human skin in vivo and found that EGCG prevented the formation of UVB-induced cyclobutane pyrimidine dimers (Katiyar 2000b). In addition, they proved that green tea polyphenols and specifically EGCG inhibited UV-induced erythema in humans and UVB-induced inflammatory responses and infiltration of human leukocytes in human skin, respectively (Mukhtar 1994 and Katiyar 2001).

There have not been any large double-blinded studies assessing green tea polyphenols and skin cancer prevention. However, the evidence is sufficient that green tea polyphenols exhibit immunoprotective, antioxidant, and anti-inflammatory effects. More research is needed on conflicting results reported on oral and topical therapy and the effect of caffeine on oral ingestion of green tea polyphenols.

LIMONENE

Hakim and colleagues evaluated 404 patients with a history of squamous cell carcinoma and conducted a retrospective analysis of citrus intake. They found no correlation with the consumption of citrus fruits and skin cancer. However, those that reported citrus peel consumption had a statistically significant reduction in squamous cell carcinoma risk (Hakim et al. 2000). D-Limonene is a monocyclic monopterpene and is found in the oil from citrus peels. D-Limonene may have a cancer chemoprotective effect, but more studies with larger sample sizes are needed.

POLYPODIUM LEUCOTOMOS

The plant extract polypodium leucotomos has been shown to have significant antioxidant properties (Gonzales et al. 1996). In addition, the plant extract can decrease UV-light-induced lipid peroxidation (Gonzales et al. 1997). Only two studies have assessed its effects and clearly more studies are needed.

POLYPHENOLS

Polyphenols are attractive as chemopreventive agents because of their multiple functions including anti-inflammatory, antimutagenic, antiproliferative, signal transduction, antioxidant, and synergistic relationships with other antioxidants such as vitamin C (Yuting et al. 1990, Craig 1996, Cody et al. 1988). Due to their multiple physiologic functions, polyphenols in certain foods (such as tea, apples, onions, eggplant, and prunes and other dried fruit) have been reported to account for a significant protective effect against oxidative stress/chronic actinic damage in skin (Purba et al. 2001).

The isoflavone 4', 5, 7-trihyroxyisoflavone, more commonly known as genistein, is a component of soybeans that has been studied in mice and humans. It is the most commonly studied polyphenol in relation to the skin. Barnes first reported the possible anticancer effects of genistein on mice models (Barnes 1995). Cai and Wei found that genistein administered for 30 days to SENCAR mice resulted in antioxidant activity. Genistein increased the activity of superoxide dismutase, glutathione peroxidase, and glutathione reductase in the skin (Cai et al. 1996, Wei et al. 1998). Wang showed that genistein inhibited the ultraviolet b-induced c-fos and c-jun in mouse skin. They concluded that this most likely occurred through the inhibition of tyrosine protein kinase and the down-regulation of epidermal growth factor receptors (Wang et al. 1998). In 7, 12-dimethyl-benz[a]anthracene (DMBA) and 12-0-tetradecanoyl phorbol-13-acetate (TPA)-treated mice, genistein was shown to inhibit tumor incidence and multiplicity (Wei et al. 1998). The authors thought this was due to the inhibition of DMBA-induced DNA adduct formation and suppressing TPA-induced H_2O_2 and inflammatory responses. Widyarini and colleagues found that an isoflavone derivative from red clover applied topically to hairless mice resulted in photoprotection (Widyarini et al. 2000). Specifically, the isoflavone reduced UV-induced erythema, the induction of ornithine decarboxylase, and the suppression of contact hypersensitivity. In addition, mice treated chronically (50 days) with the isoflavone topical lotion had significant reduction in photocarcinogenesis. Shyong and colleagues reported recently that genistein inhibits psoralen plus ultraviolet radiation (PUVA)-induced photodamage (Shyong et al. 2002). Middleton and Kandaswami suggested that the flavonoids enhance the activity of the immune system (Middleton et al. 1992). Human studies are needed; however, mouse models suggest that genistein may be an important piece of the puzzle in the defense of skin cancer with diet.

Conclusion

Tables 6.1 and 6.2 summarize current dietary and nondietary recommendations for preventing chronic actinic skin damage and skin cancer. The positive effects of vitamins C and E, carotenoids, omega-3 fatty acids, and polyphenols have been documented to show

Table 6.1. Foods Rich in Micronutrients Important for Skin Cancer Prevention

Nutrient	Foods
Beta-carotene	Carrots, mango, pumpkin, sweet potato, cantaloupe, spinach, apricots
Lutein	Kale, spinach, swiss chard, collards, parsley
Lycopene	Tomato sauces, paste, and juice; watermelon, grapefruit (pink)
Alpha-carotene	Pumpkin, carrots, squash (butternut), collards
Beta-cryptoxanthin	Tangerine, mango, orange juice, peppers (sweet, red), persimmons, cilantro
Vitamin C	Kiwi fruit, peppers (sweet, red, green), citrus, broccoli, papaya, strawberries
Vitamin E	Kale, sweet potato, wheat germ, almonds, hazelnuts, sunflower seeds, blueberries, green peas, asparagus, spinach
Polyphenols	Green/black tea, dark grape juice, flax seed, raspberries, blueberries, strawberries, blackberries, boysenberries, pomegranates, dark grapes, eggplant, whole grains, legumes
Omega-3 fatty acids	Salmon, sardines, albacore tuna, mackerel, herring, trout, wheat germ, flax seed, canola oil, soy, herring, walnuts
Isoflavones	Miso, soybeans, soymilk, soy nuts, soy flour, tempeh, tofu
Coenzyme Q	Peanuts, sardines, salmon, chicken, spinach
Zinc	Oysters, crab, wheat germ, sardines, sirloin (lean), turkey breast, pumpkin/sunflower seeds
Selenium	Brazil nuts, tuna, flounder, shrimp, turkey breast, wheat germ
Cruciferous vegetables	Kale, broccoli, cabbage, brussels sprouts, collards, cauliflower

Table 6.2. Recommendations for Optimum Skin Health

Photoprotection	Avoid blistering sunburns.
	Try to avoid sun exposure between 10 A.M. and 3 P.M.
	Beware of cloudy days, the sun is still able to burn your skin.
	The suns rays can penetrate through 3 feet of water so use "sport" lotions that are water resistant.
	Beware of reflective surfaces such as snow and sand.
	Wear a broad-brimmed hat.
	Wear protective lip balm.
	Always wear lotion that blocks UVA and UVB.
	Sunscreen should be applied 20 minutes prior to UV exposure with a minimum SPF of 15, frequent reapplications; sport lotions provide the longest protection.
	Wear sunglasses.
	Topical application of antioxidants (vitamins C, E, and polyphenols) may be useful as a modality against sun-related skin damage.
	There is no such thing as a healthy tan unless one uses sunless tanning products containing dihydroxyacetone; avoid tanning beds.
	Use common sense in your sun protection regimen.
Avoid smoking	Cigarettes and cigars cause wrinkles.
	Cigarettes/cigars decrease the blood level of vitamin C, vitamin E, and carotenoids) (beta-carotene, lutein, etc.).
	Cigarettes are associated with an increased incidence of squamous cell carcinoma.
	Avoid second-hand smoke.
Dietary	Eat fresh vegetables, fruits, grains, legumes (beans), soy, fish with omega-3 fatty acids, complex carbohydrates, and low-fat or nonfat dairy products.
	Eat a minimum daily of 7 servings of fruits and vegetables for men and 4 for women.
	Eat a diet high in vitamin C and carotenoids (see Table 14.1 for list of foods).
	Increase your consumption of vitamin E-rich foods (see Table 14.1).
	Increase your intake of coenzyme Q-rich foods (see Table 14.1).
	Drink green tea, concord grape juice, cherry juice. Make berries (blackberries, blueberries, raspberries, and boysenberries), prunes, and raisins part of your "core" diet.
	Decrease dietary fat to 20–25% of total calories and limit your saturated fat intake to no more than 10% of your total number of "fat calories" eaten.
	Decrease consumption of omega-6 polyunsaturated fat (such as, corn oil, safflower oil), while increasing your intake of omega-3 polyunsaturated fat (such as, salmon,flaxseed, albacore tuna, sardines) and monounsaturated fat (such as, extra virgin olive oil, canola oil)
	A significant increase in skin melanin concentration can be achieved by taking a combination of the following antioxidants: beta carotene, lycopene, vitamin E, and vitamin C.
	Take a multi-vitamin-mineral-antioxidant supplement two to three times daily
Preventive	Do regular skin self-exams.
	Persons who have had one or more skin cancers should see a dermatologist yearly.
	Use common sense when outdoors to protect yourself from sunburns and excessive UV exposure.

modest photoprotective effects. It appears that the topical use and oral intake of certain nutrients and phytochemicals can boost the natural SPF of our skin. There are undoubtedly other phytochemicals that will be shown to help validate a primary prevention approach to the epidemic of skin cancer that we are now experiencing (Wise 2001). A synergistic approach using all of the listed recommendations should produce a measurable decrease in the incidence of skin cancer. Well-designed clinical trials are urgently needed to validate this statement! Clinical scenarios where dietary "supplementation" might be beneficial include persons with fair skin, those with a past history of skin cancer, those with a genetic predisposition to skin cancer, and immune-compromised patients. Sunscreen and sun protection remain the cornerstone in a preventive maintenance plan; however, a well-balanced diet rich in fresh fruits and vegetables and vitamin/mineral/antioxidant/phytonutrient supplements offer an internal (and at times external) mechanism of photoprotection. Most important, mom was right when she said, "Eat your fruits and vegetables!" We would add to this, "don't forget your whole grains, legumes, and omega-3 fatty acids."

References

Ahmad N, et al. 1999. Green tea polyphenols and cancer: biologic mechanisms and practical implications. Nutr Reviews 57(3):78–83.

Barnes S. 1995. Effect of genistein on in vitro and in vivo models of cancer. J Nutr 125(3 Suppl):777s–783s.

Barthelman M, et al. 1998. (-)Epigallocatechin-3-gallate inhibition of ultraviolet B-induced AP-1 activity. Carcinogenesis 19(12):2201–4.

Beyer RE. 1994. The role of ascorbate in antioxidant protection of biomembranes, interaction with vitamin E, and coenzyme Q. Archives of Bioengineering Biomembranes 26:349–58.

Black H, et al. 1994. Effect of a low fat diet on the incidence of actinic keratosis. NEJM 330(18):1272–75.

Block G, et al. 1992. Fruit, vegetables, and cancer prevention: a review of the epidemiological evidence. Nutr Cancer 18:1–29.

Cabelli DE, et al. 1983. Kinetics and mechanism for the oxidation of ascorbic acid/ascorbate by HO_2/O_2 radicals: a pulse radiolysis and stopped flow photolysis study. J Phys Chem 87:1805–12.

Cai Q, et al. 1996. Effect of dietary genistein on antioxidant enzyme activities in SENCAR mice. Nutr Cancer 25(1):1–7.

Chou PT, et al. 1983. L-ascorbic acid quenching of singlet delta molecular oxygen in aqueous media: generalized antioxidant property of vitamin C. Biochem Biophys Res Commun 115:932–7.

Cody V, et al. 1988. *Plant flavonoids in biology and medicine. II: Biochemical, cellular and medicinal properties*. New York: Alan R Liss, Inc; 1988.

Correa P. 1981. Epidemiological correlations between diet and cancer frequency. Cancer Res., 41:3685–90.

Craig W. 1996. Phytochemicals: Guardians of our health. Veg Dietetics 5(3): 6–8.

Darr D, et al. 1992. Topical vitamin C protects porcine skin from ultraviolet radiation-induced damage. British Journal of Dermatology 127:247–53.

Dinehart SM, Pollack SV. 1989. Metastases of squamous cell carcinoma of the skin and lip. J Am Acad Dermatol 2:241.

Eberlein-Konig B, et al. 1998. Protective effect against sunburn of combined systemic ascorbic acid (vitamin C) and d-alpha tocopherol (vitamin E). J Am Acad Dermatol 38:45–8.

Fitzpatrick, Thomas. 1999. *Dermatology in general medicine*, 5th ed. New York: McGraw-Hill.

Frisch M, et al. 1996. Risk for subsequent cancer after diagnosis of basal-cell carcinoma. A population-based, epidemiological study. An Int Med 125(10):815–21.

Fuchs J, et al. 1998. Modulation of UV-light induced skin inflammation by D-alpha-tocopherol and L-ascorbic acid: a clinical study using solar stimulated radiation. Free Radical Biol Med 25:1006–12.

Funasaka AK, et al. 1999. The depigmenting effect of alpha-tocopherol ferrulate on human melanoma cells. Brit J Dermatol 141:20–29.

Garmyn M, et al. 1995. Effect of beta-carotene supplementation on the human sunburn reaction. Exp Dermatol 4:104–11.

Gensler HL, et al. 1996. Prevention of photocarcinogenesis by topical administration of pure epigallocatechin gallate isolate from green tea. Nutr Cancer 26(3):325–35.

Gollnick HPM, et al. 1996. Systemic beta-carotene plus topical UV-sunscreen are an optimal protection against harmful effects of natural UV-sunlight: results of the Berlin-Eilath study. Euro J Dermatol 6:200–5.

Gonzales S, et al. 1996. Inhibition of ultraviolet-induced formation of reactive oxygen species, lipid peroxidation, erythema, and skin photosensitization by Polypodium leucotomos. Photodermatol Photoimmunol Photomed 12:45–6.

Gonzales S, et al. 1997. Topical or oral administration with an extract of Polypodium leucotomos prevents acute sunburn and psoralen induced phototoxic reactions as well as depletion of Langerhans cells in human skin. Photodermatol Photoimmunol Photomed 13:50–60.

Greenberg E, et al. 1990. A clinical trial of beta-carotene to prevent basal cell and squamous cell carcinomas of the skin. NEJM 323:789–95.

Greenway H, Pratt S. Skin tissue levels of carotenoids, vitamin A, and antioxidants in photodamaged skin. Unpublished data. Contact Hugh Greenway, M.D. (1-858-554-9000), or Steven Pratt, M.D. (1-858-457-3010).

Greenway H, et al. 2001a. *Vitamins and micronutrients in aging and photoaging skin in vegetables, fruits, and herbs in health promotion*. New York: CRC Press.

Greenway H, et al. 2001b. Unpublished data. Contact Hugh, M.D. (1-858-554-9000) or Steven Pratt, M.D. (1-858-457-3010).

Hakim I, et al. 2000. Citrus peel use is associated with reduced risk of squamous cell carcinoma of the skin. Nutr Cancer 37(2):161–8.

Heinonen O, et al. 1994. The effect of vitamin E and beta-carotene on the incidence of lung cancer and other cancers in male smokers. NEJM 330:1029–35.

Heinrich U, et al. 1998. Photoprotection from ingested carotenoids. Cosmetic Toil 113:61–70.

Huang MT, et al. 1997. Effects of tea, decaffeinated tea, and caffeine on UVB light-induced complete carcinogenesis in SKH-1 mice: demonstration of caffeine as a biologically important constituent of tea. Cancer Res 57(13):2633–9.

Jacob, R. 1995. The integrated antioxidant system. Nutr Res 15(5):755–766.

Jeffrey, E, et al. 2001. *Cruciferous vegetables and cancer prevention in handbook of nutraceuticals and functional foods*, ed. Robert E. L. Wildman. New York: CRC Press.

Kastan MB, et al. 1998. Participation of p53 protein in the cellular response to DNA damage. Cancer Res 51:6304.

Katiyar SK, et al. 2000a. Green tea and the skin. Arch of Dermatol 136:989–94.

Katiyar SK, et al. 2000b. Green tea polyphenol treatment to human skin prevents formation of ultra-violet B-induced pyrimidine dimers in DNA. Clin Cancer Res 6(10):3864–9.

Katiyar SK, et al. 2001. DNA photodamage and photoimmunology. Annu Rev Pharmacol Toxicol 42:25–54.

Kligman AM, et al. 1986. Topical tretinoin and photoaged skin. J Am Acad Dermatol 15:836.

Knekt P. 1992. Vitamin E and cancer: epidemiology. An NY Acad Sci 669:269.

Kohlmeir L, et al. 1997. Cruciferous vegetables consumption and colorectal cancer risk: meta analysis of the epidemiological evidence. FASEB J 11:A369.

Kune GA. 1990. Eating fish protects against some cancers: epidemiological and experimental evidence for a hypothesis. J Nutr Med 1:139–144.

Kune GA. 1992. Diet, alcohol, smoking, beta-carotene, C and Vitamin A in male nonmelanoma skin cancer patients and controls. Nutr Cancer 18(3):237–44.

Kurilich A, et al. 1999. Carotene, tocopherol, and ascorbate contents in subspecies of Brassica oleracea. J Agric Food Chem 47:1576–81.

Landis SH, et al. 1998. Cancer statistics, 1998. Am Cancer J 48:6, 1998.

La Ruche G, Cesarini JP. 1991. Protective effects of oral selenium plus copper associated with vitamin complex on sunburn cell formation in human skin. Photodermatol Photoimmunol Photomed 8:232–5.

Lee J, et al. 2000. Carotenoid supplementation reduces erythema in human skin after simulated solar radiation exposure. Proc Soc Exp Biol Med 223:170–4.

Lee J, et al. 2001. *Vegetables, fruits, and herbs in health promotion.* New York: CRC Press.

Lou YR, et al. 1999. Effects of oral administration of tea, decaffeinated tea, and caffeine on the formation and growth of tumors in high-risk SKH-1 mice previously treated with ultraviolet B light. Nutr Cancer 33(2):146–53.

Marghood A, et al. 1993. Risk of another basal cell carcinoma developing after treatment of basal cell carcinoma. J Am Acad of Dermatol 28:22.

Matthews-Roth MM, et al. 1977. Beta-carotene therapy for erythropoietic protoporphyria and other photosensitivity diseases. Arch Dermatol 113: 1229–32.

Middleton E, et al. 1992. Effects of flavonoids on immune and inflammatory cell functions. Biochem Pharmacol 67:1167.

Miller DL, Weinstock MA. 1994. Non-melanoma skin cancer in the United States: Incidence. J Am Acad Dermatol 30:774.

Mukhtar H, et al. 1994. Green tea and skin-anticarcinogenic effects. J Invest Dermatol 102(1):3–7.

Murray J, et al. 1991. Topical vitamin C treatment reduces ultraviolet B radiation induced erythema in human skin (abstract). J Invest Dermatol 96: 587.

Orengo IF, et al. 1992. Influence of fish oil supplementation on the minimal erythema dose in humans. Arch Dermatol Res 284:219–21.

Peto R, et al. 1981. Can dietary beta-carotene materially reduce human cancer rates? Nature 290:201–8.

Pinnell SR, et al. 1988. Vitamin C and collagen metabolism. In Kligman AM, Takase Y, eds. *Cutaneous aging.* Tokyo: University of Tokyo Press, pp. 275–92.

Podda M, et al. 1996. Simultaneous determination of tissue tocopherols, tocotrienols, ubiquinols, and ubiquinones. J Lipid Q 37:893–901.

Postaire E, et al. 1997. Evidence for anti-oxidant nutrients-induced pigmentation of the skin: results of a clinical trial. Biochem Mol Biol Int 42:1023–33.

Purba M, et al. 2001. Skin wrinkling: Can food make a difference. J Am Coll Nutr 20:71–80.

Rhodes LE, et al. 1994. Dietary fish oil supplementation in humans reduces UVB-erythemal sensitivity but increases epidermal lipid peroxidation. J Invest Dermatol 103:151–4.

Rhodes LE, et al. 1995. Dietary fish oil reduces basal and ultraviolet B-generated PGE2 levels in skin and increases the threshold to provocation of polymorphic light eruption. J Invest Dermatol 105:532–5.

Rhodes LE, et al. 2002. Systemic eicosapentanoic acid reduces UVB-induced erythema and p53 induction in skin, while increasing oxidative stress, in a double blinded randomized study. Brit J Dermatol (in press).

Ribaya-Mercado JD, et al. 1995. Skin lycopene is destroyed preferentially over beta-carotene during ultraviolet irradiation in humans. J Nutr 125(7): 1854–9.

Riou JP, et al. 1995. The association between melanoma, lymphoma, and other primary neoplasms. Arch Surg 130(10): 1056–61.

Rossa S, et al. 1996. The multicentre south European study "Helios" I: Skin characteristics and sunburns in basal cell carcinoma and squamous cell carcinoma of the skin. Brit J Cancer 73:1447.

Scarpa M, et al. 1983. A superoxide ion as active intermediate in the autooxidation of ascorbate by molecular oxygen: effect of superoxide dismutase. J Biol Chem 258:6695–7.

Serrano M, et al. 1993. A new regulatory motif in cell-cycle causing specific inhibition of cyclic D/CDK4. Nature 366:704.

Shyong EQ, et al. 2002. Effects of the isoflavone 4',5,7-trihydroxyisoflavone (genistein) on psoralen plus ultraviolet A radiation (PUVA)-induced photodamage. Carcinogenesis 23(2):317–21.

Slaper H, et al. 1996. Estimates of ozone depletion and skin cancer incidence to examine the Vienna Convention Achievements. Nature 384:256, 1996.

Stahl W, et al. 2000. Carotenoids and carotenoids plus vitamin E protect against ultraviolet-light induced erythema in humans. Am J Clin Nutr 71:795–8.

Stahl W, et al. 2001. Dietary tomato paste protects against ultraviolet light-induced erythema in humans. J Nutr 131(5):1449–51.

Thomas WR, et al. 1974. Recovery of immune system after cigarette smoking. Nature 243: 240–1.

Verhoeven D, et al. 1996. Epidemiological studies on brassica vegetables and cancer risk. Cancer Epidemiol Biomarkers Prev 5:733–48.

Wang Y, et al. 1998. Inhibition of ultraviolet B(UVB)-induced c-fos and c-jun expression in vivo by a tyrosinase kinase inhibitor genistein. Carcinogenesis 19(4):649–54.

Wang ZY, et al. 1989. Protection against polycyclic aromatic hydrocarbon-induced skin tumor initiation in mice by green tea polyphenols. Carcinogenesis 10(2):411–5.

Wang ZY, et al. 1991. Protection against ultraviolet B radiation-induced photocarcinogenesis in hairless mice by green tea polyphenols. Carcinogenesis 12(8):1527–30.

Wei H, et al. 1998. Isoflavone genistein inhibits the initiation and promotion of two-stage skin carcinogenesis in mice. Carcinogenesis 19(8):1509–14.

Wei Q, et al. 1994. Vitamin supplementation and reduced risk of basal cell carcinoma. J Clin Epid 47: 829.

Werninghaus K, et al. 1994. Evaluation of the photoprotective effect of oral vitamin E supplementation. Arch Dermatol 130(10):1257–61.

White W, et al. 1988. Ultraviolet light-induced reductions in plasma carotenoid levels. Am J Clin Nutr 47:879–83.

Widyarini S, et al. 2000. Protective effect of isoflavone derivative against photocarcinogenesis in a mouse model. Redox Rep 5(2-3):156–8.

Wise J. 2001. Vegetables, fruits, and herbs in health promotion. New York: CRC Press.

Wolf C, et al. 1988. Do oral carotenoids protect human skin against ultraviolet erythema, psoralen phototoxicity, and ultraviolet-induced DNA-damage? J Invest Dermatol 90:55–7.

Wu D, et al. 1999. Antioxidant status, diet, nutrition, and health. New York: CRC Press.

Yuting C, et al. 1990. Flavonoids as superoxide scavengers and antioxidants. FRBM 9:19–21.

Zhang Y, et al. 1994. Anticarcinogenic activities of organic isothiocyanates: chemistry and mechanisms. Cancer Res (Suppl) 54:1976s–1981s.

7

Nutritional Strategies for the Prevention of Cervical Cancer

Paula Inserra and
Brent P. Mahoney

INTRODUCTION

Cervical cancer has declined over the past several decades as a result of Pap smear screening (Miller 1995). Despite such a dramatic decline, cervical cancer still remains the second most common cancer in women worldwide (Passani et al. 1999). In many developing countries, it remains the leading cause of cancer death in women (Passani et al. 1999). Although these high rates are mainly due to a lack of Papanicolaou (Pap) smear screening programs, in developed countries like the United States where Pap screening is widely available, high rates of cervical cancer are still observed in Black and Hispanic populations. Infection with the human papillomavirus (HPV) has been shown to be the cause of cervical cancer, as greater than 99% of cervical cancers contain oncogenic HPV DNA (Walboomers et al. 1999). Screening programs are now beginning to incorporate HPV testing along with Pap testing in order to better identify women who are likely to develop cancer. Infection with certain types of HPV, so named oncogenic HPV types (HPV 16, HPV 18, HPV 31, and HPV 45) are more likely to progress to cancer than infection with nononcogenic HPV types (HPV 6 and HPV 11). Interestingly, the vast majority of HPV infections, including the oncogenic infections, resolve spontaneously and never progress to cancer. Many investigators have therefore been focusing on the role other risk factors play in allowing the virus to persist and progress to invasive cancer. Identifying modifiable risk factors will improve cancer prevention programs in two ways: (1) by complementing current screening programs, such as Pap and HPV testing, which have already been implemented in developed countries, or (2) by offering a cost-effective means of preventing disease in developing countries where screening programs are not yet in place. Age at first intercourse, number of sexual partners, smoking, and low intakes of certain nutrients have all been associated with increased risk of cervical cancer. The focus of this chapter is to review the evidence that supports the role nutrients have in preventing cervical dysplasia, carcinoma *in situ*, and invasive cervical cancer.

VITAMIN A

Vitamin A is widely recognized as a promoter of cellular differentiation, the mechanism by which it is thought to protect against cancer. Some evidence supports a role for vitamin A intakes as well as serum retinol levels in protecting against the development of cervical cancer. Additionally, derivatives of retinol are used clinically as a treatment for cervical cancer. Early case-control studies have shown that dietary intake, as well as blood levels of vitamin A, are protective against the development of cervical cancer and cervical dysplasia.

As early as 1981, Romney et al. noticed that low dietary levels of vitamin A were significantly associated with severity of dysplasia as well as cervical carcinoma *in situ*. They also observed an inverse correlation between retinol binding protein and dysplasia. This work was later followed up by Marshall et al. (1983). Five hundred and thirteen cervical cancer cases and 490 hospitalized control subjects were enrolled. These authors found that vitamin A, mainly derived from fruits and vegetables, was a protective agent against cervical cancer. In addition, a case-control study conducted in 1984 studied 87 cases with either severe dysplasia or carcinoma *in situ* and 82 matched controls. Cases were found to have lower vitamin A intakes as compared to controls, which corresponded to a threefold increase in risk (Wylie-Rosett et al. 1984). Numerous case-control studies following these, however, failed to find an association with either dietary (Brock et al. 1988, La Vecchea et al. 1988, Verreault et al. 1989, Ziegler et al. 1990, Ziegler et al. 1991, Buckley et al. 1992) or serum (Brock et al. 1988, Cuzick et al. 1990, Potischman et al. 1994) levels of vitamin A and various indicators of cervical cancer risk. No associations were detected in cross-sectional study designs evaluating vitamin A status and cervical dysplasia and cancer (Palan et al. 1991) or cervical cancer mortality (Guo 1994). The main drawback to these investigations was that the main causative agent for cervical cancer, namely, HPV, was not measured, let alone carefully controlled for. The first investigation that controlled for HPV 16 and 18 infections, the two HPV types responsible for the vast majority of cervical cancers, was a study conducted by Herrero and colleagues in 1991. Seven hundred and forty-eight cases of invasive cervical cancer and 1411 controls participated, however they too did not observe any association between dietary retinol and invasive cervical cancer. Interestingly, when they looked at serum levels of retinol, they observed a slight trend for decreasing levels of retinol with cervical cancer stage (Potischman et al. 1991). In the remaining case-control studies controlling for HPV status, mixed results were obtained, although the majority could not detect any associations when looking at blood level indicators of vitamin A status (Goodman et al. 1998, Ho et al. 1998) or diet (Wideroff et al. 1998). In a case-control study by Kanetsky, in 32 women with dysplasia and 113 controls, women with the highest levels of dietary vitamin A were 25% less likely to have cervical dysplasia (Kanetsky et al. 1998). Two prospective studies were conducted and they too yielded different results. The first was carried out in 1998 by Palan and colleagues. In this study, 69 subjects were randomized to receive either beta-carotene or placebo and were followed for 9 months. They found no associations with plasma levels of retinol and either HPV persistence, or with the development of dysplasia. In the prospective study design by Nagata and co-authors in 1999, 134 women with dysplasia were followed for approximately 7 years. They found the rate of progression to more severe dysplasia, or to invasive cancer, to be 4.5 times as great in women with the lowest levels of serum retinol.

In view of these controversial results obtained between studies before, and even after

HPV testing was conducted, the role of vitamin A in preventing cervical dysplasia and cancer is still up to debate. The need for long-term prospective studies is apparent and until they are conducted and completed, vitamin A as a chemo preventative agent for cervical cancer cannot be recommended.

ANTIOXIDANTS

Vitamin E

Vitamin E is thought to protect against the development of many types of cancers early in the carcinogenic process due to its potent antioxidant properties. Being lipid soluble, vitamin E is the most important antioxidant found in cell membranes and functions mainly to protect and maintain these membranes from the damaging effects generated by free radical chain reactions. Similar to the vitamin A studies, the initial studies examining the association between cervical disease and vitamin E did not measure or control for HPV status of the women of the study participants. Nevertheless, three case-control studies found protective effects for vitamin E status (Verreault et al. 1989, Palan et al. 1991, Buckley et al. 1992) and two failed to show associations (Cuzick et al. 1990, Potischman et al. 1994). In the study conducted by Verreault and coworkers, women with high intakes of vitamin E were less likely to have invasive cervical cancer (Verreault et al. 1989). Palan and colleagues, detected reduced plasma levels of alpha-tocopherol in women with either cervical dysplasia or cancer (Palan et al. 1991). Similarly, Buckley et al. found that women with low intakes of vitamin E were at a significantly increased risk of developing dysplasia (Buckley et al. 1992). On the other hand, Cuzick et al. and Potischman et al. (1994) both found no significant difference in serum levels of vitamin E and risk for grade of dysplasia (Cuzick et al. 1990). A cross-sectional study that was conducted before HPV testing was widely available, failed to observe an association with dietary vitamin E and cervical cancer mortality (Guo et al. 1994).

Unlike studies conducted with vitamin A, once HPV status was addressed and controlled for, the majority of investigations were able to show protective effects for high serum levels of vitamin E. Goodman et al.'s case-control study designed to determine the association between plasma micronutrient levels and risk of cervical dysplasia in a population of women in Hawaii, enrolled 147 cases with squamous intraepithelial lesions (SIL) and 191 controls with normal cytology. These authors demonstrated an inverse dose-response association between alpha-tocopherol levels and dysplasia (Goodman et al. 1998). In 1997, Giuliano and coworkers followed a cohort of women for 9 months. They were able to show that alpha-tocopherol levels were approximately 25% lower amongst women positive for HPV at two time points as compared to women who were either negative at two time points, or HPV positive at only one time point. These results implicate a role for alpha-tocopherol in preventing persistent HPV infection (Giuliano et al. 1997). In another study, 378 women with cervical intraepithelial neoplasia (CIN) were compared to 366 control women with normal Pap smears. Inverse correlations were detected for plasma alpha-tocopherol levels in cases as compared to controls (Ho et al. 1998). A different study conducted in 1997 compared 168 HPV-negative women with normal Pap results, with 228 HPV-positive women with CIN. Significantly lower levels if alpha-tocopherol were found in sera of cases as compared with controls (Kwasniewska et al. 1997). In the one study looking at dietary vitamin E, 146 HPV-DNA-negative women who had either equivocal Pap results or SIL were compared to 683 women negative for HPV with normal Pap results. These authors found a slight protective effect for dietary vitamin E (Wideroff et al. 1998). No associations between vitamin E level and invasive cancer were observed in the case-control study conducted by Potischman et al. (1991) when HPV 16 and 18 infections were controlled. Last, in Palan et al.'s randomized placebo controlled trial, they supplemented 69 CIN cases with beta-carotene for 9 months. These authors measured plasma levels of micronutrients including vitamin E and found no associations with either HPV persistence or with CIN in placebo or supplemented groups of women (Palan et al. 1998).

Although still up to debate, the evidence for vitamin E appears to support its role as a protective agent in the development of cervical cancer and may warrant further investigation. The current evidence supports studying whether increased vitamin E intake either from food sources or from supplements could prevent progression of HPV-related disease. It is essential to stress the importance of appropriate study design when investigating vitamin E and other antioxidants. These agents protect against early carcinogenic events and trials enrolling women already diagnosed with dysplasia may not yield meaningful results.

Vitamin C

Analogous to vitamin E, vitamin C's role in the prevention of cancer is primarily due to its role as an antioxidant. Vitamin C not only has the potential for directly interacting and quenching free radicals, but also can function to recycle vitamin E. In terms of cervical cancer, vitamin C or ascorbic acid, has been studied extensively. About half of the investigations to date have not controlled for HPV, the main cause of cervical cancer, and six of them were case-control studies. In the case-controlled studies described in previous sections, dietary vitamin C demonstrated protective effects against the development of *in situ* and invasive cervical cancer as well as dysplasia (Romney et al. 1981, Brock et al. 1988, Verreault et al. 1989, Ziegler et al. 1990, Buckley et al. 1992). However, no associations were observed for dietary intake of vitamin C and development of invasive cancer or dysplasia (Ziegler et al. 1990). In the cross-sectional investigation conducted by Guo et al. (1994), decreased mortality was not related to vitamin C intake. In the studies where HPV status was measured, similar results were obtained. In the case-control study by Herrero et al. where HPV 16 and 18 statuses were controlled for, a decreased risk of invasive cervical cancer was found for increased vitamin C intake (Herrero et al. 1991). In the case-control study by Goodman et al., these authors found weak associations between plasma levels of vitamin C and risk of cervical dysplasia. Results were similar to those obtained by Ho and Van Eenwyk (Goodman et al. 1998, Ho et al. 1998, Van Eenwyk et al. 1991). The remaining case-control studies did not observe any associations between dietary vitamin C intake (Wideroff et al. 1998, Kjellberg et al. 2000) or serum vitamin C levels (Liu et al. 1995). Overall, the effect of vitamin C on the progression of cervical cancer is still highly debatable although it does appear to offer some degree of protection when all the evidence is weighed. Future studies not only need to be designed carefully, but also need to follow women prospectively for longer periods of time, as results from case-control studies are giving us equivocal results.

Carotenoids

Carotenoids are vitamin A-like compounds found in dark green leafy vegetables and bright orange and yellow vegetables, which function as antioxidants. An impressive amount of literature has been published addressing the protective role various carotenoids have in the development of cervical cancer. It is interesting to note that the vast majorities of case-control studies conducted either before HPV testing was implemented, or after, have consistently shown a protective effect of dietary beta-carotene in the development of cancer as well as its precursor lesions (Romney et al. 1981, Wylie-Rosett et al. 1984, Brock et al. 1988, LaVecchia et al. 1988, Verreault et al. 1989, Ziegler et al. 1990, Herrero et al. 1991). Protective effects were shown for other carotenoids as well (Ziegler et al. 1990, Herrero et al. 1991). Beneficial effects are also observed for serum beta-carotene levels and HPV persistence (Giuliano et al. 1997). In other case-control studies serum levels of lycopene (Potischman et al. 1994, Goodman et al. 1998, Kanetsky et al. 1998, Van Eenwyk et al. 1991), lutein (Potischman et al. 1994, Giuliano et al. 1997), and alpha, beta, or total cryptoxanthin (Giuliano et al. 1997, Goodman et al. 1998) were inversely associated with cervical cancer, dysplasia, or persistent HPV infection. Although the vast majority of case-control studies demonstrated inverse associations with risk of cervical cancer, a few failed to corroborate these findings. The investigations of dietary intake of carotenoids that did not control for HPV status (Ziegler et al. 1990, Buckley et al. 1992, Guo et al. 1994) did not find inverse associations with carotenoid intake and cancer-related disease. Additionally, Liu et al. did not find any correlations when measuring serum carotenoid levels while controlling for HPV (Liu et al. 1995). Despite the majority of case-control studies illustrating promise for beta-carotene as a chemopreventative agent, two beta-carotene randomized placebo controlled trials conducted in women with dysplasia failed to offer protection against progression of dysplasia (Romney et al. 1997, Palan et al. 1998).

Although disappointing, it is important to keep in mind that carotenoids tend to be present in the same food items and beta-carotene intake may disguise other important carotenoids (i.e., lycopene, lutein, or cryptoxanthin), which have more potent actions. Additionally, these compounds may have synergistic effects and need to be consumed in conjunction with one another to produce maximum health benefits. Although conducting trials with supplements is an easier endeavor, better results may be obtained if we look at the effects of high intakes of fruits and vegetables, which are good sources of these carotenoids. Continuing to investigate the effects of other carotenoids in addition to beta-carotene, is still warranted, particularly in long-term prospective studies. The carotenoids, like vitamins C and E, may also exert their effects early in the carcinogenic process and supplementing women who already have dysplasia may be a futile venture.

Nutrients Involved in Methylation

Methylation of the upstream regulatory region of HPV has been shown to prevent viral transcription in vitro (Rosl et al. 1993). Methylation could therefore prevent proliferation of HPV, which would allow the host to clear the virus. Several nutrients are integral to the process of methylation, namely folate, vitamin B_6, and vitamin B_{12}. These nutrients are required for the synthesis of S-adenosylmethionine (SAM). SAM's function is to donate methyl groups and, thereby, is responsible for DNA and RNA methylation. Deficiencies of these nutrients, even marginal ones, could potentially result in a lack of HPV methylation subsequently leading to viral proliferation.

About half of the literature examining the role of these nutrients in the development of cervical cancer did not control for HPV status. The case-control studies that assessed the association between dietary intake of folate and *in situ* (Brock et al. 1988) or invasive cervical cancer (Verreault et al. 1989, Ziegler et al. 1990, Herrero et al. 1991) failed to demonstrate a protective effect. Two case-control studies did find an inverse association between dietary folate and *in situ* cervical cancer (Ziegler et al. 1990) and cervical dysplasia (Buckley et al. 1992). In the following case-control studies HPV status was assessed. Goodman et al. compared 150 women with SIL to 179 control women with normal Pap smears. They not only observed in these women an inverse association between dietary intake of folate, vitamins B_6 and B_{12}, and SIL, but also they demonstrated that the C677T methylenetetrahydrofolate reductase polymorphism, in conjunction with low folate intake, significantly elevated risk of SIL compared to women without the polymorphism who had higher intakes of folate (Goodman et al. 2001). Sedjo et al. conducted a prospective study assessing the association between HPV persistence and dietary folate, vitamins B_6 and B_{12}, and circulating levels of folate and B_{12} in 201 women. They demonstrated protection against persistent HPV infection for circulating levels of B_{12}, but no associations were found for circulating or dietary levels of folate or for dietary levels of vitamins B_6 and B_{12} (Sedjo et al. 2002). Liu et al.'s study assessed the association between blood levels of folate, vitamin B_6, vitamin B_{12}, and dysplasia, and failed to show a protection for these nutrients (Liu et al. 1995). Two randomized placebo controlled trials of folic acid supplementation were conducted for a duration of 6 months. Butterworth et al. enrolled 235 subjects with CIN and supplemented with 10 mg folic acid per day controlling for HPV 16 infection only. Folic acid supplementation failed to effect progression of cervical dysplasia (Butterworth et al. 1992). In the trial conducted by Childers et al., 331 women with CIN were enrolled and supplemented with 5 mg folic acid or placebo; HPV status was not assessed. These authors also failed to demonstrate a protective effect of folate on dysplasia progression (Childers et al. 1995). In retrospect, these results are not surprising.

The nutrients involved in methylation pathways are theorized to prevent viral proliferation, and adequate intakes and levels should be important early in the infection process. The two trials supplemented women already diagnosed with dysplasia, a point in the disease process where HPV infection has already been established. A more appropriate study design would assess the effect of folate status or supplementation on infection rates of women initially negative for HPV. This type of design does have the drawback of lengthy and extensive follow-up limiting its feasibility. Folate and other nutrients involved in DNA methylation still need to be examined, especially in view of some promising studies recently conducted where HPV status was measured.

Fats

There is extensive evidence demonstrating a wide variety of health benefits from consumption of omega-3 fatty acids particularly with respect to CVD and hypertension (Simopoulos 1991). Dietary omega-3 fat has also been shown to be protective against cancer (Noguchi et al. 1997, Narisawa et al. 1994, Cave 1991, Ito et al. 1999, Yang et al. 1999, Harvel et al. 1997, Pandalai et al. 1996, Chen and Auborn 1999, Madhavi and Das 1994, Sagar and Das 1995). Recently, omega-3 fatty acids have been shown to have direct anti-cervical cancer effects, demonstrated by both in vitro (Chen and Auborn 1999, Madhavi and Das 1994, Sagar and Das 1995) and in vivo (Hursting et al. 1990) studies. In vitro, the omega-3 fatty acid metabolites, docosahexaenoic acid (DHA) and eicosapentaenoic acid (EPA) were shown to have direct cytotoxic action against the HeLa human cervical carcinoma cell line (Chen and Auborn 1999, Madhavi and Das 1994) as well as growth-inhibiting effects on HPV immortalized keratinocytes (Sagar and Das 1995). The in vivo evidence from Hursting et al. (1990) shows a trend between higher dietary intake of omega-3 fatty acids and lower incidence of cervix cancer; however it did not reach statistical significance. They measured fatty acid intake by estimating the per capita disappearance of fatty acids as compared to the incidence of cervical cancer by country. This assessment of fatty acid intake is crude and utilization of more accurate dietary measures or biomarkers may result in more pronounced effects. Hirose et al. conducted a case-control study in 556 cervical cancer cases and 2675 controls. These authors demonstrated that less-frequent intake of boiled or broiled fish (food sources high in omega-3 fatty acids) was significantly associated with cervical cancer risk (Hirose et al. 1996). The effects of omega-3 fatty acids are just beginning to be investigated with respect to cervical cancer. Initial results look promising and thereby warrant further research.

CONCLUSION

In conclusion, each of the nutrients reviewed, vitamins A, C, and E, carotenoids, nutrients involved in DNA methylation, and omega-3 fatty acids are all potential chemopreventative agents that warrant continued study. Although much research has been undertaken in this area already, many of the results are confounded due to the recent evidence implicating HPV in the pathogenesis of cervical cancer. Since it is now established as the causative agent in the development of cervical cancer, HPV status of study participants must be considered in data analysis in order to prevent biased conclusions. Future investigations should take caution to implement proper designs for the hypothesis being tested. Most of the above-mentioned nutrients act early in the disease process rendering case-control studies less effective at addressing these vital questions. Additionally, numerous case-control investigations have already been completed and results still remain inconclusive.

REFERENCES

Brock KE, Bery G, Mock PA, MacLennan R, Truswell AS, Brinton LA. 1988. Nutrients in diet and plasma and risk of *in situ* cervical cancer. *Journal of the National Cancer Institute* 80:580–585.

Buckley DI, McPherson S, North CQ, Becker TM. 1992. Dietary micronutrients and cervical dysplasia in southwestern American Indian women. *Nutrition and Cancer* 17:179–185.

Butterworth CE, et al. 1992. Oral folic acid supplementation for cervical dysplasia: a clinical intervention trial. *American Journal of Obstetrics and Gynecology* 166:803–809.

Cave WT. 1991. Dietary omega-3 polyunsaturated fatty acid effects on animal tumorigenesis. *Federation of the Academy of Science and Experimental Biology Journal* 5:2160–2166.

Chen D, and Auborn K. 1999. Fish oil constituent docosahexaenoic acid selectively inhibits growth of human papillomavirus immortalized keratinocytes. *Carcinogenesis* 20:249–254.

Childers JM, et al. 1995. Chemoprevention of cervical cancer with folic acid: a phase III Southwest Oncology Group Intergroup study. *Cancer Epidemiology, Biomarkers and Prevention* 4:155–159.

Cuzick J, De Stavola BL, Russell MJ, Thomas BS. 1990. Vitamin A, vitamin E and the risk of cervical intraepithelial neoplasia. *British Journal of Cancer* 62:651–652.

Giuliano AR, Papenfuss M, Nour M, Canfield LM, Schneider A, Hatch K. 1997. Antioxidant nutrients: associations with persistent human Papillomavirus infection. *Cancer Epidemiology, Biomarkers and Prevention* 6:917–923.

Goodman MT, Kiviat N, McDuffie K, Hankin JH, Hernandez B, Wilkens LR, Franke A, Kuypers J, Kolonel LN, Nakamura J, Ing G, Branch B, Bertram CC, Kamemoto L, Sharma S, Killeen J. 1998. The association of plasma micronutrients with risk of cervical dysplasia in Hawaii. *Cancer Epidemiology, Biomarkers and Prevention* 10:537–544.

Goodman MT, McDuffie K, Hernandez B, Wilkens LR, Bertram CC, Killeen J, Marchand LL, Selhub J, Murphy S, Donlon TA. 2001. Association of methylenetetrahydrofolate reductase polymorphism *C677T* and dietary folate with the risk of cervical dysplasia. *Cancer Epidemiology, Biomarkers and Prevention* 10:1275–1280.

Guo W, Hsing AW, Li J, Chen J, Chow W, Blot WJ. 1994. Correlation of cervical cancer mortality with reproductive and dietary factors, and serum markers in China. *International Journal of Epidemiology* 23(6): 1127–1132.

Harvel S, Bjerve KS, Tretli S, Jellum E, Robsahm TE, Vatten L. 1997. Prediagnositic level of fatty acids in serum phospholipids: omega-3 and omega-6 fatty acids and the risk of prostate cancer. *International Journal of Cancer* 71:545–551.

Herrero R, Potischman N, Brinton LA, Reeves WC, Brenes MM, Tenorio F, de Britton RC, Gaitan E. 1991. A case-control study of nutrient status and invasive cervical cancer. American Journal of Epidemiology 134:1335–1346.

Hirose K, Tajima K, Hamajima N, Takezaki T, Minoue M, Kuroishi T, Nakamura S, Tokudome S. 1996. Subsite (cervix/endometrium)-specific risk and protective factors in uterus cancer. *Japanese Journal of Cancer Research* 87:1001–1009.

Ho GYF, Palan PR, Basu J, Romney SL, Kadish AS, Mikhail M, Wassertheil-Smoller S, Runowicz

C, Burk RD. 1998. Viral characteristics of human Papillomavirus infection and antioxidant levels as risk factors for cervical dysplasia. *International Journal of Cancer* 78:594–599.

Hursting SD, Thornquist M, Henderson MM. 1990. Types of dietary fat and the incidence of cancer at five sites. *Preventative Medicine* 19:242–253.

Ito Y, Shimizu H, Yoshimuro T, Ross RK, Kabuto N, Takatsuka N, Tokui N, Suzuki K, Shinohara R. 1999. Serum concentrations of carotenoids, alpha-tocopherol, fatty acids, and lipid peroxides among Japanese in Japan, and Japanese and Caucasians in the US. *International Journal of Vitamin Research* 69:385–395.

Kanetsky PA, Gamon MD, Mandelblatt J, Zhang Z, Ramsey E, Dnistrian A, Norkus EP, Wright TC. 1998. Dietary intake and blood levels of lycopene: Association with cervical dysplasia among Non-Hispanic, Black Women. *Nutrition and Cancer* 31(1):31–40.

Kjellberg LK, Hallmans G, Ahren AM, Johansson R, Bergman F, Wadell G, Angstrom T, Dillner J. 2000. Smoking, diet, pregnancy and oral contraceptive use as a risk factor for cervical intra-epithelial neoplasia in relation to human Papillomavirus infection. *British Journal of Cancer* 82(7):1322–1338.

Kwasniewska A, Tukendorf A, Semczuk M. 1997. Content of alpha-tocopherol in blood serum of human Papillomavirus-infected women with cervical dysplasias. *Nutrition and Cancer* 28(3):248–251.

La Vecchia C, Decarlo A, Fasoli M, Parazzini F, Franceschi S, Gentile A, Negri E. 1988. Dietary Vitamin A and the risk of intraepithelial and invasive cervical neoplasia. *Gynecologic Oncology* 30:187–195.

Liu T, Soong S, Alvarez RD, Butterworth CE. 1995. A longitudinal analysis of human Papillomavirus 16 infection, nutritional status, and cervical dysplasia prognosis. *Cancer Epidemiology, Biomarkers and Prevention* 4(4): 373–380.

Madhavi N, Das UN. 1994. Effect of n-6 and n-3 fatty acids on the survival of vincristine sensitive and resistant human cervical carcinoma cells *in vitro*. *Cancer Letters* 83:31–41.

Marshall JR, Graham S, Byers T, Swanson M, Brasure J. 1983. Diet and smoking in the epidemiology of cancer of the cervix. *Journal of the National Cancer Institute* 70(5):847–851.

Miller AB. Failures of cervical screening. 1995. *American Journal of Public Health* 85:795.

Nagata C, Shimizu H, Higashiiwai H, Sugahara N, Morita N, Komatsu S, Hisamichi S. 1999. Serum retinol level and risk of subsequent cervical cancer in cases with cervical dysplasia. *Cancer Investigations* 17(4): 253–258.

Narisawa T, Fukaura Y, Yazawa K, Ishikawa C, Isoda Y, Nishizawa Y. 1994. Colon cancer prevention with a small amount of dietary perilla oil high in alpha-linolenic acid in an animal model. *Cancer* 73:2069–2075.

Noguchi M, Minami M, Yagasaki R, Kinoshita K, Yearashi M, Kitagawa H, Taniya T,, Miyazaki I. 1997. Chemoprevention of DMBA–induced mammary carcinogenesis in rats by low–dose EPA and DHA. *British Journal of Cancer* 75:348–353.

Palan PR, Chang CJ, Mikhail MS, Ho GYF, Basu J, Romeny SL. 1998. Plasma concentrations of micronutrients during a nine-month clinical trail of beta-carotene in women with precursor cervical cancer lesions. *Nutrition and Cancer* 30(1):46–52.

Palan PR, Mikhail MS, Basu J, Romney SL. 1991. Plasma levels of antioxidant beta-carotene and alpha-tocopherol in uterine cervix dysplasias and cancer. *Nutrition and Cancer* 15:13–20.

Pandalai PK, Pilat MJ, Yamazaki K, Naik H, Pienta KJ. 1996. The effect of omega-3 and omega-6 fatty acids on *in vitro* prostate cancer growth. *Anticancer Research* 16:815–820.

Passani P, Parkin DM, Bray F, Ferlay J. 1999. Estimates of the worldwide mortality from 25 cancers in 1990. *International Journal of Cancer* 83:18–29.

Potischman N, Herrero R, Brinton LA, Reeves WC, Stacewicz-Sapuntzakis M, Jones CJ, Brenes MM, Tenorio F, de Britton RC, Gaitan E. 1991. A case-control study of nutrient status and invasive cervical cancer. *American Journal of Epidemiology* 134:1347–1355.

Potischman N, Hoover RN, Briton LA, Swanson CA, Herrero R, Tenorio F, de Briton LA, Gaitan E, Reeves WC. 1994. The relations between cervical cancer and serological markers of nutritional status. *Nutrition and Cancer* 21:193–210.

Romney SL, Ho GYF, Palan PR, Basu J, Kasish AS, Klein S, Mikhail M, Hagan RJ, Chang CJ, Burk RD. 1997. Effects of beta-carotene and other factors on outcome of cervical dysplasia and human Papillomavirus infection. *Gynecologic Oncology* 65:483–492.

Romney SL, Palan PR, Duttagupta C, Wassertheil-Smoller S, Wylie J, Miller G, Slagle NS, Lucido S. 1981. Retinoids and the prevention of cervical dysplasia. *American Journal of Obstetrics and Gynecology* 141:890–894.

Rosl F, Arab A, Klevenz B, zur Hausen H. 1993. The effect of DNA methylation on gene expression of human papillomavirus. Journal of Genetic Virology 74:791–801.

Sagar PS, Das UN. 1995. Cytotoxic action of cis-unsaturated fatty acids on human cervical carcinoma (HeLa) cells *in vitro. Prostaglandins, Leukotrienes and Essential Fatty Acids* 53:287–299.

Sedjo RL, Inserra P, Abrahamsen M, Harris RB, Roe DJ, Baldwin S, Giuliano AR. 2002. Human papillomavirus persistence and nutrients involved in the methylation pathway among a cohort of young women. *Cancer Epidemiology, Biomarkers and Prevention* 11:353–359.

Simopoulos AP. 1991. N-3 fatty acids in health and disease and in growth and development. *American Journal of Clinical Nutrition* 54:438–463.

Van Eenwyk J, Davis FG, and Bowen PE. 1991. Dietary and serum carotenoids and cervical intraepithelial neoplasia. *International Journal of Cancer* 48:34–38.

Verreault R, Chu J, Mandelson M, Shy K. 1989. A case-control study of diet and invasive cervical cancer. *International Journal of Cancer* 43:1050–1054.

Walboomers JMM, Jacobs MV, Manos MM, Bosch FX, Kummer JA, Shah KV, Snijders PJ, Peto J, Meijer CJ, Munoz N. Human papillomavirus is a necessary cause of invasive cervical cancer worldwide. 1999. *Journal of Pathology* 189:12–19.

Wideroff L, Potischmann N, Glass AG, Greer CE, Manos MM, Scott DR, Burk RD, Sherman ME, Wacholder S, Schiffman M. 1998. A nested case-control study of dietary factors and the risk of incident cytological abnormalities of the cervix. *Nutrition and Cancer* 30(2):130–136.

Wylie-Rosett JA, Romney SL, Slagle S, Wassertheil-Smoller S, Miller GL, Palan PR, Lucido DJ, Duttagupta C. 1984. Influence of Vitamin A on cervical dysplasia and carcinoma *In Situ. Nutrition and Cancer* 6(1):49–57.

Yang YJ, Lee SH, Hong SJ, Chung BC. 1999. Comparison of fatty acid profiles in the serum of patients with prostate cancer and benign prostatic hyperplasia. *Clinical Biochemistry* 32:405–409.

Ziegler RG, Brinton LA, Hamman RF, Lehman HF, Levine RS, Mallin K, Norman SA, Rosenthal JF, Trumble AC, Hoover RN. 1990. Diet and the risk of invasive cervical cancer among White women in the United States. *American Journal of Epidemiology* 132:432–445.

Ziegler RG, Jones CJ, Brinton LA, Norman SA, Mallin K, Levine RS, Lehman HF, Hamman RF, Trumble AC, Rosenthal JF, Hoover RN. 1991. Diet and the risk of *in situ* cervical cancer among White women in the United States. *Cancer Causes and Control* 2:17–29.

Part II

Fruits, Vegetables, and Herbs in Cancer Prevention

8

Tomato and Cancer

Patrizia Riso,
Antonella Brusamolino,
and Marisa Porrini

INTRODUCTION

The typical diet of the southern European area has always been based on a high consumption of cereals, legumes, fruits and vegetables, olive oil plus milk and its derivatives, eggs, fish, and poultry. This dietary model has been accepted as having positive properties, due to its elevated content of complex carbohydrates, fiber, antioxidants, and a low amount of animal fats.

For some years, scientists have been investigating these positive "disease preventing" properties and have begun to identify specific food components, called phytochemicals, that may better explain the role of some foods in the prevention and treatment of diseases. Although phytochemicals are not yet classified as *nutrients*, they are substances that can positively affect human function and reduce the risk of disease.

Recently, scientists have been reconsidering the properties of whole foods rather than single compounds. This new way of thinking has arisen from the results of many epidemiological studies that have shown that there is a link between a reduced risk of cancer and a high intake of fresh fruits and vegetables, not just a high intake of any specific antioxidant. At the same time it is important to note that there is no evidence that a low intake of a specific antioxidant could be considered as a cause of cancer development.

All these considerations have generated interest in the so-called functional foods, or foods for a specific health use, that is, foods that determine a physiological effect when consumed as part of the habitual diet. Tomato could justifiably be considered a functional food for its antioxidant content. Different studies have already provided important data regarding the lower incidence of chronic disease and, in particular, of several type of cancers in populations with a regular intake of tomato and tomato products (Franceschi et al. 1994, La Vecchia 1998, Giovannucci 1999). Whether this protection is to be attributed to specific compounds present in tomato should be further evaluated.

NUTRITIONAL CHARACTERISTICS OF TOMATO

Tomato is a vegetable, with a high water content (94%), rich in antioxidant compounds. Its characteristic color derives from the presence of a considerable amount of lycopene, a carotenoid with high antioxidant potential (Di Mascio et al.1989, Stahl and Sies 1996).

Other minor sources of lycopene are watermelon (23–72 µg/g wet weight), pink guava (54.0 µg/g wet weight), pink grapefruit (33.6 µg/g wet weight), and papaya (20–53 µg/g wet weight) (Rao and Agarwal 1999). However, tomato products are the main sources of the carotenoid within the daily diet and generally tomatoes are strictly identified with lycopene. For this reason the beneficial effects of tomatoes are often attributed to this carotenoid. Nevertheless tomatoes also contain considerable quantities of different antioxidants like other carotenoids, polyphenols, and vitamin C.

In recent years a considerable number of authors have determined and published their results regarding lycopene and carotenoid content in tomato, so contributing to the update of composition tables (Hart and Scott 1995, Rao et al. 1998, U.S. Department of Agriculture 2002, Holden et al. 1999, Shi and Le Maguer 2000, Grolier et al. 2001, Djuric and Powell 2001). From these data it is clear that lycopene content in tomato is extremely variable because many factors may influence its concentration (ripening stage, light, temperature, but also technological processing and storage conditions). Furthermore, the different and sometimes not homogeneous analytical methods employed may affect results present in literature. Nevertheless. an average lycopene content of fresh red variety tomatoes is generally estimated between 1.5 and 5.6 mg/100g (Shi and Le Maguer 2000). Other carotenoids present in tomato contribute 35–40% of the total carotenoid content, in particular, most representative are beta-carotene (1–2%) phytoene (10–12%), phytofluene (4–5%), and neurosporene (7–9%) (Clinton 1998). Tomato products such as sauce and paste contain generally more lycopene (from 6.5 to 19 mg/100g for sauce and 51 to 59 mg/100 g for paste) and a variable amount of the other carotenoids.

Another important constituent that improves tomato antioxidant properties is vitamin C. Its content in fresh tomato has been estimated at about 19-25 mg/100g (USDA composition tables, Grolier et al. 2001). In other tomato foods, like tomato paste, vitamin C content is reported to be about 42 mg/100 g (USDA composition tables), while in tomato sauce, it is lower (13 mg/100 g); however, it varies greatly depending on processing. Although tomato is not a main source of vitamin C, it can significantly contribute to the daily intake by considering the frequency of consumption within the diet.

Other antioxidants in tomato and tomato products include a small amount of vitamin E (present in seeds). Its content, by USDA composition tables, is about 0.4 mg/100 g in fresh tomato, 4.2 mg/100 g in tomato paste, and 1.4 mg/100 g in tomato sauce expressed as alpha-tocopherol equivalent. Even if tomato is not a good source of this vitamin, it can gain in importance as it is often consumed regularly with oils rich in vitamin E. This aspect is important also because it has been demonstrated that the intake of oil is fundamental for carotenoid absorption (Stahl and Sies 1992, Yeum and Russell 2002).

Folates may also contribute to beneficial properties of tomato products (Kim 1999), even if tomato is not the primary source of this vitamin. Their amount in fresh tomatoes is about 15 µg/100 g, in tomato paste about 22 µg/100 g, and in tomato sauce 9 µg/100 g (USDA composition tables).

As regards the content in polyphenolic substances, accurate data are not easily available because of the complexity of analysis and the variability of the compounds present in the various species of tomatoes. Total polyphenols content, evaluated as Folin assay, is about 4–25 mg/100g (Minoggio et al. 2002) and so may represent an important contribution to total antioxidant properties of the whole tomato. Tomato polyphenols consist mainly of flavonoids and phenolic acids (Grolier et al. 2001). The contribution of each component to food antioxidant properties has been underlined by recent studies that evaluated the total antioxidant capacity of aqueous and organic extracts of different tomato products (Pellegrini et al. 1999, Lavelli et al. 1999). Djuric and Powell (2001) showed that the tomato products with the highest antioxidant capacity per serving (tomato soup) did not have the highest lycopene content. Lavelli et al. (1999) demonstrated that the antioxidant activity of tomato products, evaluated by three methods, was dependent both on hydrophilic and lipophilic fractions. This was confirmed by Takeoka et al. (2001), who observed a significant antioxidant activity in both the hexane and methanol fractions obtained from fresh tomato and tomato paste. They suggested that polyphenols may also be important in conferring protective antioxidant effects.

It is difficult to extrapolate the potential impact of each compound in vivo because it depends on the bioavailability of the compound itself and its relative absorption and metabolism in the human organism. This consideration must be kept in mind also when using data from tables of food composition to analyze epidemiological data or planning experimental protocols. It is in fact widely demonstrated that lycopene bioavailability is unpredictable and differs among different tomato sources. For example, it is reported that the intake of tomato paste or tomato sauce may have a more consistent impact on plasma lycopene levels with respect to raw fresh tomato (Gartner et al. 1997, Porrini et al. 1998).

Furthermore, we have not enough knowledge about lycopene metabolism and tissue distribution. It is known that its concentration in plasma depends strictly on the intake of tomatoes with the diet and that, although it easily reaches a plateau after daily consumption of one rich source, it decreases rapidly when the intake is suspended even for a short time. This implies that there is not a real depot of the carotenoid in the organism. There is a little literature (Furr and Clark 1997, Rao and Argawal 1999) on lycopene tissue concentration stating that it is stored mainly in testes (4.3–21.4 nmol/g wet wt), adrenal gland (1.9–21.6 nmol/g wet wt), liver (1.3–5.7 nmol/g wet wt), and also in lung (0.2–0.6 nmol/g wet wt), ovary (0.3 nmol/g wet wt), colon (0.3 nmol/g wet wt), stomach (0.2 nmol/g wet wt), skin (0.4 nmol/g wet wt), and prostate gland (0.8 nmol/g wet wt). In this last tissue, the presence of lycopene in relevant amounts has suggested a possible role of the carotenoid in the prevention of cancer (Clinton et al. 1996). At this regard, Rao et al. (1999) found that levels of serum and prostate tissue lycopene were lower in cancer patients than in controls.

EPIDEMIOLOGICAL STUDIES ON TOMATO AND CANCER

Over the last few years numerous studies have reported the association between tomato consumption and protection from degenerative diseases like cancer. However, it is difficult to come to a definite and sure conclusion about the strong effect of lycopene-containing foods on disease prevention, because of the differing study designs and outcome evaluations. Indeed, there are several problems linked to the analysis of epidemiological data involving the measurement of many different parameters. Appropriate and sensitive tools are required in order to limit potential errors and avoid misinterpretation of results.

Recently Gerber et al. (2001) made an exhaustive review of the evidence accumulated about the association between tomato consumption and cancer development within a European-funded concerted action. In this review (which is suggested for further reading and a reference for most of the literature on this topic) are reported the conclusions of four reference books (CNERNA 1996, WCRF 1997, COMA 1998, IARC 1998) updated with further studies published up to 2000. These data have been examined thoroughly for consistency of the results, strength of the association, dose response, analogy, and biological plausibility. What has come out is that the protective effect of tomato is convincing only for specific types of cancers: upper aero-digestive tract (particularly esophagus but also oral cavity, pharynx, and larynx), lung, and stomach. Until now, there have been no other publications contradicting such data.

Recent results showed that human buccal mucosa cells are able to retain lycopene but also phytofluene and beta-carotene present in tomato products (Paetau et al. 1999), and this may provide a rationalization for the higher protection in the upper digestive tract.

There aren't many data available about the effect of tomato intake on other types of cancer (particularly colon-rectum, pancreas, liver, breast, ovary, endometrium, cervix, kidney, bladder, and thyroid), and what is reported does not explain a reduced risk of such cancers (Gerber et al. 2001). This is also true when considering the analysis of the relationship between lycopene concentrations in plasma and the different types of cancer. The results coming from the few reports available are inconclusive, leading to an inconsistent or insufficient level of evidence on the specific role of lycopene in the protection from cancer development. The explanations for these results could be (1) the limited available data on carotenoids in food composition tables, and (2) the difficulties in analyzing lycopene in plasma and interpreting the results. On the other hand, it could also be that lycopene itself is not the essential or the main component in tomatoes that exerts the protective effect.

This is in contrast to what has recently been reported in a case-control study developed in Uruguay (De Stefani et al. 2000) where the effect of tomatoes, tomato products, and lycopene intake on cancer of the upper aero-digestive tract was analyzed. The authors, in fact, found a strong and dose-response protective effect of both tomato products and lycopene. The adjustment of tomato intake for other compounds such as vitamin C, folate, potassium, flavonoids, and phytosterols attenuated the effect of tomatoes even if the reduction of risk remained significant. On the contrary, the adjustment for lycopene intake resulted in a marked attenuation of the protective effect suggesting that lycopene was responsible for most of the protective effect of tomatoes and tomato products, the remaining (21%) being due to the combined effect of the other compounds (vitamin C, phytosterols, flavonoids).

The link between tomato products and/or lycopene intake and prostate cancer risk is without doubt one of the most interesting and controversial. In fact, there are a few studies reporting a significant association (Mills et al. 1989, Giovannucci et al. 1995, Tzonou et al. 1999, Gann et al. 1999, Lu et al. 2001), others reporting a not significant inverse relation (Schuman et al. 1982, Hsing et al. 1990, Norrish et al. 2000), and those that do not find any association at all (Le Marchand et al. 1991, Nomura et al. 1997, Schuurman et al. 1998).

Giovannucci and coworkers are among the most interested researchers involved in this topic and they strongly support the role of consumption of tomato products on prostate cancer prevention.

Recently they (Giovannucci et al. 2002) evaluated additional data (further 2481 case patients) from their Health Professionals Follow-up Study (HPFS), first published in 1995 (Giovannucci et al. 1995). They critically reanalyzed all the data collected taking into account an updated database for carotenoid content of tomato-based food products. From this review of data, they noticed an increase in lycopene intake of the population with respect to that reported earlier underlying the importance of the accuracy of the database in this type of analysis. The results confirmed a link between tomato sauce intake and the risk of prostate cancer. The association was observed for men of both southern European ancestry and Caucasian ancestry and remained consistent when controlled for olive oil consumption as a marker of Mediterranean diet. Furthermore, a strong correlation was found between dietary lycopene intake and circulating levels probably due to the use of more-accurate data on lycopene content of foods. The effect of tomato products was not confounded with fruit and vegetable consumption that has not been generally related to prostate cancer. The authors also provide a wide discussion on the possible reasons for different results found in literature regarding the role of tomato products and lycopene on this type of cancer. First, the size of the study may be fundamental. In fact, they maintain that small studies can fail to find a correlation as the magnitude of the association is generally moderate. Second, the assessment of the real intake of lycopene with the diet, together with its bioavailability, is another important factor of error. Moreover, in the studies analyzing lycopene plasma levels, the sampling (generally a single assessment) is not enough to describe the intake in the medium term. The results that Giovannucci et al. (2002) obtained from the update suggest that a recent intake is more important than the remote intake in explaining carotenoid plasma levels. We found a similar result analyzing the carotenoid plasma levels of a group of women who filled in a questionnaire developed for the analysis of carotenoid intake from fruit and vegetables (unpublished data). Lycopene levels did not reflect the long-term intake (the last 3 months) but just the intake of the last few days.

Concerning the plausibility of the main role of lycopene in the protection from prostate cancer development, even Giovannucci et al. (2002) admit that other components present in tomato may interact or be responsible for the protection. Furthermore, the mechanism of action involved may be different and not only the simple antioxidant effect.

MECHANISTIC STUDIES EVALUATING A POTENTIAL PROTECTIVE ROLE OF TOMATO IN CANCER DEVELOPMENT

There are many aspects of cancer etiology that have still not been clarified, because there's a long latent period between the first biological cancer event and the first clinical symptoms of malignant disease. Furthermore, every type of cancer has a different cause related to the activity of the specific organ where cancer has its origin.

Actually, three fundamental steps of cancer, progressing from the molecular level to clinical evidence, are well-recognized (Gerster 1995). (1) During the first stage of carcinogenesis (initiation), an irreversible damage of cellular DNA occurs that does not lead necessarily to cancer. This DNA alteration is due to some substances called "initiators" that become reactive after a metabolic activation. (2) In the second stage (promotion), there are a series of chain reactions that transform normal cells into tumoral ones by affecting cell differentiation, phenotypic expression, and increasing cell proliferation. (3) In the final stage (progression), an uncontrolled proliferation of mutagen cells begins, with clinical consequences.

Research has not established entirely the mechanisms by which compounds present in tomato and/or other vegetables can reduce the risk of disease development. The actual major hypothesis is that antioxidants present in these foods can safely interact with free radicals and terminate the chain reaction before vital molecules are damaged. However, other possible mechanisms, that can be interrelated with oxidative damage, are involved in the different stages of the carcinogenic process. Reactive oxygen species (ROS), in fact, can influence gene regulations or the immune system altering the normal body functions.

Some of the potential mechanisms that could support the protective effect of antioxidant compounds present in tomato products are briefly described in this section and are shown in Figure 8.1.

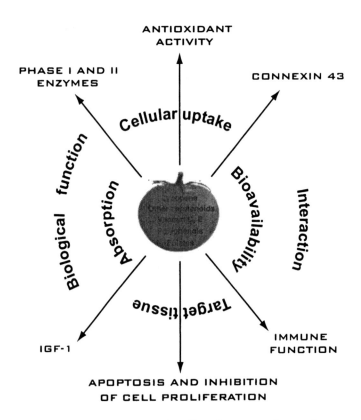

Figure 8.1. Representation of the potential protective effect of tomato products against cancer development. Each mechanism of action is strictly dependent on numerous dietary and physiological factors that together contribute to the final effect.

Antioxidant Action

Most scientific evidence agrees that there are distinct oxidative reactions that play a key role during the phases of initiation and promotion of carcinogenesis.

Oxidative damage is a process depending on the formation of ROS; produced in normal cell metabolism or formed from exogenous events like smoke or radiation, ROS can react with susceptible biomolecules, mainly protein, lipids, and DNA, producing extensive cell damage (Davies 1995, Niki 1997).

Free radical damage to proteins provokes protein radicals that cause adverse reactions such as cross-linking, polypeptide chain scission, and oxidation and modification of aminoacids with a consequent loss of biological function. In diseases involving oxidative stress status, oxidized protein generated may be not easily replaced and this is critical for normal cell functions.

Lipid peroxidation is a better characterized process with respect to protein oxidation: oxygen can react with lipids to form lipid radicals that propagate the peroxidation chain reactions in cell membranes. Peroxyl radicals formed can react with aminoacid residues provoking inhibition of enzyme function and altering the protein function compromising integrity and biochemical characteristics of membranes. Furthermore, water-soluble lipid peroxidation products (aldehydes) have been shown to diffuse from membranes into other subcellular compartments and may react with nucleic acids forming DNA adducts thus giving rise to mutations and altered patterns of gene expression (Marnett 1999).

The oxidative modification of DNA is probably the most direct and significant cause of the development of cancer disease. In normal cells, DNA damage is continuously produced by ROS attack, and a balance normally exists between oxidative products and antioxidant systems. However, the entity of damage is very consistent: it has been estimated that oxygen radicals can cause about one base modification per 130,000 bases in nuclear DNA (Davies 1995). The modifications that concern DNA can be of a different nature and the chemistry is very complicated (Wiseman et al. 1995).

Animal model studies and in vitro cell culture experiments have described the ability of carotenoids to protect against carcinogenesis thanks to their antioxidant properties. Lycopene is considered the most potent singlet oxygen quencher (Di Mascio et al. 1989) but it seems to be active also against NO_2 (Böhm et al. 2001), CCl_3O_2 (Yaping et al. 2002), H_2O_2 (Riso et al. 1999a), and UV radiation (Ribaya-Mercado et al. 1995, Stahl and Sies 2002).

The antioxidant action has been demonstrated also for other compounds present in tomato products such as flavonoids (Pietta 2000), vitamin C (Carr and Frei 1999), and vitamin E (Landvik et al. 2002). It has also been suggested that the antioxidant activity is better performed when different compounds are involved as a network.

This was supported by Stahl et al. (2000a), who investigated in vivo the ability of carotenoid supplementations (mainly beta-carotene), with or without vitamin E, to protect human dorsal skin of volunteers from UV-induced damage. The authors obtained a greater suppression of erythema with the combinations of carotenoids and vitamin E (43% versus 30% after 8 weeks). In a further study, the supplementation of a group of volunteers with 40 g tomato paste (that provided about 16 mg/day lycopene) and 10 g of olive oil (a source of vitamin E) decreased erythema formation by about 40% after 10 weeks of treatment (Stahl et al. 2001).

In a very recent study (Offord et al. 2002) on the photoprotective potential of lycopene in UVA-irradiated human fibroblasts, it was put forward that lycopene and beta-carotene did not protect the cells on their own but in the presence of vitamin E, supporting the importance of a synergic effect of lycopene and vitamin E.

Gene Expression

The new frontier for research is the understanding of the possible involvement of antioxidant compounds in the modulation of gene expression. It has been shown that ROS can activate intracellular signaling that is involved in cell protection acting as second messengers in cytokine and some growth factor signal transduction pathways that in turn regulate further transcription factors. It could be that antioxidant compounds together with other dietary factors may affect this mechanism (Lopaczynski and Zeisel 2001, Greenwald et al. 2001).

An example of gene-nutrient interaction is provided by genetic polymorphisms involved in the metabolism and detoxification of carcinogenic substances including the P450 genes for the cytochrome P450 phase I enzymes, and the genes for the phase II enzymes (Greenwald et al. 2001). The effect of compounds present in tomato on the modulation of these genes has not been clearly established; however, few studies report a potential role of carotenoids (Bilton et al. 2001).

Effect on Cell Growth

Antioxidant compounds such as carotenoids, but also vitamin E, vitamin C, and flavonoids, can inhibit significantly the development of several tumors (Gerster 1995, Bilton et al. 2001). This is confirmed also in cellular models as demonstrated for lycopene against mammary, endometrial, lung, leukemic, and prostate cancer cell growth (Wang et al. 1989, Levy et al. 1995, Pastori et al. 1998, Amir et al. 1999). Generally the combination of more than one antioxidant produces better effect, due probably to a concerted action between the compounds (Pastori et al. 1998, Amir et al. 1999).

Different mechanisms have been hypothesized, such as the inhibition of cell cycle progression at the G1 phase via reduction in the cyclin D level (Nahum et al. 2001), the modulation of IGF-1 activity or expression (Sharoni et al. 2000), and the modulation of connexin 43, which is involved in gap-junction communication (Bertram 1999).

It is also important to consider that antioxidants seem to be involved in programmed cell death, called apoptosis. Apoptosis is a physiological mode of cell death involving morphological and biochemical changes (DNA fragmentation, cell shrinkage, etc.) that occur in response to different effectors. For example, it is induced by ROS and is common to many different pathological conditions. Recently, Nara et al. (2001) showed that lycopene and other acyclic carotenoids (phytoene, phytofluene, etc.) present in tomatoes and, above all, their oxidation products were able to inhibit HL-60 cancer cells through a mechanism of apoptosis induction. On the other hand, it is important to consider that antioxidant compounds reducing ROS may inhibit apoptosis interfering with the elimination of precancerous and cancerous cells. This is potentially dangerous for people at risk of or with cancer (Lopaczynski and Zeisel 2001). Thus, further studies are necessary to understand the antioxidant doses necessary to increase protection against oxidative damage without suppressing apoptosis of cancer cells.

Connexin 43

An important mechanism proposed for the protective effect of lycopene and other carotenoids is the upregulation of gap-junction communication by increasing the gene expression of connexin 43.

Gap junctions are aqueous pores that connect adjacent cells in most organs of the body. They consist of 12 molecules of a single major protein called connexin: 6 formed in a hexagonal cylinder in one plasma membrane joined to 6 arranged in the same array in the adjacent cell membrane.

Through gap junctions, cells can exchange nutrients, waste products, and signaling molecules such as cAMP or calcium ions. Molecules such as mRNA and protein are kept out maintaining the genetic identity of the cells. Tumor cells communicate poorly with their normal counterparts and in some cases this is owing to lack of expression of the connexin gene.

Bertram (1999) reviewed exhaustively all the evidence on the effect of carotenoids on cellular gap-junction communication also reporting the rationale for their possible mechanism of action. Based on the hypothesis first formulated by Lowenstein (1979), he concluded that when junctional communication is improved by compounds such as retinoids and carotenoids and the colony size is small, cells communicate adequately, and transformation is suppressed. In contrast, cells in the center of a large colony are more susceptible to transformation due to the possible lack of communication with the normal surrounding cells.

Recently, some studies have been conducted to investigate the role of lycopene on this type of mechanism. Stahl et al. (2000b) compared the stimulation of gap-junction communications induced by lycopene and retinoids in human fetal skin fibroblasts. Results showed that lycopene was more effective than acyclo-retinoic acid. In fact, a lower amount was necessary (0.1 µmol/L versus 1 µmol/L, respectively) to obtain a comparable stimulation. More recently, Kucuk et al. (2001) supplemented with lycopene (15 mg twice daily) for 3 weeks human patients with prostate cancer before radical prostatectomy. The results obtained confirmed a significant effect of lycopene on the enhancement of expression of connexin 43 in cancerous prostate tissue when compared to the control group. However, no firm conclusions on the capacity of lycopene to reduce the growth of prostate cancer were drawn because of the small size of the sample analyzed.

Insulin-like Growth Factor (IGF)-1

Insulin-like Growth Factor (IGF)-1 is considered one of the most important factors of the IGF system. It is a molecule that acts as a growth factor in different types of cancer cells (LeRoith et al. 1995). In particular, it has been suggested that a high plasma IGF-1 level is an important risk factor for breast and prostate cancer (Hankinson et al. 1998, Chan et al. 1998). The possible role of carotenoids on IGF system modulation has been recently reviewed (Sharoni et al. 2000). It has been suggested that lycopene may both decrease IGF-1 level in blood or interfere with IGF-1 activity in cancer cells. The supplementation of human endometrial (Ishikawa), mammary (MCF-7), and lung (NCI-H226) cells with physiological concentrations of lycopene hampered the growth of IGF-1-stimulated cells demonstrating its important role in IGF-1 signaling pathway (Levi et al. 1995). Furthermore, recently Amir et al. (1999) found a synergistic effect of lycopene and $1,25(OH)_2D_3$ in the inhibition of cancer cell proliferation, hypothesizing that lycopene, or better its metabolites, may act as ligands for a nuclear receptor, thus acting as a hormone.

The results of intervention studies are still insufficient to confirm the efficacy of lycopene. Kucuk et al. (2001) supplemented 15 patients with prostate cancer with 30 mg/day lycopene for 3 weeks before prostatectomy, while 11 patients acted as control. The authors confirmed that lycopene supplementation was able to decrease the growth of prostate cancer. They found a decrease of plasma prostate-specific antigen levels and a decrease of the expression of connexin 43 in supplemented subjects, while IGF-1 decreased in both groups. Differently, in a recent case-control study involving 112 men, it was found that the consumption of cooked tomatoes was inversely associated with IGF-1 levels (Mucci et al. 2001).

Immune Function

Another aspect of the anticarcinogenic properties of carotenoids is their ability to modulate the immune function.

Oxidative stress is implicated in the loss of cell-mediated immune response, which is associated with increased risk of cancer development (Hennekens et al. 1986, Bendich 1993). Carotenoid-containing foods may act through the protection of cell integrity, limiting membrane damage and so avoiding modifications of membrane-bound receptors that are necessary for cell to cell communications (Hughes 2001, Deming et al. 2002). Recently, Hughes (2001) made an interesting report of the main results obtained in this field. Most of the work conducted focused on beta-carotene effect on immune function; however, some research has been carried out on other carotenoids such as lutein, astaxanthin, and canthaxanthin (Bendich and Shapiro 1986, Jyonuchi et al. 1994, Jyonouchi et al. 1995). Most of the studies reported a positive effect of these compounds.

Hughes et al. (1997) found that the supplementation with 15 mg beta-carotene could enhance the immune response in middle-aged subjects and suggested that it could be due to the increase of surface-molecule expression and possibly also to the alteration of the activation of the arachidonic acid cascade involved in prostaglandin E synthesis. However, the supplementation with 15 mg lycopene or lutein did not affect the expression of most of the monocyte-surface molecules studied (Hughes et al. 2000). Also, the supplementation with relatively low concentration of beta-carotene and lycopene in a group of older volunteers (over 65 years) failed to demonstrate any beneficial or detrimental effect on immune function (Corridan et al. 2001). This was supported by other authors who enriched the diet of elderly people with tomato juice for 8 weeks (Watzl et al. 2000). In a previous study, Watzl et al. (1999) reported that a low carotenoid diet was able to reduce

T-lymphocyte functions that were restored after 2 weeks' consumption of tomato juice but not carrots and spinach. This confirms that each carotenoid may act differently depending on the target cell considered.

INTERVENTION STUDIES

Large-scale intervention trials with vegetables are insufficient or do not exist at all. This is because they are much too expensive and need large resources for the follow-up, for people support, and for the analysis of data. In the past, few intervention trials have been conducted supplementing subjects with pure compounds, and the results obtained have often been contradictory and sometimes negative (Hennekens et al. 1996, Omenn et al. 1996). As regards tomato or lycopene, most of the data in literature come from small intervention trials on groups of healthy people carried out to evaluate the effect of the intake of this food for short periods of time on different variables of oxidative stress. These studies help in understanding the possible role of tomato products, but need to be confirmed with long-term studies on a large number of subjects with different characteristics and health states. Recently, Chen et al. (2001) investigated the feasibility of the addition to the diet of tomato sauce-based products in 32 patients diagnosed with prostate cancer. They analyzed lycopene cellular uptake, oxidative DNA damage, and prostate-specific antigen (PSA) levels before and after a 3-week intervention period (30 mg lycopene per day). They found a significant increase of both serum (about two times) and prostate (about three times) lycopene concentrations and consequently a significant decrease in leukocyte (about 21%) and prostate (about 28%) oxidative DNA damage (evaluated as the ratio of 8-OH dG/dG concentration). Also PSA levels showed a reduction (about 17%) after the intervention, suggesting that tomato products may be used as dietary treatment in patients with prostate cancer. The increase in lycopene concentration in the prostate was in accordance with what Clinton et al. (1996) found in a previous study where a potential role of lycopene was hypothesized in the protection of this tissue.

An interesting consideration coming from Chen et al. (2001) is the possibility "to use oxidative damage to leukocyte DNA as a surrogate marker for oxidative damage to prostate tissue to monitor the effectiveness of an antioxidant intervention." They in fact found a correlation between leukocyte and prostate DNA damage. This is extremely important if considering that it is necessary to identify possible target cells and easy to use for routine analysis of markers related to oxidative stress implicated in disease development. White blood cells have been widely used for this purpose (Anderson et al. 1994, Duthie et al. 1996, Pool-Zobel et al. 1997). We have always considered these cells in our studies as they can be easily collected. Moreover, we noticed that they respond to rapid changes in antioxidant plasma concentrations in a measurable way. We studied, in particular, lymphocyte resistance to oxidative damage following intervention with tomato products in healthy subjects. In our experience, the addition to a basal diet of one or more tomato products always involves an improvement of the antioxidant defense system of the organism evaluated by the measure of lymphocyte resistance against DNA oxidative stress (comet assay) (Riso et al. 1999b, Porrini and Riso 2000, Porrini et al. 2002). Comparable results were also found by other authors analyzing the effect of tomato consumption on DNA damage evaluated by 8-OHdG (Rao and Agarwal 1998, Chen et al. 1999) or comet assay (Pool-Zobel et al. 1997, Rehman et al. 1999). Pool-Zobel et al. (1998) suggested that tomato consumption may reduce lymphocyte DNA damage thanks to a modulation of gene expression as they found an increase of cytosolic GSTP1 and DNA repair proteins. The hypothesis of an effect of carotenoids on stimulation of DNA repair was not demonstrated by Torbergsen and Collins (2000). Other authors found that carotenoids could not be the cause of antioxidant protection (Borel et al. 1998, Collins et al. 1998).

Our recent results (Porrini and Riso 2000) showed that the correlation between cell protection and lycopene concentration we found in previous works (Porrini et al. 2002) could be misleading, with lycopene probably being only a marker of tomato intake rather than the main compound responsible for the protection. This observation was confirmed by the analysis of other antioxidants in the cells, such as vitamin C, which increased significantly during one of the interventions with tomato products (Riso et al., unpublished data). This could mean that the more the lycopene increases in the cell, the better the vitamin C may be preserved, demonstrating that any important antioxidant action may derive from an interaction between compounds available in plasma or tissues. It has recently been suggested (Brennan et al. 2000) that a protective action of vitamin C and vitamin E supplementation on H_2O_2 induced lymphocyte DNA damage.

Flavonoids could also play a role in the protective effect against DNA damage (Noorozi et al. 1998, Anderson et al. 2000) and we demonstrated that tomato puree consumption was able to increase plasma level of rutin, a well-known flavonoid (Mauri et al. 1999).

An important consideration is that in all our experimentation, the reduction of fruit and vegetables consumption requested before the period of tomato supplementation caused a rapid (about 1 week) decrease in cell protection from oxidative stress that was restored or improved by the subsequent intake of tomato products. It is obvious that tomato cannot substitute for any other food, but the integration of the diet with one or more vegetables is fundamental to help the endogenous antioxidant defense system. To further support this conclusion, in a recent study (Porrini et al. 2002), we found that the integration of the diet with spinach rich in lutein caused a significant protection from lymphocyte DNA damage, yet this protection was not improved by the contemporaneous intake of tomato puree.

It is plausible that the different cells can use the different antioxidants, exploiting them to their maximum yet depending on the mechanism and relative promptness of action of each one. The question now arises as to whether we could get the same results on other types of cells, for example, on prostate tissue (where lycopene is mainly accumulated) or the macula (where lutein is the main carotenoid).

Another interesting question regards the feasibility of potential biomarkers believed to be involved in cancer development and sensitive to dietary interventions. One example is oxidative DNA damage widely considered in this review. It is one of the most important markers in intervention studies above all because of its potential relation with cancer development. Recently, Halliwell (2002) stressed that oxidative DNA damage has not been demonstrated as being a valid biomarker of subsequent cancer development. There is also the question as to whether the levels of oxidative DNA damage may be affected more by genetic factors than as a response to diet modifications, even if most available literature supports a fundamental role of diet.

CONCLUSION

At present there are no conclusive data on the role of tomato products in cancer prevention. However, there is evidence of a potential protective effect of this food particularly if it is processed. What part carotenoids, in particular lycopene, play in this protective action has not yet been clearly established. So there are still some questions that need answers, such as, would it really be enough to improve data on lycopene intake in order to obtain more evidence on its role? Is plasma lycopene concentration a significant marker of "lycopene status" and tomato intake considering that very little is known about its metabolism and storage in tissue? Are mechanisms of action and interaction of carotenoids sufficiently recognized? Are the biomarkers available appropriate for the evaluation of the potential role of different foods in the protection from cancer development?

Another consideration to be made is that any benefit coming from the intake of a specific food can only come out of consistent long-term studies since more time is needed for the modulation of the factors taking place at the cellular levels. Consequently, the best research strategy would be for long-term intervention trials with tomato products or other functional foods (not their constituents) on population groups exposed to different risk factors.

REFERENCES

Amir, H., Karas, M., Giat, J., Danilenko, M., Levy, R., Yermiahu, T., Levy, J., Sharoni, Y. 1999. Lycopene and 1,25-dihydroxyvitamin-D_3 cooperate in the inhibition of cell cycle progression and induction of differentiation in HL-60 leukemic cells. *Nutrition and Cancer* 33:105–112.

Anderson, D., Yu, T. W., Phillips, B. J., Lowe, J. E., Szumiel, I. 1994. The effect of various antioxidants and other modifying agents on oxygen-radical-generated DNA damage in human lymphocytes in the comet assay. *Mutation Research* 307:261–271.

Anderson, R. F., Amarasinghe, C., Fisher, L. J., Mak, W. B., Packer, J. E. 2000. Reduction in free-radical-induced DNA strand breaks and base damage through fast chemical repair by flavonoids. *Free Radical Research* 33(1):91–103.

Bendich, A. 1993. Antioxidants, immune response, and animal function. *Journal of Dairy Science* 76:2789–2794.

Bendich, A., Shapiro, S. S. 1986. Effect of beta-carotene and canthaxanthin on the immune responses of the rat. *Journal of Nutrition* 116:2254–2262.

Bertram, J. S. 1999. Carotenoids and gene regulation. *Nutrition Reviews* 57(6):182–191.

Bilton, R., Gerber, M., Lowe, G., Offord, E., Porrini, M., Riso, P., Rock, E. 2001. "The role of dietary tomato products in protection against oxidative cellular injury: a review of biomarkers, mechanisms and intervention studies". In *The White Book on antioxidants in tomatoes and tomato products and their health benefits*, second revised edition. European-funded Concerted Action (FAIR CT 97-3233) on the "Role and Control of Antioxidants in the Tomato Processing Industry" edited by R. Bilton, M. Gerber, P. Grolier, C. Leoni. CMITI Sarl: Avignon Cedex.

Böhm, F., Edge, R., Burke, M., Truscott, T. G. 2001. Dietary uptake of lycopene protects human cells from singlet oxygen and nitrogen dioxide—ROS components from cigarette smoke. *Journal of Photochemistry and Photobiology B: Biology* 64:176–178.

Borel, P., Grolier, P., Boirie, Y., Simonet, L., Verdier, E., Rochette, Y., Alexandre-Gouabau, M. C., Beaufrere, B., Lairon, D., Azais-Braesco, V. 1998. Oxidative stress status and antioxidant status are apparently not related to carotenoid status in healthy subjects. *Journal of Laboratory and Clinical Medicine* 132:61–66.

Brennan, L. A., Morris, G. M., Wasson, G. R., Hannigan, B. M., Barnett, Y. 2000. The effect of vitamin C or vitamin E supplementation on basal and H_2O_2-induced DNA damage in human lymphocytes. *British Journal of Nutrition* 84:195–202.

Carr, A., Frei, B. 1999. Toward a new recommended dietary allowance for vitamin C based on antioxidant and health effects in humans. *American Journal of Clinical Nutrition* 69:1086–1107.

Chan, J. M., Stampfer, M. J., Giovannucci, E., Gann, P. H., Ma, J., Wilkinson, P., Hannekens, C. H., Pollak, M. 1998. Plasma insulin-like growth factor-I and prostate cancer risk: a prospective study. *Science* 279:563–566.

Chen, L., Bowen, P. E., Berzy, D., Aryee, F., Stacewicz-Sapuntzakis, M., Riley, R. E. 1999. Diet modification affects DNA oxidative damage in healthy humans. *Free Radical Biology & Medicine* 26:695–703.

Chen, L., Stacewicz-Sapuntzakis, M., Duncan, C., Sharifi, R., Ghosh, L., van Breemen, R., Asthon, D., Bowen, P. E. 2001. Oxidative DNA damage in prostate cancer patients consuming tomato sauce-based entrees as a whole-food intervention. *Journal of the National Cancer Institute* 93(24):1872–1879.

Clinton, S. K. 1998. Lycopene: chemistry, biology, and implications for human health and disease. *Nutrition Reviews* 56(2):35–51.

Clinton, S. K., Emenhiser, C., Schwartz, S. J., Bostwick, D. G., Williams, A. W., Moore, B. J., Erdman, J. W. 1996. *Cis-trans* lycopene isomers, carotenoids and retinal in the human prostate. *Cancer Epidemiology Biomarkers & Prevention* 5:823–833.

CNERNA. 1996. *Alimentation et cancer*. Evaluation des données scientifiques, edited by Riboli et al. Tec Doc, Lavoisier: Paris.

Collins, A. R., Olmedilla, B., Southon, S., Granado, F., Duthie, S. J. 1998. Serum carotenoids and oxidative DNA damage in human lymphocytes. *Carcinogenesis* 19(12):2159–62.

COMA. 1998. *Nutritional aspects of the development of cancer*. Report of the Working Group on Diet and Cancer of the Committee on Medical Aspects of Food and Nutrition policy. The Stationery Office: UK.

Corridan, B., O'Donoghue, M., Hughes, D. A., Morrisey, P. A. 2001. Low-dose supplementation with lycopene or beta-carotene does not enhance cell-mediated immunity in healthy free-living elderly humans. *European Journal Clinical Nutrition* 55:627

Davies, K. J. A. 1995. Oxidative stress: the paradox of aerobic life. In *Free radicals and oxidative stress: Environment, drugs and food additives*, edited by Rice-Evans, C., Halliwell, B., Lunt, G. Biochemical Society Symposium No. 61, pp. 1–35. Portland Press: London.

Deming, D. M., Boileau, T. W.-M., Heintz, K. H., Atkinson, C. A., Erdman, J. W. 2002. Carotenoids: linking chemistry, absorption, and metabolism to potential roles in human health and disease. In *Handbook of antioxidants, 2d ed., revised and expanded*. Edited by Cadenas, E., Packer, L., pp. 189–221. Marcel Dekker, Inc.: New York.

De Stefani, E., Oreggia, F., Boffetta, P., Deneo-Pellegrini, H., Ronco, A., Mendilaharsu, M. 2000. Tomatoes, tomato-rich foods, lycopene and cancer of the upper aerodigestive tract: a case-control in Uruguay. *Oral Oncology* 36(1):47–53.

Di Mascio, P., Kaiser, S., Sies, H. 1989. Lycopene as the most efficient biological carotenoid singlet oxygen quencher. *Archives of Biochemistry and Biophysics* 274(2):532–538.

Djuric, Z., Powell, L. C. 2001. Antioxidant capacity of lycopene–containing foods. *International Journal of Food Science and Nutrition* 52:143–149.

Duthie, S. J., Ma, A., Ross, M. A., Collins, A. R. 1996. Antioxidant supplementation decreases oxidative DNA damage in human lymphocytes. *Cancer Research* 56:1291–1295.

Franceschi, S., Bidoli, E., La Vecchia, C., Salamini, R., D'avanzo, B., Negri, E. 1994. Tomatoes and risk of digestive-tract cancers. *International Journal of Cancer* 59:181–184.

Furr, H. C., Clark, R. M. 1997. Intestinal absorption and tissue distribution of carotenoids. *Nutritional Biochemistry* 8:364–377.

Gann, P. H., Ma, J. Giovannucci, E., Willett, W., Sacks, F. M., Hennekens, C. H., Stampfer, M. J. 1999. Lower prostate cancer risk in men with elevated plasma lycopene levels: results of a prospective analysis. *Cancer Research* 59:1225–1230.

Gartner, C., Stahl, W., Sies, H. 1997. Lycopene is more bioavailable from tomato paste than from fresh tomatoes. *American Journal of Clinical Nutrition* 66:116–122.

Gerber, M., Amiot, M. J., Offord, E., Rock, E. 2001. The relationship between tomatoes and their constituents, and diseases. In *The white book on antioxidants in tomatoes and tomato products and their health benefits*, 2d rev. ed. European-funded concerted action (FAIR CT 97-3233), Role and Control of Antioxidants in the Tomato Processing Industry, edited by Bilton, R., Gerber, M. , Grolier, P., Leoni, C. CMITI Sarl: Avignon Cedex.

Gerster, H. 1995. Beta-carotene, vitamin E and vitamin C in different stages of experimental carcinogenesis. *European Journal of Clinical Nutrition* 49:155–168.

Giovannucci, E. 1999. Tomatoes, tomato-based products, lycopene, and cancer: review of the epidemiologic literature. *Journal of the National Cancer Institute* 91(4):317–331.

Giovannucci, E., Ascherio, A., Rimm, E. B., Stampfer, M. J., Colditz, G. A., Willet, W. C. 1995. Intake of carotenoids and retinol in relation to risk of prostate cancer. *Journal of the National Cancer Institute* 87(23):1767–1776.

Giovannucci, E., Rimm, E. B., Liu, Y., Stampfer, M. J., Willett, W. C. 2002. A prospective study of tomato products, lycopene, and prostate cancer risk. *Journal of the National Cancer Institute* 94:391–398.

Greenwald, P., Clifford, C. K., Milner, J. A. 2001. Diet and cancer prevention. *European Journal of Cancer* 37:948–965.

Grolier, P., Bartholin, G., Broers, L., Caris-Veyrat, C., Dadomo, M., Di Lucca, G., Dumas, Y., Meddens, F., Sandei, L., Schunch, W. 2001. Composition of tomatoes and tomato products in antioxidants. In *The white book on antioxidants in tomatoes and tomato products and their health benefits*, 2d rev. ed. European-funded concerted action (FAIR CT 97-3233), Role and Control of Antioxidants in the Tomato Processing Industry, edited by R. Bilton, M. Gerber , P. Grolier, C. Leoni. CMITI Sarl: Avignon Cedex.

Halliwell, B. 2002. Effect of diet on cancer development: is oxidative DNA damage a biomarker? *Free Radical Biology and Medicine* 32(10): 968–974.

Hankinson, S. E., Willett, W. C., Colditz, G. A., Hunter, D. J., Michaud, D. S., Deroo, B., Rosner, B., Speizer, F. E., Pollak, M. 1998. Circulating concentrations of insulin-like growth factor I and risk of breast cancer. *Lancet* 351:1397

Hart, D. J., and Scott, K. J. 1995. Development and evaluation of an HPLC method for the analysis of carotenoids in foods and the measurement of carotenoid content of vegetables and fruits commonly consumed in the UK. *Food Chemistry* 54:101–111.

Hennekens, C. H., Mayrent, S. L., Willett, W. 1986. Vitamin A, carotenoids, and retinoids. *Cancer* 58:1827–1841.

Hennekens, H. C., Buring, J. E., Manson, J. E., Stampfer, M., Rosner, B., Cook, N. R., Belanger, C., Lamotte, F., Gaziano, J. M., Ridker, P. M., Willett, W., Peto, R. 1996. Lack of effect of long term supplementation with beta-carotene on the incidence of malignant neoplasm and cardiovascular disease. *New England Journal of Medicine* 334:1145–1149.

Holden, J. M., Eldridge, A. L., Beecher, G. R., Buzzard, M., Bhagwat, S., Davis, C. S., Douglass, L. W., Gebhardt, S., Haytowitz, D., Schakel, S. 1999. Carotenoid content of U.S. foods: an update of the database. *Journal of Food Composition and Analysis.* 12:169–196.

Hsing, A. W., Comstock, G. W., Abbey, H., Polk, B. F. 1990. Serologic precursors of cancer. Retinol, carotenoids, and tocopherol and risk of prostate cancer. *Journal of the National Cancer Institute* 82:941–946.

Hughes, D. A. 2001. Dietary carotenoids and human immune function. *Nutrition* 17:823–827.

Hughes, D. A., Wright, A. J. A., Finglas, P. M., Peerless, A. C. J., Bailey, A. L., Astley, S. B., Pinder, A. C., Southon, S. 1997. The effect of beta-carotene supplementation on the immune function of blood monocytes from healthy male non-smokers. *Journal of Laboratory and Clinical Medicine.* 129:309–317.

Hughes, D. A., Wright, A. J. A., Finglas, P. M., Polley, A. C., Bailey, A. L., Astley, S. B., Southon, S. 2000. Effects of lycopene and lutein supplementation on the expression of functionally associated surface molecules on blood monocytes from healthy male non-smokers. *Journal of Infectious Diseases.* 182:S11–S15.

IARC handbooks of cancer prevention. 1998. Carotenoids, eds Press IARC: Lyon.

Jyonouchi, H., Sun, S., Gross, M. 1995. Effects of carotenoids on in vitro immunoglobulin production by human peripheral blood mononuclear cells: astaxanthin, a carotenoid without vitamin A activity, enhances in vitro response to a T-dependent stimulant antigen. *Nutrition and Cancer* 23:171–183.

Jyonouchi, H., Zang, L., Gross, M., Tomita, Y. 1994. Immunomodulating actions of carotenoids: enhancement of in vitro and in vivo antibody production to T-dependent antigens. *Nutrition and Cancer* 21:47–58.

Kim, Y-I. 1999. Folate and carcinogenesis: evidence, mechanisms, and implications. *Journal of Nutritional Biochemistry* 10:66–88.

Kucuk O., Sarkar, F. H., Skar W., Djuric, Z., Pollak, M. N., Khachik, F., Li, Y. W., Banerjee, M., Grignon, D., Bertram, J. S., Crissman, J. D., Pontes, E. J., Wood, D. P., Jr. 2001. Phase II randomised clinical trial of lycopene supplementation before radical prostatectomy. *Cancer Epidemiology, Biomarkers & Prevention* 10 (8) 861–8.

Landvik, S. V., Diplock, A. T., Packer, L. 2002. Efficacy of vitamin E in human health and disease. In *Handbook of antioxidants, 2d ed., revised and expanded,* edited by Cadenas, E., Packer, L., pp. 75–97. Marcel Dekker, Inc.: New York.

La Vecchia, C. 1998. Mediterranean epidemiological evidence on tomatoes and the prevention of digestive-tract cancers. *Proceedings of the Society for Experimental Biology and Medicine* 218:125–128.

Lavelli, V., Hippeli, S., Peri, C., and Elstner, E. F. 1999. Evaluation of radical scavenging activity of fresh and air-dried tomatoes by three model reactions. *Journal of Agricultural and Food Chemistry* 47:3826–3831.

Le Marchand, L., Hankin, J. H., Kolonel, L. N., Wilkens, L. R. 1991. Vegetable and fruit consumption in relation to prostate cancer risk in Hawaii: a reevaluation of the effect of dietary beta-carotene. *American Journal of Epidemiology* 133:215–219.

LeRoith, D., Werner, H., Beitner-Johnson, D., Roberts, C. T., Jr. 1995. Molecular and cellular aspects of the insulin-like growth factor I receptor. *Endocrine Review* 16:143–159.

Levy, J., Bosin, E., Feldman, B., Giat, Y., Miinster, A., Danilenko, M., Sharoni, Y. 1995. Lycopene is a more potent inhibitor of human cancer cell proliferation than either alpha-carotene or beta-carotene. *Nutrition and Cancer* 24:257–267.

Loewenstein, W. R. 1979. Junctional intercellular communication and the control of growth. *Biochemical and Biophysical Acta* 560:1–65.

Lopaczynski, W., and Zeisel, S. H. 2001. Antioxidants, programmed cell death, and cancer. *Nutrition Research* 21:295–307.

Lu, Q. Y., et al. 2001. Inverse association between plasma lycopene and other carotenoids and prostate cancer. *Cancer Epidemiology, Biomarkers & Prevention* 10:749–756.

Marnett, L. J. 1999. Lipid peroxidation-DNA damage by malondialdehyde. *Mutation Research* 424:83–95.

Mauri, P. L., Iemoli, L., Gardana, C., Riso, P., Simonetti, P., Porrini, M., Pietta, P. G. 1999 Liquid chromatography/electrospray ionization mass spectrometric characterization of flavonol glycosides in tomato extracts and human plasma. *Rapid Communication in Mass Spectrometry* 13:924–931.

Mills, P. K., Beeson, W. L., Phillips, R. L., Fraser, G. E. 1989. Cohort study of diet, lifestyle, and prostate cancer in Adventist men. *Cancer* 64:598–604.

Minoggio, M., Bramati, L., Simonetti, P., Gardana, C., Iemoli, L., Santangelo, E., Mauri, P. L., Spigno, P., Soressi, G. P., Pietta, P. G. 2002. Polyphenol pattern and antioxidant activity of different tomato lines and cultivars. *Annals of Nutrition and Metabolism.* In press.

Mucci, L. A., Tamimi, R., Lagiou, P., Trichopoulou, A., Benetou, V., Spanos, E., Trichopoulos, D. 2001. Are dietary influences on the risk of prostate cancer mediated through the insulin-like growth factor system? *BJU International* 87:814–820.

Nahum, A., Hirsch, K., Danilenko, M., Watts, C. K. W., Prall, O. W. J., Levy, J., Sharoni, Y. 2001. Lycopene inhibition of cell cycle progression in breast and endometrial cancer cells is associated with reduction in cyclin D levels and retention of p27^{Kip1} in the cyclin E-cdk2 complexes. *Oncogene* 20:3428–3436.

Nara, E., Hayashi, H., Kotake, M., Miyashita, K., Nagao, A. 2001. Acyclic carotenoids and their oxidation mixtures inhibit the growth of HL-60 human promyelocytic leukaemia cells. *Nutrition and Cancer* 39(2):273–283.

Niki, E. 1997. Free radicals in chemistry and biochemistry. In *Food and free radicals*, edited by M. Hiramatsu, T. Yoshikawa, M. Inoue, pp. 1–10. Plenum Press: New York and London.

Nomura, A. M., Stemmermann, G. N., Lee, J., Craft, N. E. 1997. Serum micronutrients and prostate cancer in Japanese Americans in Hawaii. *Cancer Epidemiology & Biomarkers Prevention* 6:487–491.

Noroozi, M., Angerson, W., Lean, M. E. J. 1998. Effects of flavonoids and vitamin C on oxidative DNA damage to human lymphocytes. *American Journal of Clinical Nutrition* 67:1210–1218.

Norrish, A. E., Jackson, R. T., Sharpe, S. J., Skeaff, C. M. 2000. Prostate cancer and dietary carotenoids. *American Journal of Epidemiology* 151:119–123.

Offord, E. A., Gautier, J. C., Avanti, O., Scaletta, C., Runge, F., Krämer, K., Applegate, L. A. 2002. Photoprotective potential of lycopene, beta-carotene, vitamin E, vitamin C and carnosic acid in UVA-irradiated human skin fibroblasts. *Free Radical Biology & Medicine* 32(12):1293–1303.

Omenn, G., Goodman, G. E., Thornquist, M. D., Balmes, J., Cullen, M. R., Glass, A., Kcogh, J. P., Meyskens, F. L., Valanis, B., Williams, J. H., Barnhart, S., Hammar, S. 1996. Effects of a combination of beta-carotene and vitamin A on lung cancer and cardiovascular disease. *New England Journal of Medicine* 334:1150–1155.

Paetau, I., Rao, D., Wiley, E. R., Brown, E. D., Clevidence, B. A. 1999. Carotenoids in human buccal mucosa cells after 4 wk of supplementation with tomato juice or lycopene supplements.
American Journal of Clinical Nutrition 70:490–494.

Pastori, M., Pfander, H., Boscoboinik, D., Azzi, A. 1998. Lycopene in association with alpha-tocopherol inhibits at physiological concentrations proliferation of prostate carcinoma cells.
Biochemical and Biophysical Research Communications 250:582–585.

Pellegrini, N., Re, R., Yang, M., and Rice-Evans, C. 1999. Screening of dietary carotenoids and
carotenoid-rich fruit extracts for antioxidant activities applying 2,2' -azinobis(3-ethyleneben-
zothiazoline-6-sulphonic acid radical cation decolorization assay. *Methods in Enzymology*
299:379–389.

Pietta, P. G. 2000. Flavonoids as antioxidants. *Journal of Natural Product* 63:1035–1042.

Pool-Zobel, B. L., Bub, A., Liegibel, U. M., Treptow-van Lishaut, S., Rechkemmer, G. 1998.
Mechanisms by which vegetable consumption reduces genetic damage in humans. *Cancer
Epidemiology, Biomarkers & Prevention* 7:891–899.

Pool-Zobel, B. L., Bub, A., Muller, H., Wollowski, I., Rechkemmer, G. 1997. Consumption of vegetables reduces genetic damage in humans: first results of a human intervention trial with
carotenoid-rich foods. *Carcinogenesis* 18(9): 1847–1850.

Porrini, M., and Riso, P. 2000. Lymphocyte lycopene concentration and DNA protection from
oxidative damage is increased in women after a short period of tomato consumption. *Journal of
Nutrition* 130(2):189–92.

Porrini, M., Riso, P., Oriani, G. A. 2002. Spinach and tomato consumption increases lymphocyte
DNA resistance to oxidative stress but this is not related to cell carotenoid concentrations.
European Journal of Nutrition 41:95–100.

Porrini, M., Riso, P., Testolin G. 1998. Absorption of lycopene from single or daily portions of raw
and processed tomato. *British Journal of Nutrition* 80:353–361.

Rao, A. V., and Agarwal, S. 1998. Bioavailability and *in vivo* antioxidant properties of lycopene
from tomato products and their possible role in the prevention of cancer. *Nutrition and Cancer*
31:199–203.

Rao, A. V., and Agarwal, S. 1999. Role of lycopene as antioxidant carotenoid in the prevention of
chronic diseases: a review. *Nutrition Research* 19 (2):305–23.

Rao, A. V., Fleshner, N., Argawal, S. 1999. Serum and tissue lycopene and biomarkers of oxidation
in prostate cancer patients: a case-control study. Nutrition and Cancer 33(2):159

Rao, A. V., Waseem, Z., Agarwal, S. 1998. Lycopene content of tomatoes and tomato products and
their contribution to dietary lycopene. *Food Research International* 31(10):737–41.

Rehman, A., Bourne, L. C., Halliwell, B., Rice-Evans, C. A. Tomato consumption modulates oxidative DNA damage in humans. 1999. *Biochemical and Biophysical Research Communications*
262:828–831.

Ribaya-Mercado, J. D., Garmin, M., Gilchrest, B. A., Russel, R. M. 1995. Skin lycopene is
destroyed preferentially over beta-carotene during ultraviolet irradiation in humans. *Journal of
Nutrition* 125:1845–1859.

Riso, P., Pinder, A., Santangelo, A., Porrini, M. 1999b. Does tomato consumption effectively
increase the resistance of lymphocyte DNA to oxidative damage? *American Journal of Clinical
Nutrition* 69(4):712–718.

Riso, P., Santangelo A., Porrini, M. 1999a. The comet assay for the evaluation of cell resistance to
oxidative stress. *Nutrition Research* 19(3):325–333.

Schuman, L. M., Mandel, J. S. D., Radke, A., Seal, U., Halberg, F. 1982. Some selected features of the epidemiology of prostatic cancer.: Minneapolis-St. Paul, Minnesota case-control study, 1976–1979. In *Trends in cancer incidence: causes and practical implications*, edited by Magnus, K., Hemisphere Publishing: Washington, DC.

Schuurman, A. G., Goldbohm, R. A., Dorant, E., van den Brandt, P. A. 1998. Vegetable and fruit consumption and prostate cancer risk: a cohort study in the Netherlands. *Cancer Epidemiology & Biomarkers Prevention* 7:673–680.

Sharoni, Y., Danilenko, M., Levy, J. 2000. Molecular mechanisms for the anticancer activity of the carotenoid lycopene. *Drug Development Research* 50:448–456.

Shi, J., and Le Maguer, M. 2000. Lycopene in tomatoes: chemical and physical properties affected by food processing. *Critical Reviews in Biotechnology* 20(4):293–334.

Stahl, W., and Sies, H. 1992. Uptake of lycopene and its geometrical isomers is greater from heat-processed than from unprocessed tomato juice in humans. *Journal of Nutrition* 122:2161–2166.

Stahl, W., and Sies, H. 1996. Lycopene: a biologically important carotenoid for humans? *Archives of Biochemistry & Biophysics* 336(1):1–9.

Stahl, W., and Sies, H. 2002. Antioxidant effect of carotenoids: implication in photoprotection in humans. In *Handbook of antioxidants. 2d ed., revised and expanded,* edited by Cadenas, E., Packer, L., pp. 223–233. Marcel Dekker, Inc.: New York.

Stahl, W., Heinrich, U., Jungmann, H., Sies, H., Tronnier, H. 2000a. Carotenoids and carotenoids plus vitamin E protect against ultraviolet light-induced erythema in humans. *American Journal of Clinical Nutrition* 71:795–798.

Stahl, W., Heinrich, U., Wiseman, S., Eichler, O., Sies, H., Tronnier, H. 2001. Dietary tomato paste protects against ultraviolet light-induced erythema in humans. *Journal of Nutrition* 131:1449–1451.

Stahl, W., von Laar, J., Martin, H. D., Emmerich, T., Sies, H. 2000b. Stimulation of gap junctional communication: comparison of acyclo-retinoic acid and lycopene. *Archives of Biochemistry & Biophysics* 373(1):271–274.

Takeoka, G. R., Dao, L., Flessa, S., Gillespie, D. M., Jewell, W. T., Huebner, B., Bertow, D., Ebeler, S. E. 2001. Processing effects on lycopene content and antioxidant activity of tomatoes. *Journal of Agriculture and Food Chemistry* 49(8):3713–3717.

Torbergsen, A. C., and Collins, A. R. Recovery of human lymphocytes from oxidative DNA damage; the apparent enhancement of DNA repair by carotenoids is probably simply an antioxidant effect. 2000. *European Journal of Nutrition* 39:80–85.

Tzonou, A., Signorello, L. B., Lagiou, P., Wuu, J., Trichopoulus, D., Trichopoulus, A. 1999. Diet and cancer of the prostate: a case-control study in Greece. *International Journal of Cancer* 80:704–708.

U.S. Department of Agriculture, Agricultural Research Service. 2002. USDA National Nutrient Database for Standard Reference, Release 15. Nutrient Data Laboratory Home Page, http://www.nal.usda.gov/fnic/foodcomp.

Wang, C. J., Chou, M. Y., Lin, J. K. 1989. Inhibition of growth and development of the transplantable C-6 glioma cells inoculated in rats by retinoids and carotenoids. *Cancer letters* 48:135–142.

Watzl, B., Bub, A., Blockhaus, M. et al. 2000. Prolonged tomato juice consumption has no effect on cell-mediated immunity of well-nourished elderly men and women. *Journal of Nutrition* 130:1719–1723.

Watzl, B., Bub, A., Brandstetter, B. R. Rechkemmer, G. 1999. Modulation of human T Lymphocyte functions by the consumption of carotenoid-rich vegetables. *British Journal of Nutrition* 82:383–389.

WCRF (World Cancer Research Fund). 1997. Food, Nutrition and the prevention of Cancer: a global perspective. World Cancer Research Fund with the American Institute for Cancer Research. Menasha, WI: Banta Book Group.

Wiseman, H., Kaur, H., Halliwell, B. 1995. DNA damage and cancer: measurement and mechanism. *Cancer Letters* 93:113–120.

Yaping, Z., Suping, Q., Wenli, Y., Zheng, X., Hong, S., Side, Y., Dapu, W. 2002. Antioxidant activity of lycopene extracted from tomato paste towards trichloromethyl peroxyl radical CCl_3O_2. *Food Chemistry* 77:209–212.

Yeum, K-J., Russell R. M. 2002. Carotenoid bioavailability and bioconversion. *Annual Review of Nutrition* 22:483–504.

9

The Role of Dietary Fiber in Colon Cancer Prevention

Nancy J. Emenaker

INTRODUCTION

Colorectal cancer is the second leading cause of cancer mortalities, affecting men and women at nearly identical incidence rates in the United States (Edwards et al. 2002). Improvements in prevention strategies including colorectal screening and the removal of premalignant polyps have contributed to the recent declines in morbidity and mortality rates. Despite these advances, the 5-year overall survival rate for colorectal malignancy is 61.5% and only 5% for patients diagnosed with a stage IV colorectal cancer in the United States. At present, data collected from 1995–1999 by the National Cancer Institute, the Centers for Disease Control, and the National Center for Chronic Disease Prevention and Health Promotion among others indicated colorectal cancer occurs at a rate of 56.9 cases per 100,000 persons and claims 21.7 lives per 100,000 Americans (Edwards et al. 2002). Although an overall decline in colorectal mortality and an increase in survival rates were observed between 1992–1998, current mortality rates are still high (Ries et al. 2002).

Increased colorectal screening practices combined with increased physical activity levels and improved dietary practices are effective colorectal cancer risk-reducing health promotion strategies. It is estimated that dietary factors contribute to an estimated 35% (10–70%) of all human cancers (Willett 1995) and that colorectal cancer cases could be reduced 50–75% if Americans would adopt a series of risk-lowering behaviors (Kim 2000). Since the human diet is a complex mixture of nutrients and biologically active compounds, modifying the intake of a single nutrient is neither sufficient nor likely to prevent the development of colon cancer. Current epidemiological data support the concept of an overall cancer preventive diet. Current dietary recommendations advocate a diet low in dietary fat and high in dietary fiber, grains, vegetables, and fruits as these overall patterns appear associated with the reduction of many types of cancers, including colorectal cancer. Thus, the overall composition of the diet when combined with other health promoting lifestyle behaviors (e.g., increased physical activity and decreased smoking and alcohol consumption) may be more effective in reducing the risk of colorectal cancer than implementing a single risk-reduction factor alone.

The purpose of this brief overview is to emphasize the recent human scientific evidence investigating the potential role of dietary fiber in colorectal cancer prevention. My apologies to those colleagues who were not included in this brief review due to space limitations. In vitro established human cells, primary human colonocytes, and epidemiological studies were emphasized since colon carcinogenesis in rodents is substantially different from humans (Topping and Clifton 2001) and because these animal models may not adequately represent human carcinogenesis due to significant genetic differences between humans and rodents (Balmain and Harris 2000, Hann and Balmain 2001). This does not imply that significant findings are not found using animal model systems, but only that differences exist between animal models and humans. Since the risk of colon cancer is dependent upon many factors affecting the colonic environment, it is important to remember that humans consume intact foods and not purified single nutrients in isolation. Dietary fiber is only one of those components. That is, dietary fiber, its metabolites, and other naturally occurring phytochemicals may act synergistically with other macronutrients, micronutrients, and biologically active compounds also present in the gastrointestinal tract. Thus, it is the combination of these factors, acting in concert with the gastrointestinal contents that may impact the colonic milieu in toto and may contribute to reducing colon cancer risk.

LINKING DIETARY FIBER CONSUMPTION TO COLON CANCER

The Early Evidence

The emergence of the "dietary fiber theory" was originally conceived by Peter Cleave (Walker and Burkitt 1976) and later developed by Burkitt (Burkitt 1970, Burkitt 1971, Burkitt 1973) and Doll and Peto (1981). The initial observations of Burkitt and others provided the epidemiological foundation on which the theory that dietary fiber protected against colorectal cancer was built. These early seminal papers by Burkitt also noted that alterations in dietary fiber consumption were not the only differences in dietary consumption patterns noticed between the Ugandan and Western populations (Burkitt 1971). The Ugandan population studied consumed lower levels of meat and fat, and higher levels of complex carbohydrates compared to Western populations who experienced higher rates of colorectal cancer.

Numerous nutritional factors (excess calories, high fat intake, and low intakes of fruits, vegetables, dietary fiber, calcium, folic acid, and selenium) have been implicated as mediators of colon cancer (Shike 1999). In addition to their effects on the colonic milieu, dietary nutrients also affect carcinogenesis by directly or indirectly regulating transcription of genes (Cousins 1999) and by regulating translation, mRNA stability, mRNA localization, and post-translational regulation (Hesketh et al. 1998). The concept that dietary fibers might protect against colon cancer by interacting with dietary metabolites (e.g., bile acids and sterols) and the colonic milieu (e.g., colonic microbial populations) is not a new concept (Walker and Burkitt 1976). These potential mechanisms of action are summarized in Table 9.1.

Newly Proposed Definition of Dietary Fiber

The definition of dietary fiber varies worldwide. Previously, the definition of dietary fiber in the United States was based upon analytical parameters put forth by the

Table 9.1.   Possible Mechanisms of Action of Dietary Fiber for the Reduction of Colon Cancer

• Increases stool bulk or weight
  Improves laxation
  Reduces intracolonic pressure
  Reduces gastrointestinal transit time
• Dilutes luminal carcinogens
• Binds bile acids
  Reduces fecal bile acid concentrations
  Prevents the conversion of primary bile acids to secondary bile acids by reducing concentrations
      of 7-a-dehydroxylase
• Reduces fecal pH levels
  Reduces free bile acid solubility
  Inhibits bacterial degradation of normal fecal constituents to potential carcinogens
• Alters colonic microflora
  Alters the species composition of gut microflora
  Stimulates microfloral growth, thereby stimulating fecal bulk
  Alters gut microflora ability to synthesize carcinogens and promoters
• Ferments fecal flora to short-chain fatty acids
  Inhibits tumor cell growth in cell lines and primary human colonocytes
  Stimulates microbial brush border enzymes
  Stimulates apoptosis
  Stimulates protease inhibitors in cell lines and primary human colonocytes
  Inhibits invasive tumor cell lines and primary human malignant colonocytes
  Modulates gene expression in cell lines and primary human colonocytes
  Predominant energy source for intestinal colonocytes
• Promotes weight maintenance by encouraging early satiety
• Reduces obesity, a risk factor for colon cancer
• Prevents insulin resistance and hyperinsulinemia

Source: Adapted from "AGA Technical Review: Impact of Dietary Fiber on Colon Cancer Occurrence" by Young-In Kim in Gastroenterology 118:1236–1249, copyright 2000 by American Gastroenterological Association, reproduced with permission from W.B. Saunders, an imprint of Elsevier Science (USA).

Association of Official Analytical Chemists International (AOAC), which focused on nondigestible food sources derived from plants, but not animals. As nutrition labeling becomes more uniform worldwide, a globally unified definition of dietary fiber is required.

In an attempt to globally unify the definition of dietary fiber, the Food and Nutrition Board of the Institute of Medicine of the National Academy of Sciences has proposed, "dietary fiber consists of nondigestible carbohydrates and lignin that are intrinsic and intact in plants" (Food and Nutrition Board 2001). This definition recognizes that dietary fiber sources also contain macronutrients and micronutrients that may also affect colonic health. These updated definitions also include nonabsorbable compounds such as resistant starch including raffinose, stachyose, verbacose, and fructans. In addition, definitions were also proposed for the terms "added fiber" and "total fiber." "Added fiber consists of isolated, nondigestible carbohydrates that have beneficial physiological effects in humans [while] total fiber is the sum of dietary fiber and added fiber" (Food and Nutrition Board 2001).

Intestinal Microflora and Dietary Substrates

Since digestion and absorption of dietary substrates from the small intestine is not 100% complete, dietary substrates reaching the colonic lumen can influence the production of carcinogens, their promoters and inhibitors by the intestinal microflora. These carcinogens include N-nitroso compounds, volatile phenols and carcinogenic aglycones. Dietary intake dramatically affects the microflora colonizing the colon. Over four hundred species of microflora inhabit the human colon; with bifidobacteria, lactobacilli, streptococci, eubacteria, and bacteroides identified as the dominant colonic anaerobes. Bacteroides comprise 30% of the total colonic microflora and are capable of metabolizing a wide variety of polysaccharides. Enterobacteria are also present at lower levels (Topping and Clifton 2001).

The proximal colon appears to be the major metabolic site of dietary substrates by the intestinal microflora as demonstrated in colectomy and ileostomy patient populations.

Total colectomy patients appear to lack the capacity to produce urinary volatile phenolic compounds and cyclic secondary amines while stable ileostomy patients demonstrate increased levels of intestinal bacteroides and clostridium (Hill 2001). When Hill altered the dietary fat, protein, bran, and pectin intakes of these patients for 3 weeks, significant changes in the colonic microbial population were noted. For example, Hill reported when patients received increasing concentrations of dietary fat (from 50 g/day to 150 g/day), bacteroides and clostridium counts were significantly increased. Moreover, when dietary protein consumption was increased from 40 g/day to 120 g/day, significant increases in facultative bacteria were also reported. Similarly, Hill also reported increases in all bacterial microflora when these patients increased their bran consumption while the addition of 30 g/day of a pectin supplement stimulated changes in sentinel enzymes (Hill 2001).

Hence, undigested insulin-type fructans (e.g., garlic, bananas, breakfast cereals, chocolate) entering the colon may act as prebiotics—compounds that stimulate the *in vitro* growth of beneficial colonic microflora such as *Bifidobacteria.*. These data and others suggest that nonabsorbable carbohydrates, resistant starches, resistant proteins, phytic acid, lignans, and flavonoids reach the colonic lumen undigested and may metabolically affect the colonic microenvironment including the colonic epithelium as shown in Table 9.2.

Many of the microbes present in the colon metabolize dietary fibers, by-products of fiber fermentation, dietary proteins and their intermediate by-products of metabolism. Hence, a wide variety of dietary substrates may influence colon carcinogenesis based on their effects on intestinal microflora carcinogen production (Hill 2001).

Short-chain Fatty Acids

Dietary fibers may directly affect colon health as shown above. The proximal colon is the site where dietary fiber exerts its predominant effect since the proximal region of the colon is a watery environment that allows the microflora ready access to undigested dietary substrates in the colonic lumen. Fermentation of dietary fibers by the anaerobic microflora results primarily in the production of carbon dioxide, hydrogen gas, methane, and short-chain fatty acids (acetate, propionate, and butyrate). Contrary to early hypotheses, short-

Table 9.2.   Biologically Active Compounds Associated with Dietary Fiber

Classification
Nonstarch polysaccharides:
Cellulose
Noncelluloses
Hemicellulose, pectins, gums, and mucilages
Nonpolysaccharides:
Lignins
Minor components:
Phytates, cutin, saponins, lectins, protein, waxes, and silicon
Related components:
Resistant starch and resistant protein
Lignans
Metabolic by-products:
Short-chain fatty acids (acetate, propionate, and butyrate)

Source: Adapted from "AGA Technical Review: Impact of Dietary Fiber on Colon Cancer Occurrence" by Young-In Kim in Gastroenterology 118:1236–1249, copyright 2000 by American Gastroenterological Association, reproduced with permission from W.B. Saunders, an imprint of Elsevier Science (USA).

chain fatty acid production ratios differ across the wide variety of dietary fibers fermented by the colonic microflora (Ehle et al. 1982, Weaver et al. 1992, Mortensen et al. 1992, Kapadia et al. 1995).

Although short-chain fatty acids are produced in the proximal colon, they may be carried to the distal regions of the colon by the fecal stream. Hence, differential effects of short-chain fatty acids are observed between the proximal and distal regions of the colon since short-chain fatty acids, which affect luminal pH, are absorbed prior to reaching the distal colon. Butyrate metabolism constitutes the dominant energy source for healthy colonocytes. Approximately 72% of the butyrate reaching the colon is metabolized by the surrounding healthy colonocytes (Cummings 1994) to CO_2 and ketones (Roediger 1994). However, dietary fiber is not the sole metabolic source of butyrate. Although dietary fiber fermentation serves as the primary contributor of butyrate to human colonocytes, undigested starches and proteins can also contribute to luminal butyrate concentrations (Macfarlene and Gibson 1995) and the production of ammonia, amines, indoles, and other volatile organic compounds.

IMPACT OF DIETARY FIBER ON COLON CARCINOGENESIS

Epigenetic Events

The malignant transformation of normal colonic epithelium to adenoma and potentially carcinoma is linked to several acquired epigenetic events. Over 11,782 active genes are present in the colon including the 892 genes unique to the human colon (National Institutes of Health 1999). Key genetic mutations or chromosomal losses in k-ras, APC (chromosome 5q), p53 (chromosome 17p), and DCC/DPC/JV18 (chromosome 18q) are associated with molecular and chromosome instabilities predisposing one to cancer (Fearon and Vogelstein 1990, Vogelstein and Kinzler 1993, Lengauer et al. 1998). The loss of the APC gene is among the earliest epigenetic events, potentially predisposing individuals to germ line mutations in the colonic mucosa. Genetic mutations occur predominantly in one of three classifications of genes: the "gatekeepers" (tumor suppressor genes, e.g., p53 and APC), the "caretaker" genes (DNA mismatch repair genes, e.g. hMSH1, hMSH2, and DNA-PKCs) (Ochiai et al. 2001), and the "landscaper" genes (e.g., PTEN) (Kinzler and Vogelstein 1998, Podsypanina et al. 1999). Not all genetic mutations lead to neoplastic transformation. Conversely, not every tumor requires that all epigenetic events occur or occur in a specific order. However, those mutations favoring malignant transformation typically result in either gain of function mutations (increased cell growth by mutating the protooncogene to the abnormal gene form, the oncogene) and/or the loss of function mutations in gatekeeper genes (prevent transcription of abnormal genes).

Genetic mutations detected in colorectal cancers can be inherited or sporadic in nature. Approximately 75% of all colorectal cancers are identified as sporadic in nature (National Cancer Institute 2002); that is, there is no prior family history of colorectal cancer or inherited genetic disorder that increases their cancer risk. The remaining 25% of colorectal cancer cases suggest an inherited genetic component. Inherited genetic disorders have been identified in some high-risk families. Persons with ulcerative colitis, polyposis syndrome, hereditary nonpolyposis colon cancer, and either family histories of colon cancer or previous colon cancer are at high risk for colon cancer. Edelstein et al. have shown that nonmalignant mucosa adjacent to malignant tissues displays abnormalities or "field defects" in intracellular pH and calcium ion transport (Edelstein et al. 1991). This suggests that an increased susceptibility to colorectal cancer is linked to an autosomal dominant inherited genetic mutation.

The most common inherited forms of colorectal cancer are Familial Adenomatous Polyposis (FAP) and Hereditary Nonpolyposis Colorectal Cancer (HNPCC). In FAP, mutations occur on chromosome 5q21-22 in the APC tumor suppressor gene altering epithelial cell-catenin interactions resulting in a nearly 100% lifetime risk of developing colorectal adenocarcinoma (Potter 1996). Mutations to the APC gene are common and probably constitute one of the earliest genetic mutations responsible for colorectal carcinogenesis. Inherited mutations can occur across several different genes. In HNPCC, the mutation occurs in the DNA mismatch repair proteins MSH2 and MLH1 carrying a 70% lifetime risk of developing colorectal cancer. These genetic mutations are linked with only 5–6% of all colorectal cancer cases. Mutations in MSH2 induce microsatellite instabilities that cannot easily be distinguished from sporadic forms of colorectal cancers. In advanced colorectal cancers, mutations have also been observed in p53 and DCC (tumor suppressor genes), while mutations in MCC (tumor suppressor gene), k-ras (membrane-associated G protein), c-myc (transcription factor), and c-erb-2 are found in more than 50% of colorectal carcinomas (Cross et al. 1995). Future studies may explain the particular functions of these active and unique genes providing detailed glimpses into their roles in the development and the progression of colon carcinogenesis.

Gene-Nutrient Interactions

Since colon cancers are predominantly sporadic in nature and do not present with a clear etiology of inherited genetic mutations, this suggests that environmental factors such as diet may affect genetic and biologic factors. A lack of genetic predisposition might suggest that environmental factors such as dietary consumption patterns may be associated with the incidence of sporadic cancer via gene-nutrient interactions. Previous studies have shown that a variety of nutrients (e.g., retinoic acid, retinal, zinc, long and short fatty acids, and vitamin D) regulate gene transcription by binding to DNA control sites (Hesketh et al. 1998, Cousins 1999).

Dietary fiber indirectly mediates gene expression via short-chain fatty acids functioning as secondary mediators. Butyrate interacts with a number of human gene expressions of over one thousand gene fragments involved in a variety of regulatory functions (Basson et al. 2000) including cell differentiation markers, regulators of the cell cycle, cell death regulators, GTP binding proteins, proteases and their inhibitors, tyrosine kinases, transcription factors, and tumor suppressors genes as shown in Table 9.3.

Butyrate appears to mediate the cell cycle through both classes of cyclins: G_1 and G_2/M checkpoints phase regulators. Cyclins C, D, and E are G_1 phase regulators controlling cell cycle events prior to DNA synthesis, while Cyclins A, B, and F regulate G_2/M checkpoints. Cyclins only allow cells to proceed from checkpoint to checkpoint if all conditions of the respective phase(s) have been met. This prevents, in theory, the proliferation of damaged or abnormal cells. Butyrate down-regulates or decreases the transcriptional induction of Cyclin D1 (necessary for entry in S phase of the cell cycle), A, and E, thereby controlling growth factor responses, cell adhesion, and DNA replication, respectively (Vaziri et al. 1998). Cell cycle and cell death (apoptosis) regulators are also affected by butyrate. Cells that are unable to proceed through the entire cell cycle and proliferate are destroyed through apoptosis. Butyrate has been shown in vitro to inhibit DNA synthesis (Emenaker and Basson 2001) and arrest neoplastic colon cell growth by modulating the activities of the cyclin-dependent kinases and Bcl-2, Bax, and Bak genes that regulate cell death (Velazquez et al. 1996, Giuliano et al. 1999). Specific tyrosine kinases p56 Lck and pp60 Src and GTP binding proteins c-ras and N-ras are down-regulated with physiologically relevant concentrations of butyrate. In addition, the transcription factors c-myb, c-myc, c-fos, c-jun, and WT1 levels (Thompson et al. 1998, Archer et al. 1998, Menssen et al. 2000, Emenaker and Basson 2001) are also mediated along with p53, RB1, PCNA, and E-cadherin (Barshishat et al. 2000; Emenaker et al. 2001).

OVERVIEW OF THE SCIENTIFIC EVIDENCE

Established Cell Line and Primary Human Cell Culture Evidence

Butyrate exerts numerous genetic and biologic effects on human colon cancer cells as shown above. Although much of the scientific evidence is congruent, not all in vivo reports support the in vitro findings. Several aspects should be considered when examining con-

Table 9.3. Biologic and Genetic Effects of Butyrate on Established and Primary Human Colon Cancer Cells

---

Biologic effects

Cell differentiation
↑ Intestinal alkaline phosphatase
↑ MUC3

Cell motility
↓ Cellular motility   ↓ Cellular adhesion
↓ Cellular invasion   ↓ Cellular proliferation

Extracellular matrix proteolytic enzymes
↓ uPA   ↓ MMP-2
↓ uPAR   ↓ MMP-9

Proteolytic inhibitors
↑ PAI   ↑ TIMP-1
↑ TIMP-2   ↑ MMP/TIMP complex formation

Genetic effects

Tyrosine kinases
↓ Lck   ↓ Erk
↓ Src

Transcription factors
↓ c-myb   ↑ COX-2
↑↓ c-myc   ↓ c-fos
↑ Cdx2   ↑ c-jun phosphorylation

Tumor suppressor genes
↓ p53   ↓ WT1
↓ RB1   ↑ E-cadherin

GTP binding proteins
↓ c-ras
↓ n-ras

Cell death regulators/inducers
↑↓ Bcl-2   ↑ Bak
↑↓ Bax   ↑ Caspase-3

Cell cycle regulators
↓ Cyclin A   ↑ p21/Waf-1/CIP-1
↓ Cyclin D1   ↓ PCNA
↓ Cyclin E   ↓ Ha-p21

Source: Adapted from Velcich et al. 1995, Basson et al. 1996, Velazquez et al. 1996, Emenaker and Basson 1998, Basson et al. 1998, Thompson et al. 1998, Archer et al. 1998, Vaziri et al. 1998, Giuliano et al. 1999, Basson et al. 2000, Barshishat et al. 2000, Menssen et al. 2000, Emenaker and Basson 2001, Emenaker et al. 2001.

flicting data reports before a conclusion can be rendered. A few of these discrepancies are briefly discussed below, as not all readers may be familiar with the arguments presented by both sides of the scientific community. First, differential responses to luminal nutrients such as short-chain fatty acids, in particular the oxidation of butyrate, occur between normal healthy colonocytes and those cells undergoing neoplastic transformation to cancer cells. Neoplastic transformation of colonocytes favors anaerobic metabolism of butyrate thereby reducing the ability of the neoplastic colonocytes to oxidize butyrate (Velazquez et al. 1997). This may be further compounded by segmental response differences to carcinogens that might require differing dietary factors with chemoprotective activity (Greenwald et al. 1987). This could account for some of the conflicting data reported in the scientific literature. Second, differential short-chain fatty acid responses may differ across species (e.g., human and rodents). Previous studies have shown that rodent models may not be appropriate for evaluating human carcinogenesis or for evaluating therapeutic strategies (Balmain and Harris 2000, Hann and Balmain 2001). Although animal models provide the opportunity to evaluate carcinogenesis in vivo, these models are not human models and should not be confused as such. On the other hand, cell culture models, although they represent human cells, are cultured in a highly defined artificial environment that does not mimic in vivo human physiology. Hence, neither animal nor cell culture models represents a full and accurate overall picture of human carcinogenesis. This is not to say that animal models and cell culture models do not provide useful insight into the carcinogenic process, but that all scientific evidence must be heavily scrutinized realizing the benefits and limitations of each model system utilized. Keeping these limitations in mind, let us review some of the current data on in vitro human cell culture models.

The effects of short-chain fatty acids on various parameters of cell differentiation and carcinogenesis have previously been evaluated using a variety of in vitro human colon cancer models. Several groups, including our own, have shown that physiological levels of short-chain fatty acids exert differential potency effects on colon cell differentiation, cell apoptosis, cell motility, cell invasion, protease and protease inhibitor production and gene expression. Butyrate directly increases the level of primary human colonocytes intestinal alkaline phosphatase (Emenaker and Basson 2001), a brush border marker of enzymatic activity, as well as induces the expression of MUC3, a gene involved in cellular differentiation (Velcich et al. 1995). Although most studies support the genetic and biologic effects of butyrate on colon cancer cells, contrasting results were reported between in vitro human colon cancer cell line studies and those conducted in vivo using rodent animal models. In vitro, butyrate is a pro-apoptotic agent stimulating cell apoptosis and cell differentiation in established human colon cancer cell lines (Basson et al. 1998; Hinnebusch et al. 2002). Short-chain fatty acids such as butyrate were later identified as potent mediators of histone acetylation (Hinnebusch et al. 2002). Yet, in vivo rodent studies suggest otherwise. Singh et al. (1997) suggest these conflicting reports are dependent upon the presence of alternative energy sources (e.g., glucose and pyruvate) and low concentrations of butyrate (0.5M and 2M). An alternative hypothesis might suggest that animal models might not accurately reflect human pathophysiology due to biological and genetic species differences between rodents and humans.

The effects of butyrate on cellular motility have revealed important differences between different short-chain fatty acids. In particular, butyrate treatment significantly decreased cell proliferation, cell adhesion, and cell motility relative to acetate and propionate treatments in metastatic human colon cancer cells (Basson et al. 1996, Basson et al. 1998). We previously reported that butyrate substantially inhibits colon cancer cell invasion in established invasive human colon cancer cells (Emenaker and Basson 1998) as well as in primary malignant invasive human colonocytes (Emenaker et al. 2001). Although butyrate, a by-product of colonic fiber fermentation, down-regulates serine and threonine kinase activities, the effects of butyrate on other degradative enzymes were relatively unknown. We found that short-chain fatty acids mediate both proteolytic and antiproteolytic enzymes during cell invasion. Butyrate is a highly potent inhibitor of cell invasion not because it inhibits the production of matrix metalloproteases, but because butyrate inhibits the secretion of uPA, a proteolytic enzyme, while also stimulating the secretion of TIMP-1 and TIMP-2, which protects the basement membrane against proteolysis. We found that a physiologic 10 mM level of butyrate was a potent inhibitor of cell invasion in both established human colon cancer cells (Emenaker and Basson 1998) and invasive primary malignant human colonocytes (Emenaker et al. 2001). In additional immunofluorescence confocal microscopy studies, we also found that short-chain fatty acids differentially mediated mutant p53, Bcl-2, Bax, p21, and PCNA protein expression levels in invasive primary malignant human colonocytes. These gene-nutrient interactions might contribute to the protection of the basement membrane against invasive cancer cells, and also to mediating apoptosis, proliferation, and tumor suppression by differing mechanisms of action.

Epidemiological and Dietary Intervention Studies

The vast majority of human colon cancer cases are sporadic in nature, suggesting a strong susceptibility to environmental factors such as diet. Internationally, migrant data show a 20-fold difference in colon cancer incidence rates. These data show immigrants typically acquire the colon cancer incidence risk rates of their host nation within two or three generations or as early as within the immigrating generation (Potter 1996). The chemoprotective use of dietary fiber and its metabolic by-products has been extensively studied, however, scientific consensus has not been reached (Ghadirian et al. 1997, Honda et al. 1999, Fuchs et al. 1999, Alberts et al. 2000).

The importance of lifelong dietary habits in reducing the risk of cancer was evaluated by Tsuji et al. (1996) and Alberts et al. Looking at trend data, Tsuji et al. reported that a decrease in total dietary fiber consumption in the Japanese population coupled with an increase in fat consumption has resulted in acceleration in colorectal cancer mortalities. They reported that a decline in total dietary fiber from 27 grams to 18 grams from 1947 to 1960 has resulted in an increase in colorectal cancer mortalities with a 23–24 year lag. However, short-term dietary intervention clinical trials (Alberts et al. 2000) showed that the addition of high levels (13.5 grams) of wheat bran for 34 months did not prevent the recurrence of additional colorectal adenomas in subjects with a history of these lesions. High dietary fiber consumptions over an extended time period may be protective since genetic mutations favoring colorectal carcinogenesis occur over time, but may not prevent genetic mutations in mucosa exhibiting field defects (Alberts et al. 2000).

The most compelling evidence supporting the association of high dietary fiber consumption and the reduction of colon cancer incidence comes from the EPIC (European Prospective Investigation into Cancer and Nutrition) multicenter prospective study, which began collecting dietary intake data and blood samples from 1993 to 1998. EPIC researchers gathered dietary intake data from 484,042 participants from nine European countries while intake data and blood specimens were collected from 387,256 subjects (Riboli 2000). Riboli (2001) reported a 50% decrease in colon cancer incidence when subjects consumed 30 grams or more of dietary fiber per day. The EPIC data confirm previous epidemiological evidence suggesting high consumption of dietary fiber decreases the risk of colorectal carcinogenesis (Giacosa et al. 1993, Meyer and White 1993) and the development of invasive colorectal cancer in humans (Giacosa et al. 1993). However, many epidemiological studies suggest that dietary fiber alone is not sufficient to reduce the incidence of colon cancer, but instead suggest that dietary fiber may act in concert with other nutrients to reduce the risk of colon cancer. The Nurses Health Study shows that colorectal cancer incidence is lowest in women consuming diets high in calcium, vitamin D, phosphorus, and dietary fiber and low in alcohol and animal fat (Martinez et al. 1996).

Establishing cause and effect associations between dietary fiber consumption patterns and the colorectal cancer incidence is difficult to prove as most studies differ in design, dietary intake evaluation methodologies, and intervention strategies. Many of these studies have associated a reduction in colon cancer risk with an increased consumption of high-fiber foods such as vegetables and whole grains (Potter 1996). These conflicting differences in outcomes suggest that overall macronutrient and micronutrient dietary compositions, food habits, and food patterns may also play an important role in chemoprevention in addition to the role type and source of dietary fibers consumed. It is unlikely that a single nutrient is the "magic bullet," however, most epidemiological studies suggest an overall dietary pattern contributes to colon cancer risk.

CURRENT DIETARY FIBER CONSUMPTION GUIDELINES

Current Recommendations

Studies by Tsuji et al. (1996) suggest that the long-term overall quality of the diet may play an important role in colon cancer prevention. Howe et al. suggest a 13-grams-per-day increase in dietary fiber consumption could reduce the risk of colorectal cancer by 31% overall in the American population (Howe et al. 1992). Americans typically consume suboptimal daily levels (14–15 grams) of dietary fiber relative to the dietary fiber public health recommendations by the American Cancer Society (Byers et al. 2002), the American Dietetic Association (American Dietetic Association 1997), the American Gastroenterological Association (Kim 2000), and the National Cancer Institute (NCI 2002). At present, the dietary fiber recommendations for Americans on average range from 20 to 35 grams of dietary fiber per day. A summary of dietary fiber consumption recommendations proposed by several public health oriented organizations appears in Table 9.4.

Table 9.4.   Guidelines for Dietary Fiber Consumption

American Cancer Society[1]

Recommendations for adults include the consumption of a variety of plant based foods to provide a wide variety of nutrient in addition to dietary fiber.
- Eat a variety of healthful foods, with an emphasis on plant sources. Eat 5 or more servings of a variety of vegetables and fruits each day.
- Choose whole grains in preference to processed (refined) grains and sugars. Whole grains are an important source of many vitamins and minerals that have been associated with lower risk of colon cancer, such as folate, vitamin E, and selenium. Whole grains are higher in fiber, certain vitamins, and minerals than processed (refined) flour products. Although the association between fiber and cancer risk is inconclusive, consumption of high-fiber foods is still recommended. Since the benefits grain foods impart may derive from their other nutrients as well as from fiber, it is best to obtain fiber from whole grains—and vegetables and fruits—rather than from fiber supplements.
- Beans are excellent sources of many vitamins and minerals, protein, and fiber. Beans are legumes, the technical term for the family of plants that includes dried beans, pinto beans, lentils, and soybeans, among many others. Beans are especially rich in nutrients that may protect against cancer and can be a useful low-fat, high-protein, alternative to meat.

American Dietetic Association[2]

Recommendations for adults range between 20 and 35 grams/day or 10–13 grams dietary fiber per 1000 kcal. Recommendations for children over the age of 2 years is to increase dietary fiber intake to an amount equal to or greater than their age plus 5 grams/day to achieve intakes of 25–35 grams/day after the age of 20 years.
- Consumption of a dietary pattern consistent with the Food Guide Pyramid.
- High fiber pediatric diets may not be sufficient to meet the caloric requirements of normal growth patterns.
- Consumption of 1–2 servings of high-fiber foods (legumes, whole grains, cereals, etc.) daily may be required to obtain an adequate intake in some patient populations (elderly, hospitalized, or long-term care).
- Use of concentrated dietary fiber sources to treat chronic constipation when adequate dietary intakes of dietary fiber consumption are not achieved.
- Incorporation of new sources of dietary fiber for diet therapy when health benefit claims are thoroughly documented and overall diet is consistent with disease-appropriate treatment plans for medical nutrition therapy.

American Gastroenterological Association[3]

Recommendations for adults range between 30 and 35 grams/day.
- Consumption of dietary fiber from all food sources including fruits, vegetables, cereals, grains, and legumes.
- Consumption of 5–7 servings of fruits and vegetables daily.
- Consumption of generous portions of whole grain cereals as recommended by the World Health Organization and the National Cancer Institute.

Table 9.4. (*Continued*)

National Cancer Institute[4]

Recommendations for adults range between 20 and 30 grams/day with an upper limit of 35 grams/day.
• Consumption of 5–9 servings of fruits and vegetables daily including at least one serving of a vitamin A-rich fruit or vegetable a day, at least one serving of a vitamin C-rich fruit or vegetable a day, and at least one serving of a high-fiber fruit or vegetable a day.

USDA Food and Nutrition Information Center[5]

Advice for today: Eat more vegetables, including dry beans and peas; fruits; and breads, cereals, pasta, and rice. Increase your fiber intake by eating more of a variety of foods that contain fiber naturally. Recommendations for adults are as follows:
• Consumption of three servings of vegetables daily (Count as a serving: 1 cup of raw leafy greens, 1/2 cup of other kinds).
• Consumption of two servings of fruit daily (Count as a serving: 1 medium apple, orange, or banana; 1/2 cup of small or diced fruit; 3/4 cup of juice).
• Consumption of six servings of grain products daily (Count as a serving: 1 slice of bread; 1/2 bun, bagel, or English muffin; 1 ounce of dry ready-to-eat cereal; 1/2 cup of cooked cereal, rice, or pasta).

[1] American Cancer Society Guidelines on Nutrition and Physical Activity for Cancer Prevention. 2002. CA Cancer Journal Clinics 52:92–119.
[2] American Dietetic Association. 1997. Health implications of dietary fiber. Position of the American Dietetic Association: Journal of the American Dietetic Association 97:1157–1159.
[3] AGA Technical Review: Impact of Dietary Fiber on Colon Cancer Occurrence. 2000. Gastroenterology 118:1235–1257.
[4] National Cancer Institute Dietary Guidelines website. Accessed May 6, 2002, at http://www. pueblo.gsa.gov/cic_text/food/guideeat/guidelns.html; http://www.pueblo.gsa.gov/cic_text/food/eating5-aday/eat5aday. txt.
[5] USDA website. Accessed March 31, 2002, at http://www.nal.usda.gov/fnic/dga/grains.htm#breads.

Dietary Fiber Sources

Public health recommendations call for adults to consume 20–35 grams of dietary fiber per day from a wide variety of food sources. Common food sources of dietary fiber can be found in Table 9.5. Caution should be taken when increasing daily dietary fiber intake. Helpful suggestions include the gradual increase of dietary fiber over time and an increase in water consumption to reduce the risk of developing flatulence, bloating, cramping, and intestinal blockages that may occur. It is recommended that dietary fiber be consumed in the context of food products (e.g., popcorn, beans, whole grain products, etc.) rather than as supplements, as supplements lack the additional macronutrients, micronutrients, and biologically active compounds that are also found in whole foods.

SUMMARY

Dietary fiber, its metabolic by-products, and associated biologically active compounds may contribute to the reduction of colon cancer incidence rates by mediating biological and genetic factors influencing carcinogenesis. Butyrate, one such by-product of microbial dietary fiber fermentation, appears to influence a wide variety of biological (e.g., cell

Table 9.5. Common Food Sources of Dietary Fiber

Food source	Serving size	Fiber (grams/serving)
Cereals—ready to eat		
All Bran, Kellogg's	1/2 cup	9.69
Raisin Bran, Kellogg's	1/2 cup	8.17
Cheerios, General Mills	1 cup	2.64
Bagels, cinnamon-raisin	4" bagel (89g)	2.05
Fruits—fresh or frozen		
Raspberries, raw	1 cup	8.36
Blackberries, raw	1 cup	7.63
Oranges, raw	1 cup	4.32
Pears, raw	1 piece (166 g)	3.98
Strawberries, raw	1 cup	3.82
Apples, raw, with skin	1 piece (138 g)	3.73
Cherries, raw, without pits	1 cup	3.33
Bananas, raw	1 cup	3.30
Fruits—dried		
Prunes, dried	1 cup	16.37
Raisins, seedless	1 cup	5.80
Figs, dried	2 pieces	4.64
Apricots, dried	10 halves	3.15
Dates, dried	5 pieces	3.11
Grains		
Rice, brown, long-grained, cooked	1 cup	3.51
Rice, wild, cooked	1 cup	2.95
Rice, white, long-grained, cooked	1 cup	2.41
Legumes		
Kidney beans, red, canned	1 cup	16.38
Black beans, cooked, boiled	1 cup	14.96
Pinto beans, cooked, boiled	1 cup	14.71
Refried beans, canned	1 cup	13.36
Baked beans, canned	1 cup	13.16
Lima beans, cooked, drained	1 cup	13.16
Lentils, cooked, boiled	1 cup	15.64
Nuts		
Coconut, dried, shredded	1 cup	4.19
Almonds	24 pieces	3.35
Peanuts, oil-roasted, with salt	1 oz.	2.61
Walnuts, English	1 oz.	1.90
Brazil nuts, dried	1 oz.	1.53
Vegetables—fresh or frozen		
Green peas, frozen	1 cup	6.97
Brussels sprouts, frozen	1 cup	6.36
Spinach, frozen, cooked, drained	1 cup	5.70
Broccoli, frozen, cooked, drained	1 cup	5.52
Carrots, cooked, drained	1 cup	5.14
Baked potato, with crisp skin	1 piece (202 g)	4.85
Yellow corn, sweet, canned, drained	1 cup	4.20

Table 9.5. (*continued*)

Food source	Serving size	Fiber (grams/serving)
Green snap beans	1 cup	4.05
Beets, canned, drained	1 cup	2.89
Mustard greens, cooked, drained	1 cup	2.80
Kale, cooked, drained	1 cup	2.60

Source: Adapted from the USDA Nutrient Database for Standard Reference, Release 14.

differentiation, cell motility, protease production, and protease inhibitor production) and genetic factors (e.g., tyrosine kinase, transcription factors, tumor suppressor genes, GTP binding proteins, cell death regulators, and cell cycle regulators). Yet, does an increase in dietary fiber consumption alone reduce the risk of colon cancer? Current research is often conflicting and contradictory. For example, since not all dietary fibers yield the same proportions of short-chain fatty acids, thereby affecting luminal butyrate concentrations, and that dietary intake determinations may not accurately reflect a populations' fiber consumption, it is not possible to determine if dietary fiber consumption is protective against colon cancer.

The bulk of in vitro established human cell culture and primary metastatic human cell culture studies support the protect effects of dietary fiber against the development of non-invasive and invasive colon cancers. However, cell culture data is not epidemiological data. While some epidemiological studies agree with these findings, others do not. At present, the EPIC study, which is at present the world's largest prospective epidemiological study, shows that dietary fiber is associated with a protective effect at levels of consumption recommended by the American Gastroenterological Association and other health agencies. Differences across study populations and their sources of dietary fiber may be responsible for conflicting reports since the proportion of short-chain fatty acids produced from the colonic microbial fermentation of the dietary fibers varies with the source consumed. When butyrate supplies are insufficient to meet colonic epithelial energy requirements, normal epithelia may be more prone to malignant transformation since in addition to supplying energy, butyrate also appears to modulate various anticarcinogenic pathways in the colon.

Although most epidemiological data do not support the hypothesis that a single nutrient is responsible for reducing the incidence rates of colon cancer, the data do suggest that several components in the human diet may act synergistically to influence the risk of developing colon cancer. The protective value of high-fiber diets may rest with other compounds such as antioxidants, micronutrients, and phytonutrients with anticarcinogenic properties coconsumed in the diet.

ACKNOWLEDGMENTS

My appreciation goes to Norman Hord, PhD, MPH, RD, for his thoughtful comments during the preparation of this manuscript.

REFERENCES

Alberts, D. S., Martinez, M. E., Roe, D. J., Guillen-Rodriguez, J. M., Marshall, J. R., van Leeuwen, J. B., Reid, M. E., Ritenbaugh, C., Vargas, P. A., Bhattacharyya, A. B., Earnest, D. L., Sampliner, and R. E. 2000. Lack of effect of a high-fiber cereal supplement on the recurrence of colorectal adenomas. Phoenix Colon Cancer Prevention Physicians' Network. New England Journal of Medicine 342(16):1156–1162.

American Dietetic Association. 1997. Health implications of dietary fiber. Position of the American Dietetic Association: Journal of the American Dietetic Association 97:1157–1159.

Archer, S., Meng, S., Wu, J., Johnson, J., Tang, R., and Hodin, R. 1998. Butyrate inhibits colon carcinoma cell growth through two distinct pathways. Surgery 124(2):248–253.

Balmain, A., and Harris, C. C. 2000. Carcinogenesis in mouse and human cells: parallels and paradoxes. Carcinogenesis 21(3):371–377.

Barshishat, M., Polak-Charcon, S., and Schwartz, B. 2000. Butyrate regulates E-cadherin transcription, isoform expression and intracellular position in colon cancer cells. British Journal of Cancer 82(1):195–203.

Basson, M. D., Emenaker, N. J., and F. Hong. Differential modulation of human (Caco-2) colon cancer cell line phenotype by short-chain fatty acids. 1998. Proceedings for the Society for Experimental Biology and Medicine 217(4):476–483.

Basson, M. D., Liu, Y.-W., Hanley, A. M., Emenaker, N. J., Shenoy, S. G., and Gould Rothberg, B. E. 2000. Identification and comparative analysis of human colonocyte short-chain fatty acid response genes. Journal of GI Surgery 4(5):501–512.

Basson, M. D., Rashid, Z., Turowski, G. A., West, A. B., Emenaker, N. J., Sgambati, S. A., Hong, F., Perdikis, D. M., Datta, S., and Madri, J. A. 1996. Restitution at the cellular level: regulation of the migrating phenotype. Yale Journal of Biology and Medicine 69(2):119–129.

Burkitt, D. P. 1970. Relationship as a clue to causation. Lancet 12;2(7685):1237–1240.

Burkitt, D. P. 1971. Epidemiology of cancer of the colon and rectum. Cancer 1:3–13.

Burkitt, D. P. 1973. Some characteristics of modern Western civilization. British Medical Journal I:274–278.

Byers, T., Nestle, M., McTiernan, A., Doyle, C., Currie-Williams, A., Gansler, T., Thun, M., and the American Cancer Society 2001 Nutrition and Physical Activity Guidelines Advisory Committee. 2002. American Cancer Society Guidelines on Nutrition and Physical Activity for Cancer Prevention (2002). Reducing the Risk of Cancer with Healthy Food Choices and Physical Activity. CA Cancer Journal Clinics 52:92–119.

Cousins, R. J. Nutritional regulation of gene expression. 1999. American Journal of Medicine 106 (1A):20S–23S.

Cross, H. S., Hulla, W., Tong, W.-M., and Peterlik, M. 1995.Growth regulation of human colon adenocarcinomas-derived cells by calcium, vitamin D and epidermal growth factor. Journal of Nutrition 125:2004S–2008S.

Cummings, J. 1994. Quantitating short-chain fatty acid production in humans. In *Short chain fatty acids*, edited by J. Cummings, H. J. Binder and K. Soergel, pp. 11–19. Boston: Kluwer Academic Publisher.

Doll, R., and Peto, R. 1981. The causes of cancer: quantitative estimates of avoidable risks of cancer in the United States today. Journal of the National Cancer Institute 66(6):1191–1308.

Edelstein, P. S., Thompson, S. M., and Davies, R. J. 1991. Altered intracellular calcium regulation in human colorectal cancers and in "normal" adjacent mucosa. Cancer Research 51(16):4492–4494,.

Edwards, B. K., Howe, H. L., Ries, L. A. G., Thun, M. J., Rosenberg, H. M., Yancik, R., Wingo, P.

A., Jemal, A., and Feigal, E. G. 2002. Annual Report to the Nation on the status of cancer, 1973–1999, featuring implications of age and aging on U.S. cancer burden. Cancer 94(10):2766–2792.

Ehle, F. R., Robertson, J. B., and Van Soest, P. J. 1982. Influence of dietary fibers on fermentation in the human large intestine. Journal of Nutrition 1982 Jan;112(1):158–66.

Emenaker, N. J., and Basson, M. D. 1998. Short chain fatty acids inhibit human (SW1116) colon cancer cell invasion by reducing urokinase plasminogen activator activity and stimulating TIMP-1 and TIMP-2 activities, rather than via MMP modulation. Journal of Surgical Research 76(1):41–46.

Emenaker, N. J., and Basson, M. D. 2001. Short chain fatty acids differentially regulate non-malignant and malignant human colonocyte phenotypes. Digestive Diseases and Sciences 46(1):96–105, 2001.

Emenaker, N. J., Calaf, G. M., Cox, D., Basson, M. D., and Qureshi, N. 2001. Short chain fatty acids inhibit primary human colon cancer by modulating uPA, TIMP-1, TIMP-2, mutant p53, Bcl-2, Bax, p21 and PCNA protein expression in an in vitro cell culture model. Journal of Nutrition 131(11S):3041S–3046S.

Fearon, E. R., and Vogelstein, B. 1990. A genetic model for colorectal tumorigenesis. Cell 61(5):759–767.

Food and Nutrition Board, Institute of Medicine, National Academy of Sciences. 2001. *Dietary reference intakes proposed definition of dietary fiber*. National Academy Press.

Fuchs, C. S., Giovannucci, E. L., Colditz, G. A., Hunter, D. J., Stampfer, M. J., Rosner, B., Speizer, F. E., and Willett, W. C. 1999. Dietary fiber and the risk of colorectal cancer and adenoma in women. New England Journal of Medicine 340(3):169–176.

Ghadirian, P., Lacroix, A., Maisonneuve, P., Perret, C., Potvin, C., Gravel, D., Bernard, D., and Boyle, P. 1997. Nutritional factors and colon carcinoma: a case-control study involving French Canadians in Montreal, Quebec, Canada. Cancer 80(5):858–864.

Giacosa, A., Filiberti, R., Visconti, P., Hill, M. J., Berrino, F., and D'Amicis, A. 1993. Dietary fibres and cancer. Advances in Experimental Medicine and Biology 348:85–97.

Giuliano, M., Lauricella, M., Calvaruso, G., Carabillo, M., Emanuele, S., Vento, R., and Tesoriere, G. 1999. The apoptotic effects and synergistic interaction of sodium butyrate and MG132 in human retinoblastoma Y79 cells. Cancer Research 59(21):5586–5595.

Greenwald, P., Lanza, E., and Eddy, G. A. 1987. Dietary fiber in the reduction of colon cancer risk. Journal of the American Dietetic Association 87(9):1178–1188.

Hann, B., and Balmain, A. 2001. Building "validated" mouse models of human cancer. Current Opinions in Cell Biology. 13(6):778–784.

Hesketh, J. E., Vasconcelos, M. H., and Bermano, B. 1998. Regulatory signals in messenger RNA: determinants of nutrient-gene interaction and metabolic compartmentation. British Journal of Nutrition 80:307–321.

Hill, M. J. 2001. Diet-induced Changes in the Colonic Environment and Colorectal Cancer Prevention Workshop. National Cancer Institute. Assessed July 29,2002 at http://www3.cancer.gov/prevention/nutrition/colonic.pdf.

Hinnebusch, B. F., Meng, S., Wu, J. T., Archer, S. Y., and Hodin, R. A. 2002. The effects of short-chain Fatty acids on human colon cancer cell phenotype are associated with histone hyperacetylation. Journal of Nutrition 132(5):1012–1017.

Honda, T., Kai, I., and Ohi, G. 1999. Fat and dietary fiber intake and colon cancer mortality: a chronological comparison between Japan and the United States. Nutrition and Cancer 33(1):95–9

Howe, G. R., Benito, E., Castelleto, R., Cornee, J., Esteve, J., Gallagher, R. P., Iscovich, J. M., Deng-
    ao, J., and Kaaks-Kune, G. A. 1992. Dietary intake of fiber and decreased risk of cancers of the
    colon and rectum: evidence from the combined analysis of 13 case-control studies. Journal of the
    National Cancer Institute 84:1887–1896.
Kapadia, S. A., Raimundo, A. H., Grimble, G. K., Aimer, P., and Silk, D. B. 1995. Influence of three
    different fiber-supplemented enteral diets on bowel function and short-chain fatty acid produc-
    tion. Journal of Parenteral and Enteral Nutrition 19(1):63–68.
Kim, Y. I. 2000. AGA technical review: impact of dietary fiber on colon cancer occurrence.
    Gastroenterology. 118(6):1235–1257.
Kinzler, K. W., and Vogelstein, B. 1998. Landscaping the cancer terrain. Science
    80(5366):1036–1037.
Lengauer, C., Kinzler, K. W., and Vogelstein, B. 1998. Genetic instabilities in human cancers.
    Nature 396(6712):643–649.
Macfarlene, G. T., and Gibson, G. R. 1995. Microbiological aspects of the production of short-chain
    fatty acids in the large bowel. In *Physiological and Clinical Aspects of Short-Chain Fatty Acids*,
    edited by Cummings, J. H., Rombeau, J. L., and T. Sakata, pp. 87–105. New York: Cambridge
    University Press.
Martinez, M. E., Giovannucci, E. L., Colditz, G. A., Stampfer, M. J., Hunter, D. J., Speizer, F. E.,
    Wing, A., and Willett, W. C. 1996. Calcium, vitamin D, and the occurrence of colorectal cancer
    among women. Journal of the National Cancer Institute 88(19):1375–1382.
Menssen, H. D., Bertelmann, E., Bartelt, S., Schmidt, R. A., Pecher, G., Schramm, K., and Thiel, E.
    2000. Wilms' tumor gene (WT1) expression in lung cancer, colon cancer and glioblastoma cell
    lines compared to freshly isolated tumor specimens. Journal of Cancer Research Clinical
    Oncology 126(4):226–232.
Meyer, F., and White, E. 1993. Alcohol and nutrients in relation to colon cancer in middle-aged
    adults. American Journal of Epidemiology 138:225–236.
Mortensen, P. B., Clausen, M. R., Bonnen, H., Hove, H., and Holtug, K. 1992. Colonic fermenta-
    tion of ispaghula, wheat bran, glucose, and albumin to short-chain fatty acids and ammonia eval-
    uated in vitro in 50 subjects. Journal of Parenteral and Enteral Nutrition 16(5):433–439.
National Cancer Institute. 2002. Genetics of Colorectal Cancer PDQ. Assessed April 8, 2002 at
    http://www.nci.nih.gov/cancer_information/doc_pdq.aspx?viewid=A4DD5637-EDE7-47C1-
    8F75-049D2E6BD550.
National Institutes of Health. 1999. National Cancer Institute. Tumor Gene Index. Assessed June 4,
    2002 at http://www.nih.gov/news/pr/aug99/nci-10a.htm.
Ochiai, M., Ubagai, T., Kawamori, T., Imai, H., Sugimura, T., and Nakagama, H. 2001. High sus-
    ceptibility of Scid mice to colon carcinogenesis induced by azoxymethane indicates a possible
    caretaker role for DNA-dependent protein kinase. Carcinogenesis 22(9):1551–1555.
Podsypanina, K., Ellenson, L. H., Nemes, A., Gu, J., Tamura, M., Yamada, K. M., Cordon-Cardo,
    C., Catoretti, G., Fisher, P. E., and Parsons, R. 1999. Mutation of Pten/Mmac1 in mice causes
    neoplasia in multiple organ systems. Proceedings of the National Academy of Sciences USA
    16;96(4):1563–1568.
Potter, J. D. 1996. Nutrition and colorectal cancer. Cancer Causes and Control 7:127–146.
Riboli, E. 2000. The European prospective investigation into cancer and nutrition: perspectives for
    cancer prevention. Nestle Nutrition Workshop Series Clinical & Performance Program
    4:117–130.
Riboli, E. 2001. Fruit and vegetable consumption and cancer prevention: New epidemiological evi-
    dence. American Institute for Cancer Research, 11th Annual Summer Research Conference on
    Diet, Nutrition and Cancer, Washington, DC.

Ries, L. A. G., Eisner, M. P., Kosary, C. L., Hankey, B. F., Miller, B. A., Clegg, L., and Edwards, B. K. (eds). *SEER Cancer Statistics Review, 1973–1999*, National Cancer Institute. Bethesda, MD, http://seer.cancer.gov/csr/1973_1999/, 2002.

Roediger, W. E. W. 1994. Imprint of Disease on short-chain fatty acids metabolism by colonocytes. In *Short chain fatty acids*, edited by J. Cummings, H. J. Binder, and K. Soergel, pp. 195–205. Boston: Kluwer Academic Publisher.

Shike, M. 1999. Diet and lifestyle in the prevention of colorectal cancer: An overview. American Journal of Medicine 106 (1A):11S–15S.

Singh, B., Halestrap, A. P., and Paraskeva, C.1997. Butyrate can act as a stimulator of growth or inducer of apoptosis in human colonic epithelial cell lines depending on the presence of alternative energy sources. Carcinogenesis 18(6):1265–1270.

Thompson, M. A., Rosenthal, M. A., Ellis, S. L., Friend, A. J., Zorbas, M. I., Whitehead, R. H., and Ramsay, R. G. 1998. c-Myb down-regulation is associated with human colon cell differentiation, apoptosis, and decreased Bcl-2 expression. Cancer Research 58(22):5168–5175.

Topping, D. L., and Clifton, P. M. 2001. Short chain fatty acids and human colonic function: roles of resistant starch and nonstarch polysaccharides. Physiology Reviews 81(3):1031–1064.

Tsuji, K., Harashima, E., Nakagawa, Y., Urata, G., and Shirataka, M. 1996. Time-lag effect of dietary fiber and fat intake ratio on Japanese colon cancer mortality. Biomedical and Environmental Sciences 9:223–228.

U.S. Department of Agricultural Research Service. 2001. USDA Database for Standard Reference, Release 14. Nutrient Data Laboratory Home Page, http://www.nal.usda.gov/fnic/food comp.

Vaziri, C., Stice, L., and Faller, D. V. 1998. Butyrate-induced G1 arrest results from p21-independent disruption of retinoblastoma protein-mediated signals. Cellular Growth and Differentiation 9(6):465–474.

Velazquez, O. C., Lederer, H. M., and Rombeau, J. L. 1996. Butyrate and the colonocyte: Implications for neoplasia. Digestive Diseases and Sciences 41(4):727–739.

Velazquez, O. C., Lederer, H. M., and Rombeau, J. L. 1997. Butyrate and the colonocytes. In *Dietary Fiber in Health and Disease*, edited by David Kritchevsky and Charles Bonfield, pp. 123–134. New York: Plenum Press.

Velcich, A., Palumbo, L., Jarry, A., Laboisse, C., Racevskis, J., and Augenlicht, L. 1995. Patterns of expression of lineage-specific markers during the in vitro-induced differentiation of HT29 colon carcinoma cells. Cellular Growth and Differentiation 6(6):749–757.

Vogelstein, B., and Kinzler, K. W. 1993. The multistep nature of cancer. Trends in Genetics 9(4):138–141.

Walker, A. R., and Burkitt, D. P. 1976. Colonic cancer-hypotheses of causation, dietary prophylaxis, and future research. American Journal of Digestive Diseases 21(10):910–917.

Weaver, G. A., Krause, J. A., Miller, T. L., and Wolin, M. J. 1992. Cornstarch fermentation by the colonic microbial community yields more butyrate than does cabbage fiber fermentation; cornstarch fermentation rates correlate negatively with methanogenesis. American Journal of Clinical Nutrition 55(1):70–77.

Willett, W. C. 1995. Diet, nutrition, and avoidable cancer. Environmental Health Perspectives 103 (Suppl 8):165–170.

10

Soy Food and Breast Cancer

Debra Hickman

Why do Asian women get breast cancer at one-fifth the rate American women do?[1] This is a four- to sixfold lower risk of developing breast cancer. The incidence of breast cancer in Asian women approaches that of American women only after they have had several generations of residence in the United States.

Lower breast cancer risk in Asian countries is due to the environment or the diet, not the genetics. Since soy use is much greater in Asian food than in American food, what the Americans *don't* eat rather than what they do eat is affecting breast cancer rates.[2,3] The anticarcinogenic effect of soybeans is attributed to phytosterols, phytates, saponins, protease inhibitors, and isoflavones. Soy contains protein, carbohydrates, and fat as well as vitamins, calcium, folic acid, iron, and other minerals. Natural vitamin E from the soybean has been the focus of several studies looking at heart disease, cancer, Alzheimer's, diabetes, and aging.[4]

Specific isoflavones found in soybeans, plant estrogens, are unique to soy foods. Genistein and daidzein are present in high amounts in soybeans. These compounds influence sex-hormone metabolism, intracellular enzymes, protein synthesis, growth-factor action, malignant cell proliferation, and angiogenesis, making them a likely suspect in anticarcinogenic activity.[5]

High blood levels of estrogen are an established risk factor for breast cancer, whereas lower estrogen levels appear to be anticarcinogenic. Isoflavones (particularly genistein) bind to estrogen receptors and produce a weak estrogenic effect ranging between 1/1000 and 1/1,000,000 of the activity of estradiol, natural human estrogen.[5]

Genistein blocks the much more potent effect of endogenous estrogens, a factor in hormone-dependent breast cancers. High blood levels of estrogen are an established risk factor for breast cancer, whereas weak estrogen has been found to be anticarcinogenic. Genistein administered to rats during the neonatal period protects against DMBA-induced mammary tumors. In mammary gland differentiation, studies found that the mammary gland size of the mice at 21 days was significantly larger by 50 days. The gland size was not significantly different from the vehicle-treated animals. By day 50, the ratio of terminal end buds to lobules was smaller than the vehicle-treated animals and smaller than at day 21. Since terminal end buds are thought to be more susceptible and lobules less susceptible to carcinogens, then the low ratio of end buds to lobules would suggest a reduced cancer risk. Female rats treated with genistein developed almost 50% fewer tumors than control animals. Genistein's advantage over other estrogens is its low toxicity potential.

Another prevention factor associated with genistein has been its role in inhibiting unregulated angiogenesis and/or proliferation of tumor cells. Genistein was found to inhibit endothelial-cell proliferation in in vitro angiogenesis and also to inhibit the proliferation of various tumor cells. The imbalance between angiogenesis and the inhibitors needs to be understood and regulated.[6] New tumor blood vessels provide a pathway to the distant places in the body, making metastasis likely. Dietary soy compound inhibits angiogenesis, explaining to some extent the long-known preventive effect of plant-based diets on tumorigenesis. One explanation for the genistein activity points toward the molecular events affected by it. Genistein specifically inhibits the activity of the enzyme tyrosine protein kinase (TPK), which is responsible for controlling cell growth and regulation.[7] Agents that inhibit TPK activity are considered to be potential anticarcinogens. Most notably, it inhibits DNA topisomerase, which is a common target of chemotherapy.[7] To complicate matters, isoflavones are contained in two chemical forms in soy foods: aglycones and glucosides.[8] Aglycone-rich products had a higher absorption rate over the glucoside isoflavone. Therefore, the aglycones might be more useful than the glucoside isoflavone. The aglycones might be more useful than the glucosides in maintaining a high level of isoflavone concentrations in the plasma.

Protease Inhibitors and Cancer Reduction

The isoflavones may not be the only component of soy food that is providing anticarcinogenic effects. The protease inhibitor, Bowman-Birk Inhibitor, showed the greatest suppression of carcinogenesis in animal carcinogenesis assays. Colon carcinogenesis was suppressed by 100%, liver by 71%, oral epithelium by 86%, and lung by 48%. Phytoesterols and saponins are concentrated in soybeans at a high level and are structurally similar to the animal sterol cholesterol. There is little evidence to indicate that the level of saponins in soybeans poses any risk to human health.[9]

Adverse Effects of Soy

While reports on the beneficial effects of soy have been growing, there is also a growing interest in the possible adverse effects. One of the most significant health concerns is that soybean protease inhibitors contributed to pancreatic cancer and its development while suppressing cancer in other organs.[10] Genistein led to a small and erratic decrease in food consumption in rats but at very high doses, 25% of rats died with depression of body and organ weight gain.[11] Human populations with high levels of soy food in their diets show no higher incidence of pancreatic cancer and some even have lower rates of pancreatic cancer.[10] The efficacy of soy for women trying to get pregnant is high since phytoestrogens may decrease their rate of ovulation. Reproductive disorders have been reported in sheep, and male infertility in mice given genistein.[3] There is no evidence that fertility is a problem in Asia.

A recent study on tamoxifen versus genistein sheds more light on the questions surrounding the issue of phytoestrogens interfering with estrogen receptors and cancer prevention.[12] Will genistein cancel out the known beneficial effects of tamoxifen? In tamoxifen-treated rats, there was a 29% reduction in the number of tumors per rat. In genistein-treated rats, there was a 37% reduction. In the combination of tamoxifen plus soy treated rats, there was a 65% reduction.

HUMAN EPIDEMIOLOGY STUDIES: ROLE OF SOY IN CANCER PREVENTION

More than 20 human studies found that the consumption of just one serving of soy per day reduced cancer risk.[2] A recent epidemiology study examined soy food intake during adolescence when breast tissue is most sensitive to environmental stimuli.[13] During this period there is an increase in the ductal cells, cells susceptible to carcinogens. The terminal end buds that branch during adolescence into a treelike system of ducts are suspected to be the carcinogenic factor. The incomplete hollowing of these terminal end buds causes the increase in ductal cells, which ultimately allows for the carcinogenic transformation. Components of soy interfere so that the number of hollow ducts available to the carcinogens is lowered. Women whose consumption of soy foods during adolescence was in the upper fifth had only half the breast cancer risk of those in the lower fifth. Inverse associations with soy food intake and breast cancer exist for both pre- and postmenopausal women.[13] The effect of soy food intake early in life is independent from adult soy food intake. If there is a critical time period for soy intake to do its work, then it could explain why the studies on adult consumption of soy food are not impressive.[14]

A study of tofu and the risk of breast cancer in Asian-Americans was the first study on breast cancer to relate intake of soy foods among the Asian-American population. Tofu is made from cooked pureed soybeans processed into a custardlike cake and is consumed by Asian-Americans at a much higher rate than non-Asians. Although Asian-Americans' rate of breast cancer is lower than U.S. whites', it is considerably higher than rates prevailing in Asia. Tofu intake was more than twice as high among Asian-Americans born in Asia compared to those born in the United States. The results in this study showed statistically significant reduction in breast cancer risk in relation to tofu intake. Tofu intake at least once a week was associated with a significant 15% reduction in risk. The protective effect of high tofu intake was observed in pre- and postmenopausal women.

In two case-controlled breast cancer studies of diet and breast cancer in China, a high soy protein intake did not protect against breast cancer. Researchers found that it was a diet high in pork intake and low in vegetable intake, particularly green vegetables, that puts women at a high risk of breast cancer. Thus, other components of Chinese green vegetables besides soy could be responsible for the protective effect.[1] Women with breast cancer or those with high risk of breast cancer (omnivorous women living in Boston) excreted low amounts of isoflavones. Finnish subjects with medium risk of breast cancer also have low isoflavone excretion, while Japanese subjects at low risk of breast cancer have high isoflavonoid excretions.[5] Soy was also found to increase the menstrual cycle length in women, suggesting that isoflavones affect the hormonal system via the hypothalamus-physeal endocrine system.[5] Shorter menstrual length has been associated with female breast cancer patients and as expected, women in the United States have shorter menstrual cycles than women in Japan.[14]

Seventh-Day-Adventist women and nonvegetarian adolescent girls were examined for their hormone levels. The hormone difference in the two groups seemed to be explained by the wide use of soy products listed in the dietary records at the Adventist school. The more soy intake, the higher levels of hormones of follicular or luteal dehydroepiandrosteronesulfate (DHEA). In a subsequent study of older Adventist women, they found similar trends regarding the association between soy intake and DHS although it was more apparent in younger than older women.[2]

Currently, the National Institutes of Health is sponsoring a long-term follow-up study on soy infant formula. Young adults who consumed soy formula as infants are compared with young adults who consumed milk-based formulas as infants.

No study disputes the fact that breast cancer risk is significantly greater in American women than in Asian women,[15] but is soy food the critical reason for this? Most of the studies in this review reported beneficial effects of eating soy food. Are there adverse effects from eating soy? None of the studies were conclusive. Should a patient taking tamoxifen refrain from eating soy food for fear that it will inhibit the effects of the tamoxifen? On the contrary, soy food and tamoxifen together showed an even greater inverse relationship to breast cancer in animal studies.

How much soy food is needed to exert the anticancer effect? That information is not clear at this time, but recommendations are about a cup of soymilk or one-half cup of tofu a day.

What's the shortcoming of the research at this point? The rat and mice studies are promising but they have not all been replicated in humans. Human studies rely heavily on interviews and recall of dietary habits, leaving a trail of subjectivity.

Could the miracle drug of soybeans be another passing fad? Certainly. But if not soy, what is the critical factor among Asian women that reduces breast cancer rates so dramatically as compared to American women?

ACKNOWLEDGMENT

The author was supported by R25RR15670.

REFERENCES

1. Yuan, J., et al. Diet and breast cancer in Shanghai and Tianjin, China. *Brit. J. Cancer*, 71, 1353, 1995.
2. Ingram D. Case-control study of phyto-oestrogens and breast cancer. *The Lancet,* 350, 990, 1997.
3. Key T. J., et al. Soy food and breast cancer risk: a prospective study in Hiroshima and Nagasaki, Japan. *Brit. J. Cancer,* 81, 1248–1256, 1999.
4. Messina, M., et al. The role of soy products in reducing risk of cancer. *Commentary* 83, 541, 1991.
5. Herman, C., et al. Soybean phytoestrogen intake and cancer risk. *American Institute of Nutrition,* 22, 3166, 1995.

6. Fotsis, T., et al. Genistein, a dietary ingested isoflavonoid, inhibits cell proliferation and in vitro angiogenesis. *American Institute of Nutrition* 002-3166, 1995.

7. Soyfoods and cancer, www.talksoy.com/cancer1.htm.

8. Murrell, W. B., et al. Prepubertal genistein exposure suppresses mammary cancer and enhances gland differentiation in rats. *Carcinogensis*, 17, 1451, 1996.

9. Liener, I. E. Possible adverse effects of soybean anticarcinogens. *J. Nutr.*, 744, 1995.

10. Kennedy, A. R. The evidence for soy bean products as cancer preventive agents. *J. Nutr.*, 125, 733, 1995.

11. Steele, V. E., et al. Cancer chemoprevention agent development strategies for genistein. *J. Nutr.*, 125, 713, 1995.

12. Soy and tamoxifen, www.webmd.com 2001.

13. Shu, X. O., et al. Soyfood intake during adolescence and subsequent risk of breast cancer among Chinese women. *Cancer Epid Biomark & Prevent*, 10, 483, 2001.

14. Ingram, D. Phyto-estrogens and breast cancer. *Lancet*, 350, 971, 1997.

15. Wu, A. H. Tofu and risk of breast cancer in Asian-Americans. *Cancer Epid. Biomark Prevent*, 5, 901, 1996.

11

Preventive and Therapeutic Effects of Dietary Phytochemicals on Cancer Development

Ali Reza Waladkhani and
Michael R. Clemens

ABSTRACT

Phytochemicals and about 30 classes of chemicals with cancer-preventive effects that may have practical implications in reducing cancer incidence in human population have been described. Examples of plant-derived substances that might prevent or postpone the onset of cancer in vitro and in vivo experiments are genistein from soybeans, indole-3-carbinol from cruciferous vegetables such as brussels sprouts and broccoli, resveratrol from grapes, and epigallocatechin gallate from tea. Phytochemicals can inhibit carcinogenesis by induction of phase II enzymes, and inhibiting phase I enzymes, scavenge DNA reactive agents, suppress the abnormal proliferation of early, preneoplastic lesions, and inhibit certain properties of the cancer cell. Treatment of animals with phytochemicals decreases toxicity, mutagenicity, and carcinogenicity of various chemical carcinogens.

INTRODUCTION

Vegetables and fruits contain a wide array of compounds that may inhibit cancer, thus conferring a potential chemoprotective effect.[1] Examples of plant-derived substances that might prevent or postpone the onset of cancer in vitro and in vivo experiments are genistein from soybeans,[2] indole-3-carbinol from cruciferous vegetables such as brussels sprouts and broccoli,[3] resveratrol from grapes,[4] and epigallocatechin gallate from tea.[5]

About 30 classes of chemicals with cancer-preventive effects that may have practical implications in reducing cancer incidence in human population have been described.[6] Food chemists and natural product scientists have identified hundreds of phytochemicals that are being evaluated for the prevention of cancer. These include the presence in plant foods of such potentially anticarcinogenic substances as carotenoids, chlorophyll, flavonoids, indoles, polyphenolic compounds, protease inhibitors, sulfides, and terpens (Table 11.1). Phytochemicals can inhibit carcinogenesis by induction of phase II enzymes, and inhibiting phase I enzymes, scavenge DNA reactive agents, suppress the abnormal proliferation of early, preneoplastic lesions, and inhibit certain properties of the cancer

Table 11.1.   Some Dietary Sources of Phytochemicals

Carotenoide	Apricot, peach, nectarine, orange, broccoli, cabbage, spinach, pea, pumpkin, carrots, tomato
Flavonoids	Green tea, black tea, citrus fruits, onion, broccoli, cherry, wheat, corn, rice, tomatoes, spinach, cabbage, apples, olives, red wine, soy products
Polyphenole	Grapes, strawberries, raspberries, pomegranate, paprika, cabbage, walnut
Protease inhibitors	Soybean, oats, wheat, peanut, potato, rice, maize
Sulfide	Cabbage, chives, allium, onion, garlic
Terpene	Grapefruits, lemons, limes, oranges, lavender, mints, celery seeds, cherries

Source: Waladkhani and Clemens 1998.[7]

cell[8,9] (Fig. 11.1). Treatment of animals with phytochemicals that preferentially induce phase II xenobiotic-metabolizing enzymes reduces the conversion of chemical carcinogens to mutagenic metabolites and enhances their metabolic inactivation and excretion as a result of conjugate formation. Also, such treatment decreases toxicity, mutagenicity, and carcinogenicity of various chemical carcinogens.[10]

CAROTENOID

In several feeding studies, an increase in dietary intake of fruits and vegetables has been correlated with an increase in circulating plasma carotenoid concentrations.[11,12] On the other hand, intake of fruit and vegetables rich in carotenoids has a protective effect against

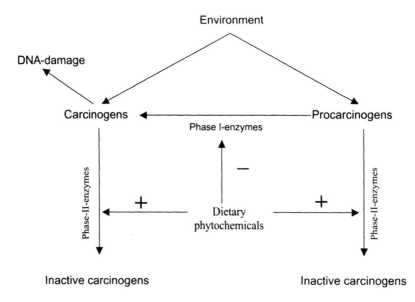

Figure 11.1.   Relationship between phytochemicals and inactivation of carcinogens.

the development of various cancers.[13] Carotenoids are a diverse group of over 600 structurally related compounds synthesized by bacteria and plants. Carotenoids, like alpha-carotene, beta-carotene, and lycopene, have been shown to have antioxidant activity in in vitro experiments.[14] Carotenoids enhance gap-junction cellular communication[15] and stimulate the immune system.[16] Several studies have shown that beta-carotene prevents DNA damage induced by carcinogenic chemicals.[17,18,19,20] Also, beta-carotene has been shown to attenuate hepatic drug-metabolizing enzymes[21] and to inhibit carcinogen activation.[19] The lack of toxicity of beta-carotene[22] allowed its safe use alone or as a dietary supplement. Recently, several studies have shown that alpha-carotene may be more effective than beta-carotene in preventing cancer.[23,24] Animal studies suggest that the administration of beta-carotene or vitamin A to mice enhanced the survival and recovery of peripheral leukocytes in mice given gamma-ray irradiation.[25] On the other side, some recent intervention trials using synthetic beta-carotene failed to show the protective effect against cancer.[26] Unfortunately, three of these studies failed to detect any protective effect of beta-carotene, or of a combination of beta-carotene and vitamin A, on the incidence of diverse cancers. In contrast to what was expected, two of these studies showed that these compounds could increase the incidence of lung cancer.[27,28] Clinical studies with lycopene indicate that lycopene supplementation in patients with prostate cancer may decrease the growth of prostate cancer.[29] Also, carotenoid-rich extracts of carrots, tomato paste, or orange juice have been shown to reduce the number of liver preneoplastic foci induced by aflatoxin B_1 in the rat, when administered together with the carcinogen.[30] Feeding rats with canthaxanthin, astaxanthin, and beta-apo-8'-carotenal inhibits the initiation of liver preneoplastic by aflatoxin B_1 and reduces in vivo aflatoxin B_1-induced liver DNA single-strand breaks and the in vivo binding of aflatoxin B_1 to liver DNA.[31]

CHLOROPHYLL

Chlorophyll is the ubiquitous pigment in green plants. Chlorophyllin, the food-grade derivative of chlorophyll, has been used historically in the treatment of several human conditions, with no evidence of human toxicity.[32] The potential carcinogenic activity of chlorophyll is of considerable interest because of its relative abundance in green vegetables widely consumed by humans. Chlorophyll and chlorophyllin have been shown to exert profound antimutagenic impact against a wide range of potential human carcinogens.[33,34] In spectrophotometry studies mutagen-inhibitor interaction (molecular complex formation) was identified. In vivo, chlorophyllin reduced hepatic aflatoxin B_1-DNA adducts and hepatocarcinogenesis when the inhibitor and carcinogen were coadministered in the diet.[35] Also, the formation of chlorophyllin:aflatoxin B_1 complex reduces systemic aflatoxin B_1 bioavailability.[36] Vibeke et al.[37] indicated that the amount of chlorophyllin required to give an overall protection against aflatoxin B_1-induced hepatocarcinogenesis was less than 1500 ppm in animal experiments. By comparison, the reported concentration of chlorophyll in spinach isolates is in the range of 1500–600,000 ppm, depending on agronomic conditions. Also spinach leaves may contain between 2.6 and 5.7% of their dry weight as chlorophylls.[38]

Chlorophyllin possesses free radical-scavenging properties. Recent studies suggest that chlorophyllin effectively protects plasmid DNA against ionizing radiation independent of DNA repair or other cellular defense mechanisms.[39] The chlorophyll-mediated reduction in dibenzo[a,1]pyrene-DNA adducts in vivo suggests a potential role for dietary chlorophylls in reducing the risk of tumor initiation by certain polycyclic hydrocarbons, mycotoxins, and heterocyclic amines present in the human diet.[40]

Chlorophyll-related compounds pheophytin a and b have been recently identified as antigenotoxic substances in the nonpolyphenolic fraction of green tea.[41] They have potent suppressive activities against tumor promotion in mouse skin.[42]

FLAVONOIDS

Over 5000 different naturally occurring flavonoids have been described,[43] and all are derivatives of the parent compound flavone (2-phenyl-benzopyrene or 2-phenylchromone) comprising a tricyclic C6-C3-C6 nucleus, varying substitutions to which give rise to nine classes of flavonoid compounds. Flavonoids may be broadly classified as phenolic or nonphenolic.[44] After consumption, the plant flavonoids undergo many metabolic conversions by intestinal bacteria, and both the metabolites and parent compounds are absorbed into the blood and then excreted, mainly in the urine.[45]

Polymethoxyflavonoids including nobiletin occur exclusively in citrus fruit, and the Dancy tangerine has the highest total, containing approximately five times the amount found in the peel of sweet orange varieties.[46] Nobiletin has previously been reported to induce differentiation of mouse myeloid leukemia cells,[47] to exhibit antiproliferative activity toward a human squamous cell carcinoma cell line,[48] to exert antimutagenic activity,[49] and to suppress the induction of matrix metalloproteinase-9.[50] Nobiletin also suppressed the expression of cyclooxygenase-2 and inducible NO synthase proteins and prostaglandin E2 release.[51] In addition, tangeretin was reported to inhibit tumor invasion and metastasis[52] and to induce apoptosis in HL-60 cells.[53] Tangeretin and nobiletin given to brain tumor cell cultures have the potential to retard motile or invasive behavior.[54]

Increased levels of estrogens in blood and urine are markers for high risk for breast cancer.[55,56] In a large prospective, case-control study, there was a significant relationship between serum estrogen levels and the risk for breast cancer in women in New York.[56] Goldin et al.[57] reported 44% lower blood levels of estrogen and androgens in Oriental women who emigrated to the United States from areas of low breast cancer risk, when compared to Caucasian Americans, who have a higher risk for breast cancer. Women newly diagnosed with breast cancer excreted substantially lower levels of urinary isoflavonoids and phenols than controls, and high excretions of these compounds were associated with a substantially reduced risk of breast cancer. In particular, high excretions of phenols and total isoflavonoids were associated with an 85% statistically significant reduced risk of breast cancer.[58] Among premenopausal women in Singapore, breast cancer risk was inversely related to soy protein intake.[59] Soy contains significant amounts of the isoflavones daidezein and genistein.[60] They may act as anti-estrogens by competing with endogenous estrogens for receptor binding, and this may reduce estrogen-induced stimulation of breast cell proliferation[61] and breast tumor formation. Some isoflavonoids have been shown to stimulate the synthesis of sex hormone-binding globulin (SHBG), decreasing blood levels of free estrogens that are more available to the target tissues[45,62] (Fig. 11.2). Certain isoflavonoids may inhibit important steroid biosynthetic enzymes, including aromatase and 17beta-hydroxysteroid dehydrogenase I, thus affecting the level of circulating estrogens.[45,62] In addition to these antiestrogenic effects, isoflavonoids have also been found to have inhibitory effects on angiogenesis, apoptosis, and tumor invasion as well as antioxidative, antiproliferative, and apoptosis-inducing activities.[45,63] Flavonoids inhibit mitogenic signaling pathway(s) and alter cell cycle regulators, albeit at different levels, leading to growth inhibition and death of advanced and androgen-independent prostate carcinoma cells.[64]

INDOLE

In ancient times cruciferous vegetables were cultivated primarily for medicinal purposes.[65] The biological active compound is glucobrassicin, a secondary plant metabolite that is abundant in cruciferous vegetables[3] (Table 11.2). Large quantities of inducers of enzymes that protect against carcinogens can be delivered in the diet by small quantities of young crucifer sprouts (e.g., 3-day-old broccoli sprouts) that contain as much inducer activity as ten to one hundred times larger quantities of mature vegetables.[66] Glucobrassicin undergoes autolysis during maceration to indole-3-carbinol, which is known to undergo acid condensation in the stomach following ingestion. Incubation of indole-3-carbinol under conditions that mimic the acid conditions in the stomach results in the production of multimeric derivatives of indole-3-carbinol.[67] Glucosinolates and glucosinolate breakdown

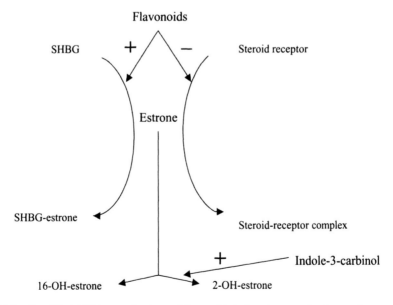

Figure 11.2.   Possible inhibiting mechanisms of flavonoids in breast cancer development.

Table 11.2.   Glucosinolate Content of Cruciferous Vegetables

Vegetable	Range µg/g)
Broccoli	450–1480
Brussels sprouts	600–3900
Cauliflower	270–830
Red cabbage	470–1240
White cabbage (kraut)	430–760
White cabbage	260–1060

Source: Fenwick et al. 1983.[65]

products are hydrophilic, and as much as 63% of the glucosinolate content of a vegetable may leach into the cooking water during boiling.[68] Steaming provides less opportunity for leaching, and stir-fried vegetables retain glucosinolate levels.[69] Light cooking may disrupt plant cell membranes without leaching of the indoles into the cooking medium, providing the opportunity for myrosinase to release these indoles for eventual conversion to indolo[3,2-b]carbazole.[68,70]

The natural indoles 3,3'-diindolylmethane, ascorbigen, indole-3-carbinol, and indolo[3,2-b]carbazole, as well as the natural isothiocyanates sulforaphane, benzyl isothiocyanate and phenethyl isothiocyanate, all possess cancer chemopreventive properties.[71] Indole-3-carbinol inhibits the growth of PC-3 prostate cancer cells by inducing G1 cell cycle arrest leading to apoptosis, and regulates the expression of apoptosis-related genes.[72] Further, blends of isoprenoids suppressed B16 and HL-60 promyelocytic leukemia cell proliferation with efficacies equal to the sum of the individual impacts.[73] Animals fed diets high in cruciferous vegetables and then exposed to various carcinogens expressed lower tumor yields and increased survival rates.[74,75] Indole-3-carbinol administration is known to induce cytochrome P_{450} and glutathione S-transferase activities, resulting in increased metabolic capacity toward chemical carcinogens.[76] These properties of indole-3-carbinol are considered to contribute to the known anticarcinogenic properties of this compound, as well as to the reduced risk of cancer associated with diets rich in cruciferous vegetables.[77] Evidence from an epidemiological case-control study of diet and cancer also suggested that consumption of cruciferous vegetables is associated with a decreased incidence of cancer.[78] Results from one cross-national study found that those countries with higher cabbage intake had a lower breast cancer mortality rate.[79] In three small human intervention studies, the daily administration of indole-3-carbinol pills (400 mg/day) or broccoli (500 g/day) significantly increased the urinary 2-hydroxyestrone: 16-hydroxyestrone value,[80,81,82] consistent with reduced breast cancer risk. Also, higher urinary 2-hydroxyestrone:16-hydroxyestrone values suggest protection from breast cancer, whereas lower urinary 2-hydroxyestrone:16-hydroxyestrone values suggest greater risk.[83] Indole-3-carbinol administration is known to induce cytochrome P_{450}.[76] P_{450} enzymes hydroxylate estrone on the second carbon, leading to greater 2-hydroxyestrone production and decreasing the pool of estrone available for conversion to 16-hydroxyestrone, thus increasing the 2-hydroxyestrone: 16-hydroxyestrone ratio[81,68,84] (Fig. 11.2). Unlike the 16-

hydroxyestrone metabolite, 2-hydroxyestrone has a low affinity for the estrogen receptor, and 2-hydroxyestrone is rapidly methylated by catechol-O-methyl transferase in the circulation.[85] In addition to a lower estrogenic potential, the 2-hydroxylated metabolites can inhibit angiogenesis.[86,87]

POLYPHENOLS

The polyphenolic components of higher plants may act as antioxidants or as agents of other mechanisms contributing to anticarcinogenic or cardioprotective action[88] (Table 11.3). Two epidemiological studies indicate that people who consume tea regularly may have a decreased risk of prostate cancer.[89] About 10% of the dry weight of green tea is catechins, which include (-)-epigallocatechin-3-gallate (EGCG), (-)-epigallocatechin (EGC), (-)-epicatechin-3-gallate (ECG), and (-)-epicatechin (EC).[90] EGCG has been shown to cause growth inhibition and regression of human prostate and breast tumors in athymic nude mice.[91] EGCG inhibits free radical formation and lipid peroxidation,[92,93,94] the inhibition of ornithine decarboxylase,[95,96] and the inhibition of DNA–carcinogen binding and adduct formation.[96] Treatment of prostate carcinoma DU145 cells with EGCG also inhibits mitogenic signaling pathway(s) and alters cell cycle regulators, albeit at different

Table 11.3.   Some Dietary Sources of Flavonoids

Flavanol	
Epicatechin	
Catechin	
Epigallocatechin	Green and black teas
Epicatechin gallate	Red wine
Flavanone	
Naringin	Peel of citrus fruits
Taxifolin	Citrus fruits
Flavonol	
Kaempferol	Endive, leek, broccoli, radish, grapefruit, black tea
Quercetin	Onion, lettuce, broccoli, cranberry, apple skin, berries, olive, tea, red wine
Myricetin	Cranberry, grapes, red wine
Flavone	
Chrysin	Fruit skin
Apigenin	Celery, parsley
Anthocyanidins	
Malvidin	Red grapes, red wine
Cyanidin	Cherry, raspberry, strawberry, grapes
Apigenidin	Colored fruit and peels
Phenyl propanoids	
Ferulic acid	Wheat, corn, rice, tomatoes, spinach, cabbage, asparagus
Caffeic acid	White grapes, white wine, olives, olive oil, spinach cabbage, asparagus, coffee
Beta-coumaric acid	White grapes, white wine, tomatoes, spinach, cabbage, asparagus
Chlorogenic acid	Apples, pears, cherries, plums, peaches, apricots blueberries, tomatoes, anis

Source: Rice-Evans et al. 1996.[88]

levels, leading to growth inhibition and death of advanced and androgen-independent prostate carcinoma cells.[64] EGCG and EGC possess growth inhibitory activities against human lung tumor cells. ECG has lower inhibitory activity and EC was much less effective.[97] Inhibition of tumorigenesis in mice could be demonstrated by the average EGCG and EGC concentrations in the range of 0.2 to 0.3 µM.[98] After ingestion of two or three cups of tea by human subjects, the average peak plasma values of EGCG and EGC were also in this range, and the highest individual values observed for EGCG and EGC were 0.65 µM.[99] In the manufacturing of black tea known as fermentation, the tea catechins are oxidized and polymerized to form the characteristic black tea polyphenols, theaflavins, and thearubigins.[90] These polyphenol compounds are known to have antioxidative activities due to their radical scavenging and metal chelating functions, as well as antimutagenic activities.[100,101] Theaflavins are responsible for the characteristic reddish color and astringency of black tea.[90,100] The astringency is due to the precipitation of the mucous glycoproteins in the mouth by polyphenols.[102] Theaflavins from black tea exhibit growth-inhibitory activities in cancer cells, although the activities are lower than those with EGC and EGCG.[97] Administration of theaflavins in A/J mice decreased both lung tumor multiplicity and volume. Also, the treatment with theaflavins inhibited the proliferation index in lung hyperplasia and adenomas.[103] Tea polyphenols in concentrations of 100 µM and 30 µM induce apoptosis, showing apoptosis indices of about 80% and 8–26%, respectively.[97]

Curcumin, a plant phenolic, has been considered as a potentially important chemopreventive agent against cancer.[104] Animal studies have demonstrated that curcumin inhibits carcinogenesis in various tissues, including skin,[105] colorectal,[106] oral,[107] forestomach,[108] and mammary cancers.[109] In mice, dietary administration of 5000–20,000 ppm curcumin reduced the incidence of intestinal tumors.[110] Further, curcumin induces apoptotic cell death in promyelocytic leukemia HL-60 cells at concentrations as low as 3.5 µg/ml.[111] Recent studies demonstrated an inhibitory effect of dietary curcumin when administered continuously during the initiation and postinitiation phases.[112,113] Administration of curcumin may retard growth and/or development of existing neoplastic lesions in the colon.[112]

Resveratrol is other polyphenol, which is synthesized by a wide variety of plant species, including aliments such as grape skins, peanuts, and mulberries, in response to injury, UV irradiation, and fungal attack.[114] Resveratrol was first detected in grapevines in 1976,[114] and then in wine in 1992.[115] It is synthesized in the leaf epidermis and the skin of grape berries, but not in the flesh.[116] Resveratol was shown to induce phase II metabolism and inhibit cyclo-oxygenase.[117]

PROTEASE INHIBITORS

Epidemiological and experimental data suggest that protease inhibitors have significant anticarcinogenic activity.[118] Several different types of protease inhibitors have been shown to inhibit the carcinogenic process, and on a molar basis those that inhibit chemotrypsin proteases have been the most effective. The content of two prominent protease inhibitors (Bowman-Birk inhibitor, BBI, and Kunitz-Trypsin inhibitor, KTI) varies considerably with species of soy,[119] and protease inhibitors (PI) content of several soy protein isolates can vary by as much as 20-fold. The BBI content in soy flour can be as high as 5.5 mg/g.[120]

Also, 1 g of textured soy protein, tofu, dry cereal, or pancake mix contains 0.48, 0.08, 0.10, or 0.38 mg of BBI, respectively.[121] BBI is a potent anticarcinogenic agent that inhibits chemical carcinogen- and radiation-induced malignant transformation in vitro and suppresses carcinogenesis in several organ systems and animal species.[118] Recent studies indicate that BBI and BBI concentrate prevent and suppress malignant transformation in vitro and carcinogenesis in vivo without toxicity.[122] BBI, in the form of BBI concentrate, has achieved Investigational New Drug status with the U.S. Food and Drug Administration. In a recently completed Phase IIa oral cancer chemoprevention trial in patients with premalignant lesions known as oral leukoplakia, treatment with BBI concentrate at daily doses of 200-1066 chymotrypsin inhibition units for 1 month led to a dose-dependent decrease in oral leukoplakia lesion size.[123]

A number of clinically important PI are found in serum, including alpha 2-protease inhibitor, alpha 2-macroglobulin, alpha 1-antichymotrypsin, alpha 1-acid glycoprotein, and so on. Many of these PI are referred to as acute-phase reactants and are active against serine proteinases.[124] Other potentially important effects of dietary PI may occur via hormonal modulation and inactivation of trypsin and chymotrypsin in the duodenum by dietary PI. For example, potato carboxypeptidase inhibitor is an antagonist of human epidermal growth factor. It competes with epidermal growth factor for binding to epidermal growth factor receptor (EGFR) and inhibits EGFR activation and cell proliferation induced by this growth factor. Potato carboxypeptidase inhibitor suppressed the growth of several human pancreatic adenocarcinoma cell lines, both in vitro and in nude mice.[125] A number of studies have, for instance, documented that dietary PI stimulate secretion of pancreatic enzymes, presumably via modulation of cholecystokinin levels.[126] Cholecystokinin release is of additional interest because cholecystokinin acts as a cocarcinogen in various models.[127]

Among other effects, PI block release of oxygen radicals and H_2O_2 from polymorphonuclear leukocyte and activated macrophages,[128] which may protect DNA from oxidative damage or from single-strand breaks. Hydroxyl radicals also appear to be involved.[129] Further, PI inhibit influx of polymorphonuclear leukocytes.[128]

SULFIDES

The *Allium* genus of vegetables includes garlic, onions, leeks, scallions, chives, and shallots. These vegetables are characterized by a composition that is high in flavonols and organosulfur compounds. The anticarcinogenic effects of sulfur-containing compounds, such as diallyl disulfide (DADS), have been demonstrated in animals.[130] The number of sulfur atoms on the molecule can influence the degree of protection, with diallyl trisulfide > diallyl disulfide > diallyl sulfide.[131,132] DADS and diallyl trisulfide (DATS) are far more effective in retarding the growth of neoplasms than were water-soluble allyl sulfur compounds such as *S*-allyl cysteine.[133] At least part of the ability of DADS to induce differentiation in DS19 mouse erythroleukemic cells might relate to its ability to increase histone acetylation.[134] Interestingly, DADS has also been reported to inhibit the growth of H-ras oncogene–transformed tumors in nude mice.[135]

Cytochrome P_{450} 2E1 (CYP2E1) appears to be one that is particularly vulnerable to the effects of allyl sulfur compounds.[136,137] An autocatalytic destruction of CYP2E1 has been demonstrated and may account for the chemoprotective effects of DAS, and possibly other allyl sulfur compounds against some chemical carcinogens.[138] Singh et al.[139] provided evidence that the efficacy of various organosulfides to suppress benzo(a)pyrene tumorigenesis correlated with their ability to suppress NAD(P)H:quinone oxidoreductase, an enzyme involved with the removal of quinones associated with this carcinogen. Depressed carcinogen bioactivation because of reduction in cyclo-oxygenase and lipoxygenase activity may also account for some of the lower incidence of tumors after treatment with some carcinogens.[140,141] In Wistar rats, DADS treatment strongly increased the activity of all the phase II enzymes examined, such as total glutathione S-transferase activity, quinone reductase activity, and epoxide hydrolase activity. Also, the antimutagenic activities of organosulfur compounds against several ultimate carcinogens are closely related to their ability to induce phase II enzymes.[142]

In rat liver supernatant ajoene and DAS affected aflatoxin B_1 metabolism and DNA binding by inhibiting phase I enzymes and may therefore be considered as potential cancer chemopreventive agents.[143] In mice, the oral application of DAS suppressed the activity of ornithine decarboxylase.[144] In the murine model, topical application of DAS and DADS, oil-soluble constituents of garlic and onion, significantly inhibited skin papilloma formation from the ninth week of promotion and significantly increased the rate of survival.[145] In an in vivo assay, intraperitoneal injection of 1 or 2 mg DADS three times a week from the day of tumor cell inoculation until the end of the experiment (after 35 days) caused growth retardation and 43% reduction in primary tumor weight.[146] In studies of the effect of DADS on the growth of transplanted human colon carcinoma cell lines in immunologically compromised nude mice, DADS was as effective as 5-FU in inhibiting tumor growth. Combining the DADS and 5-FU did not increase the effect, but concurrent DADS treatment did significantly reduce the depression of leukocyte counts and splenic weight associated with chemotherapy administration.[147]

In high doses, wild garlic can cause gastroenteritis, diarrhea, rash, and leukocytosis. Also, long-term ingestion of wild garlic or onion will block iodine uptake by the thyroid.[148]

TERPENES

Monoterpenoids are commonly produced by plants and found in many fruits and vegetables. The pharmacokinetic studies in dogs and rats revealed that p.o. administration of perillyl alcohol is rapidly absorbed from the gastrointestinal tract and metabolized to perillic acid and dihydroperillic acid.[149,150] Several monoterpenes induce phase II enzymes.[151] With regard to the mode of the chemopreventive action of perillyl alcohol, monoterpenes exhibit a diverse array of metabolic, cellular, and molecular activities, including inhibition of activation of carcinogen metabolism, inhibition of cellular proliferation, and the induction of differentiation and apoptosis.[152,153] Limonene, which is a monocyclic monoterpene found in essential oils of citrus fruits, spices, and herbs, is known to be an inhibitor of chemically induced breast, forestomach, liver, lung, and skin carcinogenesis in rodents.[154]

Limonene caused regression of DMBA-induced mammary tumors.[155] Limonene is also capable of inhibiting the development of upper digestive tract carcinomas in N-nitrosodiethylamine treated mice.[156] In humans, the three metabolic derivatives detected in plasma after single oral doses of 100 mg/kg limonene are perillic acid, dihydroperillic acid, and limonene-1,2-diol.[157] The metabolic precursors to perillic acid and dihydroperillic acid are likely perillyl alcohol and perillyl aldehyde, both of which have potent antiproliferative activities in cell culture systems.[158,159,160] In TM6 cells, perillyl alcohol causes an early G1 cell-cycle block and slows the G2–M transition.[161] Limonene impairs DNA synthesis in the human-derived myeloid leukemia cell line THP-1 and in the lymphoid leukemia cell line RPMI-8402 in a concentration-dependent manner.[160] In addition, d-limonene inhibits carcinogen activation to produce an inhibitory effect in carcinogenesis. Animal studies indicated that d-limonene administered in the diet at the 1–5% levels inhibited both DMBA- and MNU-induced rat mammary carcinogenesis in female rats.[162]

Limonene such as auraptene is found in orange peels but its amount is small. Dietary administration of auraptene could effectively suppress tumor development. Auraptene administration during the initiation phase could exert its chemopreventive action by enhancing carcinogen detoxification systems, such as glutathione S-transferase and quinone reductase.[163]

CONCLUSION

Plant foods have preventive potential, and consumption of vegetables and fruits is lower in those who subsequently develop cancer. It may be more relevant to increase the intake of intact dietary items, rather than isolated certain chemicals occurring in natural products, in order to balance chemoprotective effects.

REFERENCES

1. Steinmetz, K. A., Potter, J. D. 1991. Vegetables, fruit, and cancer II: Mechanisms. Cancer Causes Control, 2, 427.
2. Barnes, S. 1995. Effect of genistein on in vitro and in vivo models of cancer. J. Nutr., 125, 777S.
3. McDanell, R., McLean, A. E. M., Hanley, A. B., Heaney, R. K., and Fenwick, G. R. 1986. Chemical and biological of indole glucosinates (glucobrassicins): a review. Food Chem. Toxicol., 26, 59.
4. Surh, Y-J. 1999. Molecular mechanisms of chemopreventive effects of selected dietary and medicinal phenolic substances. Mutat. Res., 428, 305.
5. Kuroda, Y., Hara, Y. 1999. Antimutagenic and anticarcinogenic activity of tea polyphenols. Mutat. Res., 436, 69.
6. Wattenberg, L. W. 1997. An overview of chemoprevention: current status and future prospects. Proc. Soc. Exp. Biol. Med., 216, 133.
7. Waladkhani, A. R., Clemens, M. R. 1998. Effect of dietary phytochemicals on cancer development. Internat. J. Mol. Med., 1, 747.
8. Sipes, I. G., Gandolfi, A. J. 1993. Biotransformation of toxicants. In *Toxicology-the basic science of poisons*, Amdur, M. O., Doull, J., Klassen, C. D. (Eds.), McGraw-Hill, New York, 88.

9. Wattenberg, L. W. 1992. Chemoprevention of cancer by naturally occurring and synthetic compounds. In *Cancer chemoprevention*, Wattenberg, L. W., Lipkin, M., Boone, C. W., Kelloff, G. J. (Eds.), CRC Press, Boca Raton, FL, 19.

10. Primiano, T., Enger, P. A., Sutter, T. R., Kelloff, G. J., Roebuck, B. D., Kensler, T. W. 1995. Intermittent dosing with oltipraz: relationship between chemoprevention of aflatoxin-induced tumorigenesis and induction of glutathione S-transferase. Cancer Res., 55, 4319.

11. Martini, M. C., Campbell, D. R., Gross, M. D., Grandits, G. A., Potter, J. D., Slavin, J. L. 1995. Plasma carotenoids as biomarkers of vegetable intake: the University of Minnesota Cancer Prevention Research Unit feeding studies. Cancer Epidemiol. Biomark. Prev., 4, 491.

12. Yeum, K. J., Booth, S. L., Sadowski, J. A., Liu, C., Tang, G., Krinsky, N. I., Russell, R. M. 1995. Human plasma carotenoid response to the ingestion of controlled diets high in fruits and vegetables. Am. J. Clin. Nutr., 64, 594.

13. Peto, R., Doll, R., Buckley, J. D., Sporn, M. B. 1981. Can dietary beta-carotene materially reduce human cancer rates? Nature, 290, 201.

14. Mascio, P. D., Kaaiser, S., Sies, H. 1989. Lycopene as the most efficient biological carotenoid singlet oxygen quencher. Arch. Biochem. Biophys., 274, 532.

15. Zhang, L. X., Cooney, R. V., Bertram, J. S. 1991. Carotenoids enhance gap junctional communication and inhibit lipid peroxidation in C3H/10T1/2 cells: relationship to their cancer chemopreventive action. Carcinogenesis, 12, 2109.

16. Roe, D. A., Fuller, C. J. 1993. Carotenoids and the immune function. In *Human nutrition-A comprehensive treatise,* vol. 8. Klurfeld, MD (ed.), Plenum Press, New York, 229.

17. Aidoo, A., Lyn-Cook, L. E., Lensing, S., Wamer, W. 1995. In vivo antimutagenic activity of beta-carotene in rat spleen lymphocytes. Carcinogenesis 16, 2237.

18. Renner, H. W. 1995. Anticlastogenic effect of beta-carotene in Chinese hamster. Time and dose-response studies with different mutagens. Mutat. Res., 144, 251.

19. Sarker, A., Mukjerjee, B., Chetterjee, M. 1994. Inhibitory effect of beta-carotene on chronic 2-acetylaminofluorene-induced hepatocarcinogenesis in rat: reflection in hepatic drug metabolism. Carcinogenesis ,15, 1055.

20. Uehara, N., Iwahori, Y., Asamoto, M., et. al. 1996. Decrease levels of 2-amino-3-methylimidazol[4,5-f]quinoline-DNA adducts in rats treated with beta-carotene, alpha-tocopherol and freeze-dried aloe. Jpn. J. Cancer Res., 87, 324.

21. Basu, T. K., Temple, N. J., Ng, J. 1987. Effect of dietary beta-carotene on hepatic drug-metabolizing enzymes in mice. J. Clin. Biochem. Nutr., 3, 95.

22. Bendich, A. 1988. The safety of beta-carotene. Nut. Cancer, 11, 207.

23. Murakoshi, M., Nishino, H., Satomi, Y., et al. 1992. Potent preventive action of α-carotene against carcinogenesis: spontaneous liver carcinogenesis and promoting stage of lung and skin carcinogenesis in mice are suppressed more effectively by alpha-carotene than by beta-carotene. Cancer Res., 52, 6583.

24. Ziegler, R. G., Colavito, E. A., Hartge, P., McAdams, M. J., Schoenberg, J. B., Mason, T. J., Fraumeni, J. F. Jr. 1996. Importance of alpha-carotene, beta-carotene, and other phytochemicals in the etiology of lung cancer. J. Natl. Cancer Inst., 88, 612.

25. Seifter, E., Rettura, G., Padawer, J., Stratford, F., Weinzweig, J., Demetriou, A. A., Levenson, S. M. 1984. Morbidity and mortality reduction by supplementation vitamin A or beta-carotene in CBA mice given total-body gamma-radiation. J. Natl. Cancer Inst., 73, 1167

26. Mayne, S. T. 1996. Beta-carotene, carotenoids, and disease prevention in humans. FASEB J., 10, 690.

27. The Alpha Tocopherol, Beta Carotene Cancer Prevention Study Group. 1994. The effects of vitamin E and beta carotene on the incidence of lung cancer and other cancers in male smokers. N. Engl. J. Med., 330, 1029.

28. Omenn, G. S., Goodman, G. E., Thornquist, M. D., et al. 1996. Effects of a combination of beta-carotene and vitamin A on lung cancer and cardiovascular disease. N. Engl. J. Med., 334, 1150.

29. Kucuk, O., Sarkar, F. H., Sakr, W., Djuric, Z., Pollak, M. N., Khachik, F., Li, Y.-W., Banerjee, M., Grignon, D., Bertram, J. S., Crissman, J. D., Pontes, E. J., Wood, D. P., Jr. 2001. Phase II randomized clinical trial of lycopene supplementation before radical prostatectomy. Cancer Epid. Biom. Prev., 10, 861.

30. He, Y., Root, M. M., Parker, R. S., Campbell, T. C. 1997. Effects of carotenoid-rich food extracts on the development of preneoplastic lesions in rat liver and on in vivo and in vitro antioxidant status. Nutr. Cancer, 27, 238.

31. Gradelet, S., Le Bon, A. M., Bergès, R., Suschetet, M., Astorg, P. 1998. Dietary carotenoids inhibit aflatoxin B_1 –induced liver preneoplastic foci and DNA damage in the rat: Role of the modulation of aflatoxin B_1 metabolism. Carcinogenesis, 19(3), 403.

32. Young, R. W., Beregi, J. S. 1980. Use of chlorophyllin in the care of geriatric patients. J. Am. Geriatr. Soc., 28, 48.

33. Lai, C., Butler, M. A., Matney, T. S. 1980. Antimutagenic activities of common vegetables and their chlorophyll content. Mutat. Res., 77, 245.

34. Negishi, T., Arimoto, S., Nishizaki, C., and Hayatsu, H. 1989. Inhibitory effect of chlorophyll on the genotoxicity of 3-amino-1-methyl-5H-pyrido[4,3-b]indole (Trp-P-2). Carcinogen., 10, 145.

35. Dashwood, R., Negishi, T., Hayatsu, H., Breinholt, V., Hendricks, J., Bailey, G. 1998. Chemopreventive properties of chlorophylls towards aflatoxin B1: a review of the antimutagenicity and anticarcinogenicity data in rainbow trout. Mutat. Res., 399(2), 245.

36. Breinholt, V., Arbogast, D., Loveland, P., et al. 1999. Chlorophyllin chemoprevention in trout initiated by aflatoxin B(1) bath treatment: An evaluation of reduced bioavailability vs. target organ protective mechanisms. Toxicol. Appl. Pharmacol., 158(2), 141.

37. Vibeke, B., Hendricks, J., Pereira, C., et al. 1995. Dietary chlorophyllin is a potent inhibitor of aflatoxin B1 hepatocarcinogenesis in Rainbow Trout. Cancer Res., 55, 57.

38. Khalyfa, A., Kermasha, S., and Alli, I. 1992. Extraction, purification and characterization of chlorophyll from spinach leaves. J. Agric. Food. Chem., 40, 215.

39. Kumar, S. S., Chaubey, R. C., Devasagayam, T. P., et al. 1999. Inhibition of radiation-induced DNA damage in plasmid pBR322 by chlorophyllin and possible mechanism(s) of action. Mutat. Res., 425(1), 71.

40. Harttig, U., Bailey, G. S. 1998. Chemoprotection by natural chlorophylls in vivo: inhibition of dibenzo[a,l]pyrene-DNA adducts in rainbow trout liver. Carcinogenesis, 19(7), 1323.

41. Okai, Y., Higashi-Okai, K. 1997. Potent suppressing activity of the non-polyphenolic fraction of green tea (Camellia sinensis) against genotoxin-induced umu C gene expression in Salmonella typhimurium (TA 1535/pSK 1002)—association with pheophytins a and b. Cancer Lett., 120(1),117.

42. Higashi-Okai, K., Otani, S., and Okai, Y. 1998. Potent suppressive activity of pheophytin a and b from the non-polyphenolic fraction of green tea (Camellia sinensis) against tumor promotion in mouse skin. Cancer Lett., 129(2), 223.

43. Harborne, J. B. (ed.). 1994. *The flavonoids. Advances in research since 1986*. London: Chapman & Hall.

44. Hertog, M. G. L., Hollman, P. C. H., Katan, M. B., Kromhout, D. 1993. Intake of potentially anticarcinogenic flavonoids and their determinants in adults in Netherlands. Nutr. Cancer, 20, 219.

45. Adlercreutz, H., Mazur, W. 1997. Phyto-oestrogens and Western diseases. Ann. Med., 29, 95.

46. Chen, J., Montanari, A. M., Widmer, W. W. 1997. Two new polymethoxylated flavonoids, a class of compounds with potential anticancer activity, isolated from cold pressed Dancy tangerine peel oil solids. J. Agric. Food Chem., 45, 364.

47. Sugiyama, S., Umemura, K., Kuroyanagi, M., et al. 1993. Studies on the differentiation inducers of myeloid leukemic cells from Citrus species. Chem. Pharm, Bull., 41, 714.

48. Kandawaswami, C., Perkins, E., Soloniuk, D. S., et al. 1991. Antiproliferative effects of citrus flavonoids on a human squamous cell carcinoma in vitro. Cancer Lett., 56, 147.

49. Wall, M. W., Wani, M. C., Manukumar, G., et al. 1998. Plant antimutagenic agents, 2 Flavonoids. J. Nat. Prod. (Lloydia), 51, 1084.

50. Ishiwa, J., Sato, T., Mimaki, Y., et al. 2000. A citrus flavonoid, nobiletin, suppresses production and gene expression of matrix metalloproteinase 9/gelatinase B in rabbit synovial fibroblasts. J. Rheumatol., 27, 20.

51. Murakami, A., Nakamura, Y., Torikai, K, et al. 2000. Inhibitory effect of citrus nobiletin on phorbol ester-induced skin inflammation, oxidative stress, and tumor promotion in mice. Cancer Res., 60, 5059.

52. Bracke, M. E., Bruyneel, E. A., Vermeulen, S. J., et al., 1994. Citrus flavonoid effect on tumor invasion and metastasis. Food Technol., 48, 121.

53. Hirano, T., Abe, K., Gotoh, M., Oka, K. 1995. Citrus flavone tangeretin inhibits leukaemic HL-60 cell growth partially through induction of apoptosis with less cytotoxicity on normal lymphocytes. Br. J. Cancer, 72, 1380.

54. Rooprai, H. K., Kandanearatchi, A., Maidment, S. L., et al. 2001. Evaluation of the effects of swainsonine, captopril, tangeretin and nobiletin on the biological behaviour of brain tumour cells in vitro. Neuropath. Appl. Neurob., 27(1), 29.

55. Bernstein, L., Yuan, J. M., Ross, R. K., et al. 1990. Serum hormone levels in pre-menopausal Chinese women in Shanghai and white women in Los Angeles: results from two breast cancer case-control studies. Cancer Caus. Cont., 1, 51.

56. Toniolo, P. G., Levitz, M., Zeleniuch-Jacquotte, A., et al. 1995. A protective study of endogenous estrogens and breast cancer in postmenopausal women. J. Natl. Cancer Inst., 87, 190.

57. Goldin, B. R., Adlercreutz, H., Gorbach, S. L., et al. 1986. The relationship between estrogen levels and diets of Caucasian American and Oriental immigrant women. Am. J. Clin. Nutr., 44, 945.

58. Zheng, W., Dai, Q., Custer L. J., et al. 1999. Urinary excretion of isoflavonoids and the risk of breast cancer. Cancer Epid. Biom. Prev., 8, 35.

59. Lee, H. P., Gourley, L., Duffy, S. W., et al. 1992. Risk factors for breast cancer by age and menopausal status: a case-control study in Singapore. Cancer Caus. Cont., 3, 313.

60. Price, K. R., Fenwick, G. R. 1985. Naturally occurring oestrogens in foods: a review. Food Addit. Contam., 2, 73.

61. Martin, P. M., Horwitz, K. B., Ryan, D. S., McGuire, W. L. 1978. Phytoestrogen interaction with estrogen receptors in human breast cancer. Endocrin., 103, 1860.

62. Messina, M., Barnes, S., Setchell, K. D. 1997. Phyto-oestrogens and breast cancer. Lancet, 350, 971.

63. Uckun, F. M., Evans, E., Forsyth, C. J., et al. 1995. Biotherapy of B-cell precursor leukemia by targeting genistein to CD19-associated tyrosine kinases. Science (Washington DC), 267, 886.

64. Bhatia, N., Agarwal, R. 2001. Detrimental effect of cancer preventive phytochemicals silymarin, genistein and epigallocatechin 3-gallate on epigenetic events in human prostate carcinoma DU145 cells. The Prostate, 46(2), 98.

65. Fenwick, G. R., Heaney, R. K., Mullin, W. J. 1983. Glucosinolates and their breakdown products in food and food plants. Crit. Rev. Food Sci. Nutr.,18, 123.

66. Fahey, J. W., Zhang, Y., Talalay, P. 1997. Broccoli sprouts: An exceptionally rich source of inducers of enzymes that protect against chemical carcinogens. Proc. Natl. Acad. Sci. USA, 94(19), 10367.

67. DeKruif, C. A., Marsman, J. W., Venekamp, J. C., et al. 1991. Structure elucidation of acid reaction products of indole-3-carbinol: detection in vivo and enzyme induction in vivo. Chem.-Biol. Interact., 80, 303.

68. Sepkovic, D. W., Bradlow, H. L., Michnovicz, J., et al. 1994. Catechol estrogen production in rat microsomes after treatment with indole-3-carbinol, ascorbigen, or B-naphthoflavone: a comparison of stable isotope dilution gas chromatography-mass spectrometry and radiometric methods. Steroids, 59, 318.

69. Betz, J., Obermeyer, W. 1993. Effects of processing on the glucosinolate content of broccoli. FASEB J., 7, 863.

70. Kwon, C-S., Grose, K. R., Riby, J., et al. 1994. In vivo production of enzyme-inducing activity of indolo[3,2-b]carbazole. J. Agric. Food Chem., 42, 2536.

71. Bonnesen, C., Eggleston, I. M., Hayes, J. D. 2001. Dietary indoles and isothiocyanates that are generated from cruciferous vegetables can both stimulate apoptosis and confer protection against DNA damage in human colon cell lines. Cancer Res., 61(16), 6120.

72. Chinni, S. R., Li, Y., Upadhyay, S., et al. 2001. Indole-3-carbinol (I3C) induced cell growth inhibition, G1 cell cycle arrest and apoptosis in prostate cancer cells. Oncogene, 20(23), 2927.

73. Tatman, D., Mo, H. 2002. Volatile isoprenoid constituents of fruits, vegetables and herbs cumulatively suppress the proliferation of murine B16 melanoma and human HL-60 leukemia cells. Cancer Lett., 175(2), 129.

74. Boy, J. N., Babish, J. G., and Stoewsand, G. S. 1982. Modification by beet and cabbage diets of aflatoxin B1-induced rat plasma alpha-foetoprotein elevation, hepatic tumorigenesis, and mutagenicity of urine. Food Chem. Toxicol., 20, 47.

75. Wattenberg, L. W. 1983. Inhibition of neoplasia by minor dietary constituents. Cancer Res., 43, 2448s.

76. Morse, M. A., LaGreca, S. D., Amin, S. G., Chung, F. L. 1990. Effects of indole-3-carbinol on lung tumorigenesis and DANN methylation induced by 4-(methylnitrosamino)-1-butanone (NNK) and on the metabolism and disposition of NNK in A/J mice. Cancer Res., 50,1613.

77. Marchand, L. L., Yoshizawa, C. N., Kolonel, L. N., et al. 1989. Vegetable consumption and lung cancer risk: a population based case-control study in Hawaii. J. Natl. Cancer Inst., 81,1158.

78. Graham, S. 1983. Results of case-control studies of diet and cancer in Buffalo, NY. Cancer Res., 43, 2409s.

79. Hebert, J. R., Rosen, A. 1996. Nutritional, socioeconomic, and reproductive factors in relation to female breast cancer mortality: findings from a cross-national study. Cancer Detect. Prev., 20, 234.

80. Bradlow, H. L., Michnovicz, J. J., Halper, M., et al. 1994. Long-term responses of women to indole-3-carbinol or a high fiber diet. Cancer Epidemiol. Biomark. Prev., 3, 591.

81. Kall, M. A., Vang, O., Clausen, J. 1996. Effects of dietary broccoli on human in vivo drug metabolizing enzymes: evaluation of caffeine, estrone, and chlorzoxazone. Carcinogenesis (Lond.), 17, 793.

82. Michnovicz, J. J., Bradlow, H. L. 1991. Altered estrogen metabolism and excretion in humans following consumption of indole-3-carbinol. Nutr. Cancer, 16, 59.

83. Kabat, G. C., Chang, C. J., Sparano, J. A., et al. 1997. Urinary estrogen metabolites and breast cancer: a case-control study. Cancer Epidemiol. Biomar. Prev., 6, 505.

84. Vang, O., Jensen, H., Autrup, H. 1991. Induction of cytochrome P-450IA1, IA2, IIB1, and IIE1 by broccoli in rat liver and colon. Chem.-Biol. Interact., 78, 85.

85. Bradlow, H. L., Telang, N. T., Sepkov, D. W., Osborne, M. P. 1996. 2-Hydroxyestrone: the "good" estrogen. J. Endocrinol., 150, S256.

86. Klauber, N., Parangi, S., Flynn, E., et al. 1997. Inhibition of angiogenesis and breast cancer in mice by the microtubule inhibitors 2-methoxyestradiol and taxol. Cancer Res., 57, 81.

87. Zhu, B. T., Conney, A. H. 1998. Functional role of estrogen metabolism in target cells: review and perspectives. Carcinogenesis (Lond.), 19, 1.

88. Rice-Evans, C. A., Miller, N. J., Paganga, G. 1996. Structure-antioxidant activity relationships of flavonoids and phenolic acids. Free Rad. Biol. Med., 20(7), 933.

89. Kinlen, L. J., Willows, A. N., Goldblatt, P., Yudkin, J. 1988. Tea consumption and cancer. Br. J. Cancer, 58, 397.

90. Balentine, D. A. 1992. Manufacturing and chemistry of tea. In *Phenolic compounds in food and their effects on health I: Analysis, occurrence, and chemistry.* Ho, C. T., Huang, M. T. Lee C. Y. (eds.). American Chemical Society, Washington, DC, 102.

91. Liao, S., Umekita, Y., Guo, J., et al. 1995. Growth inhibition and regression of human prostate and breast tumors in athymic mice by tea epigallocatechin gallate. Cancer Lett., 96, 239.

92. Chan, M.-Y., Ho, C.-T., Huang, H.-I. 1995. Effects of three dietary phytochemicals from tea, rosemary and turmeric on inflammation-induced nitrite production. Cancer Lett., 96, 23.

93. Yen, G.-C., Chen, H.-Y. 1995. Antioxidant activity of various tea extracts in relation to their antimutagenicity. J. Agric. Food Chem., 43, 27.

94. Uchida, S., Edamatsu, R., Hiramatsu, M., et al. 1987. Condensed tannins scavenge active oxygen free radicals. Med. Sci. Res., 15, 831.

95. Hu, G., Han, C., Chen, J. 1995. Inhibition of oncogene expression by green tea and (–)epigallocatechin gallate in mice. Nutr. Cancer, 24, 203.

96. Katiyar, S. K., Agarwal, R., Wood, G. S., et al. 1992. (–)-Epigallocatechin-3-gallate in Camellia sinensis leaves from Himalayan region of Sikkim: inhibitory affects against biochemical events and tumor initiation in SENCAR mouse skin. Nutr. Cancer, 18, 73.

97. Yang, G., Liao, J., Kim, K., et al. 1998. Inhibition of growth and induction of apoptosis in human cancer cell lines by tea polyphenols. Carcinogenesis, 19(4), 611.

98. Yang, C. S., Chen, L., Lee, M. J., Landau, J. M. 1996. Effects of tea on carcinogenesis in animal models and humans (Edited under the auspices of the American Institute for Cancer Research). In *Dietary phytochemicals in cancer prevention and treatment.* Plenum Press, New York, 51.

99. Lee, M. J., Wang, Z. Y., Li, H., et al. 1995. Analysis of plasma and urinary tea polyphenols in human subjects. Cancer Epidemiol. Biomark. Prev., 4, 393.

100. Rafat, H. S., Cillard, J., Cillard, P. 1987. Hydroxyl radical scavenging activity of flavonoids. Phytochemistry, 26, 2489.

101. Serafini, M., Ghiselli, A., Ferro-Luzzi, A. 1996. In vivo antioxidant effect of green and black tea in man. Eur. J. Clin. Nutr., 50, 28.

102. Rider, P. J., Marderosian, A. D., Porter, J. R. 1992. Evaluation of total tannins and relative astringency in teas. In *Phenolic compounds in food and their effects on health I.* Huang, M. T., Ho, C. T., Lee, C. Y. (ed.). ACS, Washington, DC, 93.

103. Yang, G., Liu, Z., Seril, D. N., et al. 1997. Black tea constituents, theaflavins, inhibit 4-(methylnitrosoamino)-1-(3-pyridyl)-1-butanone (NNK)-induced lung tumorigenesis in A/J mice. Carcinogenesis, 18(12), 2361.

104. Kelloff, G. J., Hawk, E. T., Karp, J. E., et al. 1997. Progress in clinical chemoprevention. Semin. Oncol., 24, 241.

105. Huang, M. T., Newmark, H. L., Frenkel, K. 1997. Inhibitory effects of curcumin on tumorigenesis in mice. J. Cell. Biochem., 27 (suppl.), 26.

106. Rao, C. V., Rivenson, A., Simi, B., Reddy, B. S. 1995. Chemoprevention of colon carcinogenesis by dietary curcumin, a naturally occurring plant phenolic compound. Cancer Res., 55, 259.

107. Tanaka, T., Makita, H., Ohnishi, M., et al. 1994. Chemoprevention of 4-nitroquinoline 1-oxide-induced oral carcinogenesis by dietary curcumin and hesperidin: comparison with the protective effect of beta-carotene. Cancer Res., 54, 4653.

108. Singh, S. V., Hu, X., Srivastava, S. K., et al. 1998. Mechanism of inhibition of benzo[a]pyrene-induced forestomach cancer in mice by dietary curcumin. Carcinogenesis, 19, 1357.

109. Singletary, K., MacDonald, C., Iovinelli, M., et al. 1998. Effect of the ß-diketones diferuloyl methane (curcumin) and dibenzoylmethane on rat mammary DNA adducts and tumors induced by 7,12-dimethylbenz[a]anthracene. Carcinogenesis, 19, 1039.

110. Huang, M. T., Lou, Y. R., Ma, W., et al. 1994. Inhibitory effect of dietary curcumin on forestomach, duodenal, and colon carcinogenesis in mice. Cancer Res., 54(22), 5841.

111. Kuo, M. L., Huang, T. S., Lin, J. K. 1996. Curcumin, an antioxidant and anti-tumor promoter, induces apoptosis in human leukemia cells. Biochim. Biophys. Acta, 1317(2), 95.

112. Kawamori, T., Lubet, R., Steele, V. E., et al. 1999. Chemopreventive effect of curcumin, a naturally occurring anti-inflammatory agent, during the promotion/progression stages of colon cancer. Cancer Res., 59, 597.

113. Pereira, M. A., Grubbs, D. J., Barnes, L. H., et al. 1996. Effects of the phytochemicals, curcumin and quercetin, upon azoxymethane-induced colon cancer and 7,12-dimethylbenz[a]anthracene-induced mammary cancer in rats. Carcinogen., 17, 1305.

114. Langcake, P., Pryce, R. J. 1976. The production of resveratrol by Vitis vinifera and other members of the Vitaceae as a response to infection or injury. Physiol. Plant Pathol., 9, 77.

115. Siemann, E. H., Creasy, L. L. 1992. Concentration of phytoalexin resveratrol in wine. Am. J. Enol. Vitic., 43, 49.

116. Creasy, L. L., Coffee, M. 1988. Phytoalexin production potential of grape berries. J. Am. Soc. Hort. Sci., 113, 230.

117. Jang, M., Cai, L., Udeani, G. O., et al. 1997. Cancer chemopreventive activity of resveratol, a natural product derived from grapes. Science, 275, 218.

118. Kennedy, A. R. 1998. Chemopreventive agents: protease inhibitors. Pharmacol. Ther., 78, 167.

119. Eldridge, A., Kwolek, W. 1983. Soybean isoflavones: Effect of environment and variety on composition. J. Agr. Food Chem., 31, 394.

120. Brandon, D. L., Bates A. H., Friedman M. 1991. ELISA analysis of soybean trypsin inhibitors in processed foods. In *Nutritional and toxicological consequences of food processing*. Friedman, M. (ed.). Plenum Publishing Corp. New York, 321.

121. Di Pietro, C. M., Liener, I. E. 1989. Soybean protease inhibitors in foods. J. Food Sci., 54, 606.

122. Kennedy, A. R. 1998. The Bowman-Birk inhibitor from soybeans as an anticarcinogenic agent. Am. J. Clin. Nutr., 68(6 Suppl), 1406S.

123. Meyskens, F. L. Jr., Armstrong, W. B., Wan, X. S., et al. 1999. Bowman-Birk inhibitor concentrate (BBIC) affects oral leukoplakia lesion size, new protein levels and proteolytic activity in buccal mucosal cells. Proc. Am. Assoc. Cancer Res., 40, 432.

124. Clawson, G. A. 1996. Protease inhibitors and carcinogenesis: a review. Cancer Invest., 14(6), 597.

125. Blanco-Aparicio, C., Molina, M. A., Fernandez-Salas, E., et al. 1998. Potato carboxypeptidase inhibitor, a T-knot protein, is an epidermal growth factor antagonist that inhibits tumor cell growth. J. Biol. Chem., 273(20), 12370.

126. Ware, J. H., Wan, X. S., Rubin, H., et al. 1997. Soybean Bowman-Birk protease inhibitor is a highly effective inhibitor of human mast cell chymase. Arch. Biochem. Biophys., 344(1), 133.

127. Howatson, A. 1986. The potential of cholecystokinin as a carcinogen in the hamster-nitrosamine model. In *Nutritional and toxicological significance of enzyme inhibitors in foods.* Friedman, M. (ed.). Plenum Press, New York, 109.

128. Goldstein, B., Witz, G., Amoruso, M., and Troll, W. 1979. Protease inhibitors antagonize the activation of polymorphonuclear leukocyte oxygen consumption. Biochem. Biophys. Res. Commun., 88, 854.

129. Troll, W. 1991. Prevention of cancer by agents that suppress oxygen radical formation. Free Rad. Res. Commun., 12-13, 751.

130. Reddy, B. S., Rao, C. V., Rivenson, A., Kelloff, G. 1993. Chemoprevention of colon carcino-genesis by organosulfur compounds. Cancer Res., 53, 3493.

131. Sakamoto, K., Lawson, L. D., Milner, J. 1997. Allyl sulfides from garlic suppress the in vitro proliferation of human A549 lung tumor cells. Nutr. Cancer, 29, 152.

132. Tsai, S. J., Jenq, S. N., Lee, H. 1996. Naturally occurring diallyl disulfide inhibits the forma-tion of carcinogenic heterocyclic aromatic amines in boiled pork juice. Mutagenesis, 11, 235.

133. Sundaram, S. G., Milner, J. A. 1993. Impact of organosulfur compounds in garlic on canine mammary tumor cells in culture. Cancer Lett., 74, 85.

134. Lea, M. A., Randolph, V. M., Patel M. 1999. Increased acetylation of histones induced by dial-lyl disulfide and structurally related molecules. Int. J. Oncol., 15, 347.

135. Singh, S. V., Mohan, R. R., Agarwal, R., et al. 1996. Novel anti-carcinogenic activity of an organosulfide from garlic: inhibition of H-ras oncogene transformed tumor growth in vivo by diallyl disulfide is associated with inhibition of p21H-ras processing. Biochem. Biophys. Res. Commun., 225, 660.

136. Jeong, H. G., Lee, Y. W. 1998. Protective effects of diallyl sulfide on N-nitroso-dimethyl-amine-induced immunosuppression in mice. Cancer Lett., 134, 73.

137. Yang, C. S. 2001. Mechanisms of inhibition of chemical toxicity and carcinogenesis by dial-lyl sulfide (DAS) and related compounds from garlic. J. Nutr., 131, 1041S.

138. Jin, L., Baillie, T. A. 1997. Metabolism of the chemoprotective agent diallyl sulfide to glu-tathione conjugates in rats. Chem. Res. Toxicol., 10, 318.

139. Singh, S. V., Pan, S. S., Srivastava, S. K., et al. 1998. Differential induction of NAD(P)H:quinone oxidoreductase by anti-carcinogenic organosulfides from garlic. Biochem. Biophys. Res. Commun., 244, 917.

140. Rioux, N., Castonguay, A. 1998. Inhibitors of lipoxygenase: a new class of cancer chemopre-ventive agents. Carcinogenesis, 19, 1393.

141. Roy, P., Kulkarni, A. P. 1999. Co-oxidation of acrylonitrile by soybean lipoxygenase and par-tially purified human lung lipoxygenase. Xenobiotica, 29, 511.

142. Guyonnet, D., Belloir, C., Suschetet, M., et al. 2001. Antimutagenic activity of organosulfur compounds from Allium is associated with phase II enzyme induction. Mutat. Res., 495(1-2), 135.

143. Tadi, P. P., Lau, B. H., Teel, R. W., Herrmann, C. E. 1991. Binding of aflatoxin B1 to DNA inhibited by ajoene and diallyl sulfide. Anticancer Res., 11(6), 2037.

144. Baer, A. R., Wargovich, M. J. 1989. Role of ornithine decarboxylase in diallyl sulfide inhibition of colonic radiation injury in the mouse. Cancer Res., 49(18), 5073.

145. Dwivedi, C., Rohlfs, S., Jarvis, D., Engineer, F. N. 1992. Chemoprevention of chemically induced skin tumor development by dially sulfide and diallyl disulfide. Pharm. Res., 9(12), 1668.

146. Nakagawa, H., Tsuta, K., Kiuchi, K., et al. 2001. Growth inhibitory effects of diallyl disulfide on human breast cancer cell lines. Carcinogenesis, 22(6), 891.

147. Sundaram, S. G., Milner, J. A. 1996. Diallyl disulfide suppresses the growth of human colon tumor cell xenografts in athymic nude mice. J. Nutr., 126, 1355.

148. Saxe, T. G. 1987. Toxicity of medicinal herbal preparations. Am. Fam. Physician, 35, 135.

149. Haag, J. D., Gould, M. N. 1994. Mammary carcinoma regression induced by perillyl alcohol, a hydroxylated analog of limonene. Cancer Chemother. Pharmacol., 34, 477.

150. Phillips, L. R., Malspeis, L., Supko, J. G. 1995. Pharmacokinetics of active drug metabolites after oral administration of perillyl alcohol, an investigational antineoplastic agent, to the dog. Drug Metab. Dispos., 23, 676.

151. Zheng, G. Q., Zhang, J., Kenny, P. M., Lam, L. K. T. 1994. Stimulation of glutathione S-transferase and inhibition of carcinogenesis in mice by celery seed oil constituents. In *Food phytochemicals for cancer prevention I*. Huang, M., Osawa, T., Ho, C., Rossen, R. T. (eds.). American Chemical Society, Washington DC, 230.

152. Mills, J. J., Chari, R. S., Boyer, I. J., et al. 1995. Induction of apoptosis in liver tumors by the monoterpene perillyl alcohol. Cancer Res., 55, 979.

153. Morse, M. A., Toburen, A. L. 1996. Inhibition of metabolic activation of 4-(methylnitrosamine)-1-(3-pyridyl)-1-butanone by limonene. Cancer Lett., 104, 211.

154. Crowell, P. L., Gould, M. N. 1994. Chemoprevention and therapy of cancer by d-limonene. Crit. Rev. Oncogensis, 5, 1.

155. Elegbede, J. A., Elson, C. E., Tanner, M. A., et al. 1986. Regression of rat primary mammary tumors following dietary d-limonene. J. Natl. Cancer Inst., 76, 323.

156. Wattenberg, L. W., Sparnns, V. L., Barany, G. 1989. Inhibition of N-nitrosodiethylamine carcinogenesis in mice by naturally occurring organosulfur compounds and monoterpenes. Cancer Res., 49, 2689.

157. Crowell, P. J., Elson, C. E., Bailey, H. H., et al. 1994. Human metabolism of the experimental cancer therapeutic agent d-limonene. Cancer Chemother. Pharmacol., 35, 31.

158. Ruch, R. J., Sigler, K. 1994. Growth inhibition of rat liver epithelial tumor cells does not involve RAS plasma membrane association. Carcinogen., 15, 787.

159. Schulz, S., Buhling, F., Ansorge, S. 1994. Prenylated proteins and lymphocyte proliferation: inhibition by d-limonene and related monoterpenes. Eur. J. Immunol., 24, 301.

160. Hohl, R. J., Lewis, K. 1992. RAS expression in human leukemia is modulated differently by lovastatin and limonene. Blood, 80, 299a (Abstr.).

162. Gould, M. N. 1995. Prevention and therapy of mammary cancer by monoterpenes. J. Cell Biochem., 522, 139.

161. Shi, W., Gould, M. N. 2002. Induction of cytostasis in mammary carcinoma cells treated with the anticancer agent perillyl alcohol. Carcinogenesis, 23(1), 131.

163. Tanaka, T., Kawabata, K., Kakumoto, M., et al. 1998. Chemoprevention of 4-nitroquinoline 1-oxide-induced oral carcinogenesis by citrus auraptene in rats. Carcinogenesis, 19(3), 425.

12

Phytomedicines and Cancer Prevention

Piergiorgio Pietta

INTRODUCTION

To date some phytomedicines have been postulated to be potential cancer chemopreventive agents through their ability to prevent, inhibit, or reverse carcinogenesis. This ability is ascribed to the presence in these phytomedicines of specific chemical families, including polyphenols, polysaccharides, terpenes, and sulfur compounds, that may interfere with one or more of the mechanisms that are considered central to cancer promotion and progression (Wargovich et al. 2001; Ferguson 2001; Abdullaev 2002; Kucuk 2002).

These natural compounds may act by several ways, some of which are briefly described:

- Scavenging free radicals responsible (reactive oxygen species) for DNA mutations and genetic instability. Indeed, DNA alterations may induce abnormal gene expression that results in production of proteins involved in the transformation of healthy cells into cancer cells. Thus, errors in the p53 gene or in the Bax gene can produce proteins that fail to promote apoptosis in cells with damaged DNA. Similarly alterations in the Bcl-2 gene imply an overproduction of proteins capable of protecting malignant cells from apoptosis.
- Limiting the activity of proteins that mediate signal transduction from outside the cell toward the nucleus, such as protein tyrosine kinase (PTK), protein kinase C (PKC), and the ras proteins. Consequently, an abnormal activity of the transcription factors NF-κB (nuclear factor-kappa B) and AP-1 (activator protein 1) may be prevented, thereby devoiding cancer cells of proliferation and survival advantages.
- Inhibiting uncontrolled angiogenesis, that is, normalizing the synthesis or the activity of angiogenic factors, like the vascular endothelial growth factor (VEGF), eicosanoids from omega-6 fatty acids (PGE_2), the tumor necrosis factor (TNF), and histamine.
- Improving the immune function by activating cytotoxic T cells, macrophages, and natural killer (NK) cells and limit the ability of cancer cells to escape the immune defense.
- Inhibiting the formation/activation of carcinogens, preventing carcinogen-DNA binding, and deactivating/detoxifying carcinogens through modulation of cytochrome P450 and GSH/GST activities.
- Limiting polyamine synthesis (involved in one of the early events of cell proliferation) by inhibition of ornithine decarboxylase (ODC).

- Inhibiting hydroxymethylglutaryl-coenzyme A reductase (HMGR) and farnesyl protein transferase (FTPase) activities. Both enzymes are involved in the isoprenylation of ras and nuclear lamin proteins, which is required for cell proliferation. HMGR plays an initial role in the synthesis of all isoprenes, and FTPase catalyzes the attachment of farnesyl groups to ras and lamins to form the needed lipid tail.

REDUCING THE OXIDATIVE STRESS

Reactive oxgen species (ROS) play a primary role in promoting oxidative DNA damage. There may be as many as ten thousand oxidative hits to DNA per cell per day in the human body (Ames et al. 1993). Most of these lesions are repaired, but those remaining may progress toward abnormal gene expression.

In addition, a production of ROS overwhelming the body's antioxidant system (i.e., oxidative stress conditions) may promote cancer cell proliferation by increasing the sensitivity of growth factor receptors and kinases involved in signal transduction, and inducing the activity of NF-κB or decreasing the function of the p53 protein, that is, the guardian of the cell (Barouki and Morel 2001). For these reasons, inhibiting the excessive formation of ROS (as in the case of chronic inflammatory diseases) or scavenging them is essential to avoid persistent oxidative stress and reduce the risk of degenerative diseases, including cancer.

Antioxidant supplementation can play a preventative role in maintaining a "normal stress" status. However, to this end decreasing extracellular ROS production is a better strategy than increasing antioxidant reserves. Such a decrease can be accomplished by using:

- anti-inflammatory compounds, such as selective inhibitors of cyclooxygenase 2 (COX-2)
- compounds that chelate iron and copper, thereby reducing their levels
- compounds that prevent tissue damages, such as enzyme inhibitors and extracellular matrix protectors

Conversely, using antioxidants in cancer therapy remains a matter of much debate, and available data from in vitro and animal studies are somewhat conflicting.

Indeed, antioxidants may display a double-edged role, since they may decrease or increase cancer cell proliferation, or have limited effects on it, depending on the degree of the oxidative stress at the cancer site and on the antioxidant reserves of the individual. For example, highly oxidizing conditions in a subject with low antioxidant reserves limit cancer cell proliferation either by massive oxidative damage or by generation of lipid peroxides, which promote cancer cell death. In this case, an antioxidant supplementation (not to be confused with normal dietary intake) would increase cancer cell proliferation. On the other hand, normal to mild oxidative stress conditions combined with low antioxidant reserves will benefit from antioxidant supplementation. In this situation of ROS concentrations only moderately elevated (not sufficient to kill cancer cells), giving antioxidants should permit a shift from mild oxidative stress that can assist cancer proliferation to a normal stress status.

However, antioxidants may have other beneficial effects. They can help normal tissues function and protect them from adverse effects of chemotherapy. In addition, antioxidants can assist the immune system (which needs a certain amount of antioxidants) in inhibiting cancer.

In any case, when antioxidants are used, their effects should be maximized by including compounds that reduce ROS generation and that are anti-inflammatory agents, iron and copper chelators, and redox enzyme inhibitors; and possibly the antioxidants should be combined with compounds that inhibit cancer through nonantioxidant means. This is the case with various polyphenol-containing herbs (Pietta 2000; Kimata et al. 2000; Ross and Kasum 2002).

Indeed, phenolic compounds, and particularly flavonoids, are capable of inhibiting cancer cells through multiple means. These include:

1. reduction or inhibition of DNA oxidative damage
2. modulation of enzymes involved in the metabolism and detoxification of carcinogens
3. inhibition of kinases (PTK, PKC) involved in signal transduction, and responsible for proliferation, cell migration, angiogenesis, and reduced apoptosis
4. protection of p53 protein (a cysteine-containing protein sensitive to oxidants), thus preserving DNA repair and/or initiation of apoptosis
5. inhibition of transcriptor factors NF-κB and AP-1 required for proliferation, angiogenesis, and invasion
6. induction of p21 or p27 activity, which means reducing proliferation while maintaining DNA repair
7. reduction of detrimental eicosanoid synthesis, such as PGE_2 (COX-2 assisted), LTA_4 and 5-HETE (all derived from omega-6 PUFAs)
8. inhibition of hyaluronidase, beta-glucuronidase, elastase, and collagenase, which affect vascular permeability and extracellular matrix integrity
9. inhibition of histamine release from mast cells (i.e., reduction of vascular permeability and angiogenesis)
10. enhancement of the immune system by protecting immune cells against oxidative damages

Polyphenols Regarded as Preventive or Supportive Agents

A number of polyphenols are considered to be preventive or supportive agents. They are listed here with pertinent sources.

Anthocyanins: *Vaccinium myrtillus* and different fruits (Skrede and Wrolstad 2002; Liu et al. 2002)
Apigenin: various vegetables and herbs (Pietta 1998; Ross and Kasum 2002)
Baicalin: *Scutellaria baicalensis* (Park et al. 1998; Chang et al. 2002)
Caffeic acid esters and galangin: propolis(Banskota et al. 2001; Heo et al. 2001)
Curcumin: *Curcuma longa*(Wargovich et al. 2001; Holy 2002)

Epigallocatechingallate: green tea(Wargovich et al. 2001; Morris 2002)

Genistein: soybeans (Chang 2002)

Emodin: *Aloe* spp, *Poligonum cuspidatum* (Pecere et al. 2000; Lee et al. 2001)

Luteolin: various vegetables and herbs (Pietta 1998; Ross and Kasum 2002)

Proanthocyanidins: tea, chocolate, grapes, and herbs (Skrede and Wrolstad 2002; Bagchi et al. 2002)

Quercetin: various vegetables and herbs (Pietta 1998; Ross and Kasum 2002)

Resveratrol: wines and some herbs (Fremont 2000; Kimura and Okuda 2001)

Silymarin: *Silybum marianum* (Bathia and Agarwal 2001)

DOWN-REGULATING TRANSCRIPTOR FACTORS THROUGH INHIBITION OF PROTEIN TYROSINE KINASE AND PROTEIN KINASE C

The transcription factors p53, NF-κB, and AP-1 have an important role in the proliferation of both healthy and cancer cells. Cancer cells rely on low p53 protein activity and abnormally high NF-κB and AP-1 activity. Different compounds provided by some herbs may help in normalizing both of the last factors, whose activation may be down-regulated by inhibiting two important proteins involved in signal transduction, namely protein tyrosine kinase (PTK) and protein kinase C (PKC).

Several studies lend support for the inhibition of these kinases by the flavones apigenin and luteolin, curcumin, caffeic acid phenyl ethyl ester (CAPE), epigallocatechingallate (EGCG), genistein, hypericin, parthenolide, quercetin, proanthocyanidins, resveratrol, and emodin (Surh et al. 2000; Kapadia et al. 2002; Kobayashi et al. 2002). The chemopreventive properties of these compounds and related herbs may be ascribed to their ability to inhibit ATP-kinases interactions, which are needed for the activation of these kinases (Akiyama et al. 1987), resulting therefore in suppressed activity of transcriptor factors NF-κB and AP-1.

Concerning apoptosis, a variety of herbal extracts have been investigated for their ability to influence it. Apoptosis—the programmed cell death—is a highly conserved mechanism of self-defense, also found to occur in plants. Hence, plants should have chemicals that regulate this process in them, and these chemicals could act as apoptotic agents also in humans. The ability of herbs to influence programmed cell death in cancerous cells in an attempt to arrest their proliferation has been investigated on various cell lines like HL-60, human hepatocellular carcinoma cell line (KIM-1), HeLa cells, human lymphoid leukemia (MOLT-4B) cells, and others. Extracts or isolated compounds from *Allium sativum, Semicarpus anacardium, Trichosanthes kirilowii,* var. *japonica, Viscum album* (Thatte et al. 2000; Borek 2001; Hu et al. 2002; Kwon et al. 2002), propolis, *Curcuma longa* (Chandouri et al. 2002), *Aloe* (Furukawa et al. 2002), *Glycyrrhiza glabra* (Ma et al. 2001), *Silybum marianum* (Dhanalakshmi et al. 2002), and *Zingiber officinalis* have been found to induce apoptosis and therefore arrest proliferation. For example, caffeic acid phenyl ester (CAPE), an active component of propolis, was shown to arrest the growth of different tumor cells (Usia et al. 2002). CAPE was found to be the most active as an antiproliferative agent; benzyl and cinnamyl caffeates (also occurring in propolis), however, were less active (Banskota et al. 2002). CAPE was also found to induce apoptosis in human leukemic HL-60 cells through p53-dependent (Nomura et al. 2001) and p53-independent pathways (Chen et al., 2001b). According to Na et al. (2000), the anticancer mechanism of CAPE is partly mediated by its ability to restore gap junctional intercellular communication, whose deficiency has been shown to be a characteristic of most cancer cells. Other active compounds isolated from propolis include artepillin C, galangin, and PM-3. Artepillin C (3,5-diprenyl-4-hydroxycinnamic acid) induced marked apoptosis in various human leukemia cell lines in vitro; this effect may be partially associated with enhanced Fas antigen expression and loss of mitochondrial membrane potential (Kimoto et al. 2001). Interestingly, artepillin C was not cytocidal to normal lymphocytes. PM-3 (3-[2-dimethyl-8-(3-methyl-2-butenyl)benzopiranyl]-6-propenoic acid) isolated from Brazilian propolis markedly inhibited the growth of MCF-7 human breast cancer cells by multiple actions, including down-regulation of cyclin D1 and cyclin E proteins, both frequently overexpressed in human breast cancer cells, induction of apoptosis, and inhibition of estrogen response element (ERE) promoter activity (Luo et al. 2001). Overall, ethanolic extracts of propolis administered to male Wistar rats after treatment with the colon carcinogen 1,2-dimethylhydrazine exerted a protective influence on the process of colon carcinogenesis, suppressing the development of preneoplastic lesions (Bazo et al. 2002).

Curcumin from *Curcuma longa* was also found to inhibit tumor formation in animals (Min/+mice) bearing a germline mutation in the APC gene and spontaneously developing intestinal adenomas (adenomatous polyposis) by 15 weeks of age. Tumor prevention by curcumin was associated with increased enterocyte apoptosis and decreased expression of the oncoprotein beta-catenin in the enterocytes (Jaiswal et al. 2002). Together with curcumin, capsaicin, a pungent principle of *Capsicum annuum*, was reported to inhibit NF-κB and AP-1 activation in cultured human promyelocytic leukemia (HL-60) cells stimulated with the tumor promoter 12-O-tetradecanoylphorbol-13-acetate (Surh et al. 2000). The sesquiterpene zerumbone and the pungent vanilloids gingerol and paradol from *Zingiber officinalis* have been reported to suppress colonic adenocarcinoma cell lines and HL-60 cells by inducing apoptosis (Murakami et al. 2002; Lee and Surh 1998) .

Interestingly, the polyunsaturated fatty acid gamma-linolenic acid (GLA, C20:3, n-6), occurring in various herbs, such as *Enothera biennis, Ribes nigrum, Borago officinalis*, was found to induce apoptosis in B-cell chronic lymphocytic leukemia in vitro with minor effects on normal peripheral blood B and T cells (Mainou-Fowler et al. 2001).

The mechanisms by which the apoptosis is influenced are not clear. Likely endonuclease activation, induction of p53, and activation of caspase 3 protein via a Bcl-2-insensitive pathway are involved in the modulation of the apoptotic process (Thatte et al. 2000).

INHIBITING UNCONTROLLED ANGIOGENESIS

Like signal transduction, angiogenesis is a normal process, needed particularly during wound healing. Angiogenesis in cancer, however, is uncontrolled and ongoing. The body uses different factors to assure angiogenesis, including the vascular endothelial growth factor (VEGF), tumor necrosis factor (TNF), eicosanoids such as PGE_2 that derive from omega-6 fatty acids and histamine. These factors produce increased vascular permeability and/or inflammation, and are involved in tumor angiogenesis. A number of natural compounds may block the abnormal production or activity of these angiogenic factors. Thus, the production of VEGF by macrophages or other cells in response to growth factors (PDGF, EGF, and TNF) or hypoxia may be reduced by PTK/PKC inhibitors and leukotriene inhibitors. PTK/PKC inhibitors such as genistein (an isoflavone from soybean), curcumin (a polyphenol from *Curcuma longa*), EGCG (epigallocatechingallate from green tea), and caffeic acid phenethyl ester (CAPE from propolis) are able to reduce EGF and PDGF signaling in different cells, thereby limiting the production of VEGF, which means a lower degree of angiogenesis (Tang and Meydani 2001; Ross and Kasum 2002). In addition, PKC inhibitors may reduce angiogenesis by lowering the production of enzymes (i.e., collagenases) involved in tumor invasion or by decreasing histamine release. EGCG inhibits the binding of EGF to its receptors. Polysaccharide K (PSK), a high molecular-weight polysaccharide from *Coriolus versicolor* inhibits the binding of TGF-beta to its receptors (Matsunaga et al. 1998).

A second possible way to reduce VEGF-induced angiogenesis is to minimize vascular permeability, which is the primary effect of VEGF. *Centella asiatica,* horse chestnut, and butcher's broom are the herbs most suitable for normalizing vascular permeability. Other herbs containing anthocyanins (present in various berries, such as *Vaccinium myrtillus*) or proanthocyanidins occurring in grape seeds are reported as inhibitors of increased vascular permeability (Balentine et al. 1999).

Prostanoids (PGE_2) and leukotrienes (5-HETE) produced from omega-6 fatty acids (via the cyclooxygenase and lipoxygenase pathways, respectively) may mediate angiogenesis (Cuendet and Pezzuto 2000). Conversely, eicosanoids from omega-3 fatty acids are considered beneficial. Compounds reported to beneficially affect eicosanoid production include CAPE (Michaluart et al. 1999), curcumin (Goel et al. 2001), different flavonoids largely present in herbs (Pietta 1998; Chen 2001a), parthenolide (a sesquiterpene lactone from *Tanacetum parthenium*; Sumner et al. 1992), and resveratrol (a phytoalexin found in a variety of plants, including *Vitis vinifera* and *Polygonum cuspidatum*; Surh et al. 2001). Many of these compounds are in vitro inhibitors of COX-2, and hence of PGE_2 production. Reducing the intake of omega-6 fatty acids (common in most vegetable oils) and preferring the consumption of omega-3-rich sources (fish, algae, and various vegetable oils such as canola oil, flaxseed oil, rosa mosqueta oil, soybean oil, etc.) may also help cells use these fatty acids to make beneficial eicosanoids to the disadvantage of detrimental ones derived from omega-6 fatty acids (Das 2002).

Histamine released from mast cells in response to tissue injury is thought to increase vascular permeability and stimulate angiogenesis. Herbs used to treat allergies and asthma, which are diseases mediated by histamine release, may inhibit mast cell granulation, that is, the release of histamine from intracellular granules of mast cells (Lavens-Phillips et al. 1998).

Again, these herbs are characterized by the presence of various flavonoids, such as apigenin, luteolin, and quercetin, which are known to inhibit histamine release (Kimata et al. 2000).

IMPROVING THE IMMUNE FUNCTION

A large number of natural compounds can support the immune system. Thus, antioxidants like vitamins C and E and selenium as a crucial constituent of glutathione peroxidase may protect immune cells against an excess of reactive oxygen and nitrogen species. Besides antioxidants, various polysaccharides occurring in some mushrooms like *Astragalus membranaceous* (Mills and Bone 2000), *Ganoderma lucidum, Lentinus edodes*, and *Coriolus versicolor* (Wasser and Weis 1999; Ooi and Liu 2000) may exert immunostimulating effects. The mechanisms by which these effects are exerted are not clear. Likely these herbs and their extracts act in part by increasing production of immunostimulating cytokines (such as IL-1, IL-2, IL-6, interferons) and the responsiveness of cytokine receptors; and/or by decreasing the production or the activity of cytokines that suppress the immune system, like TGF-beta and IL-10. The resulting effect is increased proliferation and function of natural killer cells, macrophages, and T cells. For example, *Astragalus membranaceous* polysaccharides have been shown to enhance various types of immune responses, such as the production of IL-2 and gamma-interferon, and to improve the cytotoxicity of lymphokine-activated killer (LAK) cells from the impairment induced by carcinogens and/or anticancer agents (Kurashige et al. 1999). *Astragalus membranaceous* extracts increased also the in vitro toxicity of natural killer cells activated by low doses of IL-2, as a possible result of an improved binding of this cytokine to its receptors. As another example, oral administration of *Ganoderma lucidum* polysaccharides has been reported to increase the number of white blood cells in humans. This effect is ascribed to the increased production of IL-2 and interferon-gamma (Lu et al. 2002). A synergistic antimetastatic effect was seen when IL-2 was combined with lentinan (from *Lentinus edodes*) in mice. In humans, the polysaccharides PSK and PSP from the mushroom *Coriolus versicolor* was found to produce some beneficial effects, particularly in preventing recurrence after surgical removal of some tumors (Fukushima 1996).

INFLUENCING EITHER PHASE I OR PHASE II ENZYME ACTIVITIES

Modulating hepatic carcinogen-activating enzymes (e.g., CYP1A1, phase I) and/or inducing phase II detoxifying enzymes such as glutathione S-transferase and quinone reductase is a major mechanism for affording protection against reactive metabolic intermediates and carcinogens. Various polyphenols, including curcumin (*Curcuma longa*), genistein (*Glycine max*), epigallocatechingallate (*Camellia sinensis*; Sueoka et al. 2001), quercetin (occurring in numerous herbs) (Valerio et al. 2001), 8-prenyl-naringenin (*Humulus lupulus*; Henderson et al. 2000), and baicalin (*Scutellaria baicalensis*; Park et al. 1998), the organosulfur compounds from *Allium cepa* and *Allium sativum* (Munday and Munday 2001), the isoprenoids limonene and perillyl alcohol (Belanger 1998) have been proved to affect the activity of phase I and phase II enzymes, and can be viewed as potential means of chemoprevention. Galangin, a flavonol isolated from propolis and occurring in some herbs, like *Alpinia officinarum*, was also shown to modulate phase I and phase II enzyme activities, suppressing therefore the genotoxicity of chemicals (Heo et al. 2001).

LIMITING POLYAMINE SYNTHESIS

The polyamines putrescine, spermidine, and spermine are required for cell survival and their increased synthesis is thought to be one of the early events of cell proliferation. In fact, compounds that inhibit polyamine synthesis also prevent cancer cell proliferation. Polyamines are partly related to the S-adenosylmethionine (SAM) cycle in that SAM (apart from providing methyl groups for methylation of cytosine and other compounds) is also metabolized (about 1%) into polyamines. This step requires ornithine and ornithine decarboxylase (ODC) to produce the precursor polyamine, putrescine. Thus, ODC is a rate-limiting enzyme in polyamine synthesis, and its inhibition may limit cancer cell proliferation (Shantz and Pegg 1999). A number of polyphenolic compounds from some herbs already mentioned have been shown to inhibit ODC activity and reduce polyamine concentration in cancer cells. Interestingly, the ODC inhibition by the phenolics occurring in propolis (CAPE is the promoting agent), *Curcuma longa* (curcumin), *Glycine max* (genistein), *Camellia sinensis* (EGCG), and *Silybum marianum* (silymarin) is exerted together with other actions that promote a decrease in cancer proliferation. In addition to these phenolic compounds, geraniol (a monoterpene found in essential oils of fruits and herbs) caused a 50% decrease of ODC activity in a human colon cancer cell line (Caco-2), and also activated the intracellular catabolism of polyamines (Carnesecchi et al. 2001). Besides this effect on polyamines, individual isoprenoids and their blends were proved to suppress the proliferation of B16 and HL-60 promyelocytic leukemia cells with varying degrees of potency. The cell cycle arrest at the G(0)-G(1) phase and apoptosis accounted, at least partly, for the suppression (Shi and Gould 2002; Tatman and Mo 2002).

INHIBITING HYDROXYMETHYLGLUTARYL-COENZYME A REDUCTASE (HMGR) AND FARNESYL PROTEIN TRANSFERASE (FTPASE) ACTIVITIES

Hydroxymethylglutaryl-coenzyme A reductase (HMGR) and farnesyl protein transferase (FTPase) are involved in the isoprenylation of ras and nuclear lamin proteins, which is required for cell proliferation. HMGR plays an initial role in the synthesis of all isoprenes, including farnesylpyrophosphate; FTPase catalyzes the attachment of farnesyl groups to ras proteins and nuclear lamin proteins, thus providing them with the lipid tail needed for cell proliferation. The function of all isoprenylated proteins may be reduced by decreasing the synthesis of farnesylpyrophosphate (by inhibition of HMGR) and its attachment to the inactive proteins (by inhibition of FTPase). Isoprenoids, a broad class of mevalonate-derived phytochemicals largely diffused in herbs, are capable to inhibit both these enzymes. Thus, the monoterpenes limonene (occurring in various essential oils, particularly in oils of lemon, orange, mandarin, caraway, and parsley) and perillyl alcohol (a hydroxylated analogue of limonene from the essential oils of lavender, peppermint, spearmint, etc.) have been shown to inhibit HMGR activity at concentrations lower than 1 mM, and to reduce also protein farnesylation at higher concentrations (Elson et al. 1999).

In addition to terpenes, sulfur-containing compounds from *Allium sativum* have been proved to reduce HMGR activity in human cancer cells in vitro as well as in both liver and tumor tissue in vivo in mice (Gebhardt and Beck 1996).

CONCLUSIONS

Most evidence on the inhibitory effects has been attained by in vitro studies, that is, at concentrations higher than those normally achievable in the body. Nevertheless, the results are encouraging and endorse a possible role of selected polyphenols, organosulfur compounds, terpenes, polysaccharides, and related herbs in preventing or retarding the multistage process of carcinogenesis and impeding tumor progression.

ACKNOWLEDGMENT

This work was supported by a grant from the National Council of Research, Italy.

REFERENCES

Abdullaev, FI. 2002. Cancer chemopreventive and tumoricidal properties of saffron (*Crocus sativus L.*). *Exp Biol Med(Maywood)* 227(1):20–5.

Akiyama, T, J Ishida, S Nakagawa. 1987. Genistein, a specific inhibitor of tyrosine-specific protein kinases. *J Biol Chem* 262(12):5592–5.

Ames, BN, MK Shigenaga, TM Hagen. 1993. Oxidants, antioxidants and the degenerative diseases of aging. *Proc Natl Acad Sci USA* 90(9):7915–22.

Bagchi, D, M Bagchi, SJ Stohs, SR Ray, CK Sen, HG Preuss. 2002. Cellular protection with proanthocyanidins derived from grape seeds. *Ann NY Acad Sci* 957(5):260–70.

Balentine, DA, MC Albano, and MG Nair, 1999 . Role of medicinal plants , herbs, and spices in protecting human health. *Nutr Rev* 57:S41–S45 .

Banskota, AH, T Nagaoka, LY Sumioka, Y Tezuka, S Awale, K Midorikawa, K Matsushige, S Kadota. 2002. Antiproliferative activity of the Netherlands propolis and its active principles in cancer lines. *J Ethnopharmacol* 80(1):67–73.

Banskota, AH, Y Tezuka, S Kadota. 2001. Recent progress in pharmacological properties of propolis. *Phytother Res* 15:561–71.

Barouki, R, Y Morel. 2001. Oxidative stress and gene expression. *J Soc Biol* 195(4):377–82.

Bathia, N, R Agarwal. 2001. Detrimental effect of cancer preventive phytochemicals silymarin, genistein and epigallocatechingallate on epigenetic events in human prostate carcinoma DU 145 cells. *Prostate* 46(2):98–107.

Bazo, AP, MA Rodrigues, JM Sforcin, JL de Camargo, LR Ribeiro, DM Salvadori. 2002. Protective action of propolis on the rat carcinogenesis. *Teratog Carcinog Mutagen* 22(3):183–94.

Belanger, JT. 1998. Perillyl alcohol: applications in oncology. *Alter Med Rev* 3(6)448–57.

Borek, C. 2001. Antioxidant health effects of aged garlic extracts. *J Nutr* 131(3):1010S–15S.

Carnesecchi, S, Y Schneider, J Ceraline, B Duranton, F Gosse, N Seiler, F Raul. 2001. Geraniol, a component of plant essential oils, inhibits growth and polyamine synthesis in human colon cancer cells. *J Pharmacol Exp Ther* 298(1):197–200.

Chandouri, T, S Pal, ML Agarwal, T Das, G Sa. 2002. Curcumin induces apoptosis in human breast cancer cells through p53-dependent Bax induction. *FEBS Lett* 512(1–3):334–40.

Chang, SKC. 2002. Isoflavones from soybeans and soy foods. In *Functional Foods-Biochemical and Processing Aspects*, edited by J Shi, G Mazza, M Le Maguer, pp. 39–70. Boca Raton: CRC Press.

Chang, WH, CH Chen, FJ Lu. 2002. Different effects of baicalin, baicalein, wogonin on mithochondrial function, glutathione content and cell cycle progression in human hepatoma cell lines. *Planta Med* 68(2):128–32.

Chen, YC, SC Chen, WR Lee, WC Hou, LL Yang, TJ Lee. 2001a. Inhibition of cyclooxygenase-2-gene expression by rutin, quercetin, and quercetin pentaacetate in RAW 264.7 macrophages. *J Cell Biochem* 82(4):537–48.

Chen, YJ, MS Shiao, SY Wang. 2001b. The antioxidant caffeic acid phenethyl ester induces apoptosis associated with selective scavenging of hydrogen peroxide in human leukemic HL-60 cells. *Anticancer Drugs* 12(2): 143–9.

Cuendet, M, JM Pezzuto. 2000. The role of cyclooxygenase and lipoxygenase in cancer chemoprevention. *Drug Metab Drug Interact* 17(1-4):109.57.

Das, U. 2002. A radical approach to cancer. *Med Sci Monit* 8(4):RA79–92.

Dhanalakshmi, S, RP Singh, C Agarwal, R Agarwal. 2002. Silibinin inhibits constitutive and TNF alpha-induced activation of NF-κB and sensitizes human prostate carcinoma DU 145 cells to TNF alpha-induced apoptosis. *Oncogene* 21(11):1759–67.

Elson, CE, DM Peffley, P Hentosh, H Mo. 1999. Isoprenoid-mediated inhibition of mevalonate synthesis: potential application to cancer. *Proc Soc Exp Biol Med* 2221(4):294–311.

Ferguson, LR. 2001. Role of plant polyphenolics in genomic stability. *Mutat Res* 475:89–111.

Fremont, L. 2000. Biological effects of resveratrol. *Life Sci* 66(8):663–73.

Fukushima, M. 1996. Adjuvant therapy of gastric cancer: The Japanese experience. *Semin Oncol* 23(3):369–78.

Furukawa, F, A Nishikawa, T Chihaza, K Shimpo, H Beppu, H Kuruya, IS Lee, M Hirose. 2002. Chemopreventive effects of Aloe arborescens on N-nitrosbis(2-oxopropyl)amine-induced pancreatic carcinogenesis in hamsters. *Cancer Lett* 178(2):117–22.

Gebhardt, R, H Beck. 1996. Differential inhibitory effects of garlic-derived organosulfur compounds on cholesterol biosynthesis in primary rat hepatocyte cultures. *Lipids* 31(12):1269–76.

Goel, A, CR Boland, DP Chanhan. 2001. Specific inhibition of cyclooxygenase-2 expression by dietary curcumin in HT-29 human colon cancer cells. *Cancer Lett* 172(2):111–8.

Henderson, MC, CL Miranda, JF Stevens, ML Deinzer, DR Buhler. 2000. In vitro inhibition of human P450 enzymes by prenylated flavonoids from hops, *Humulus lupulus. Xenobiotica* 30(3):235–51.

Heo, MY, SJ Sohn, WW Au. 2001. Anti-genotoxicity of galangin as a cancer chemopreventive candidate. *Mutat Res* 488(2):135–50.

Holy, JM. 2002. Curcumin disrupts mitotic spindle structure and induces micronucleation in MCF-7 breast cancer cells. *Mutat Res* 518(1):71–84.

Hu, X, BN Cao, G Hu, DQ Yang, YS Wan. 2002. Attenuation of cell migration and induction of apoptosis by aged garlic extract in rat sarcoma cells. *Int J Mol Med* 9(6):641–3.

Jaiswal, AS, BP Marlow, N Gupta, S Narayan. 2002. beta-Catenin-mediated transactivation and cell-cell adhesion pathways are important in curcumin (diferuylmethane)-induced growth arrest and apoptosis in colon cancer cells. *Oncogene* 21 (55):8414–27.

Kapadia, GI, MA Azuine, H Tokuda, E Hang, T Mukainaka, H Nishino, R Srdhar. 2002. Inhibitory effect of herbal remedies on TPA-promoted Epstein-Barr virus early antigen activation. *Pharmacol Res* 45(3):231–20.

Kimata, M, N Inagaki, H Nagai. 2000. Effects of luteolin and other flavonoids on IgE-mediated allergic reactions. *Planta Med* 66(1):25–9.

Kimoto, T, M Aga, K Hino, S Koya-Miyata, Y Yamamoto, MJ Micallef, T Hanaya, S Arai, M Ikeda, M Kurimoto. 2001. *Anticancer Res* 21(1A):221–8.

Kimura, Y, H Okuda. 2001. Resveratrol isolated from *Polygonum cuspidatum* root prevents tumor growth and metastasis to lung and tumor-induced neovascularization in Lewis lung carcinoma-bearing mice. *J Nutr* 131(6):1844–9.

Kobayashi, T, T Nakata, T Kurumaki. 2002. Effects of flavonoids on cell cycle progression in prostate cancer cells. *Cancer Lett* 176(1):17–23.

Kucuk, O. 2002. New opportunities in chemoprevention research. *Cancer Invest* 20(2)237–45.

Kurashige, S, Y Akurawa, F Endo. 1999. Effects of astragali radix extract on carcinogenesis, cytokine production and cytotoxicity in mice treated with a carcinogen N-butyl-N'-butanolni-trosamine. *Cancer Invest* 17(1): 30–35.

Kwon, KB, SJ Yoo, DG Ryu, JY Yang, HW Rho, JS Kim, JW Park, HR Kim, BH Park. 2002. Induction of apoptosis by diallyl sulfide through activation of caspase-3 in human leukemia cells. *Biochem Pharmacol* 63(1):41–7.

Lavens-Phillips, SE, EH Mockford, JA Warner. 1998. The effect of tyrosine kinase inhibitors on IgE-mediated histamine release from human lung mast cells and basophiles. *Inflamm Res* 47(3):137–143.

Lee, E, YJ Suhr. 1998. Induction of apoptosis in HL-60 cells by pungent vanilloids, [6]-gingerol and [6]-paradol. *Cancer Lett* 80(1-2):163–8.

Lee, HZ, SL K Hsu. MC Liu, CH Wu. 2001. Effects and mechanisms of aloe-emodin on cell death in human lung squamous cell carcinoma. *Eur J Pharmacol* 431(3):287–95.

Liu, M, XQ Li, C Weber, CY Lee, J Brown, RH Liu. 2002. Antioxidant and antiproliferative activities of raspberries. *J Agric Food Chem* 50(10):2926–30.

Lu, H, E Kyo, T Uesaka, O Katoh, H Watanabe. 2002. Prevention of development of N,N'-dimethyl-hydrazine-induced colon tumors by a water-soluble extract of *Ganoderma lucidum* in male ICR mice. *Int J Mol Med* 9(2):113–7.

Luo, J, JW Soh, WQ Xing, Y Mao, T Matsuno, IB Weinstein. 2001. PM-3, a benzo-gamma-pyran-derivative isolated from propolis, inhibits growth of MC-7 human breast cancer cells. *Anticancer Res* 21(3B):1665–71.

Ma, J, NY Fu, DB Bang, WY Wu, AL Xu. 2001. Apoptosis induced by isoliquiritigenin in human gastric cancer MGC-803 cells. *Planta Med* 67(11):754–7.

Mainou-Fowler, T, SJ Proctor, AM Dickinson. 2001. Gamma-linolenic acid induces apoptosis in B-chronic lymphocytic leukemia cells in vitro. *Leuk Lymphoma* 40(3):393–403.

Margovich, MJ, C Woods, DM Hollis, ME Zander. 2001. Herbals, cancer prevention and health. *J Nutr* 131(11):3034S–6S.

Matsunaga, K, A Hosokawa, M Oohara. 1998. Direct action of a protein-bound polysaccharide, PSK, on transforming growth factor-beta. *Immunopharmacol* 40(11):219–30.

Michaluart, P, JL Masferrer, AJ Dannengerg. 1999. Inhibitory effects of CAPE on the activity and expression of cyclooxygenase-2 in human oral epithelial cells and in a rat model of inflammation. *Cancer Res* 59(10):2347–52.

Mills, S, K Bone. 2000. *Principles and practice of phytotherapy*. Edinburgh: Churchill Livingstone.

Morris, K. 2002. Tea chemicals confirmed as cancer-busting compounds. *Lancet Oncol* 3(5):262.

Munday, R, CM Munday. 2001. Relative activities of organosulfur compounds derived from onions and garlic in increasing tissue activities of quinone reductase and glutathione transferase in rat tissues. *Nutr Canc* 40(2):205–10.

Murakami, A, D Takahashi, T Kinoshita, K Koshizumi, HW Kim, A Yoshikiro, Y Nakamura, S Jiwajinda, J Terao, H Ohigashi. 2002. Zerumbone, a Southeast Asian ginger sesquiterpene, markedly suppressed free radical generation, proinflammatory protein production, and cancer cell proliferation accompanied by apoptosis: the alpha, beta-unsaturated carbonyl group is a pre-requisite. *Carcinogenesis* 23(5):795–802.

Na, HK, MR Wilson, KS Kang, CC Chang. 2000. Restoration of gap junctional intercellular communication by caffeic acid phenethyl ester in a ras-transformed rat liver epithelial cell line. *Cancer Lett* 157(1):31–8.

Nomura, M, A Kaji, W Ma, K Miyamoto. 2001. Suppression of cell transformation and induction of apoptosis by caffeic acid phenethyl ester. *Mol Carcinog* 31(2): 83–9.

Ooi, VE, F Liu. 2000. Immunomodulation and anticancer activity of polysaccharide-protein complexes. *Curr Med Chem* 7(7):715–29.

Park, HI, YW Lee, HH Park, IB Kwon, JH Hu.1998. Induction of quinone reductase by a methanol extract of *Scutellaria baicalensis* and its flavonoids in murine Hepa 1c1c7 cells. *Eur J Cancer Prev* 7:467–71.

Pecere, T, V Gazzola, C Mucignat, C Parolin, F Dalla Vecchia, A Cavaggioni, G Basso, A Diaspro, B Salvato, M Carli, G Palù. 2000. Aloe-emodin is a new type of anticancer agent with selective activity against neuroectodermal tumors. *Cancer Res* 60(1):2800–2804.

Pietta, P. 2000. Flavonoids as antioxidants. *J Nat Prod* 63(7):1035–42.

Pietta, P. 1998. "Flavonoids in Medicinal Plants". In *Flavonoids in health and disease*, edited by CA Rice-Evans, L Packer, pp. 61–110. New York: Marcel Dekker, inc.

Ross, JA, CM Kasum. 2002. Dietary flavonoids: Bioavailability, metabolic effects and safety. *Annu Rev Nutr* 22:19–34.

Shantz, LM, AE Pegg. 1999. Translational regulation of ornithine decarboxylase and other enzymes of the polyamine pathway. *Int J Biochem Cell Biol* 31(1):107–22.

Shi, W, MN Gould. 2002. Induction of cytostasis in mammary carcinoma cells treated with the anticancer agent perillyl alcohol. *Carcinogenesis* 23(1):131–42.

Skrede, G, RE Wrolstad. 2002. Flavonoids from berries and grapes. In *Functional Foods-Biochemical and Processing Aspects*, edited by J Shi, G Mazza, M Le Maguer, pp 71–134. Boca Raton: CRC Press.

Sueoka, N, N Sugunama, E Sueoka, S Okabe, S Matsuyama, K Imai, K Nakachi, H Fujiki. 2001. A new function of green tea: prevention of life-style related diseases. *Ann NY Acad Sci* 28(4):274–80.

Sumner, H, U Salan, DW Knight, JR Hoult. 1992. Inhibition of 5-lipoxygenase and cyclooxygenase in leukocytes by feverfew. Involvement of sesquiterpene lactones and other compounds. *Biochem Pharmacol* 43(11):2313–20.

Surh, YJ, KS Chun, HH Cha, SS Han, YS Keum, KK Park, SS Lee. 2001. Molecular mechanisms underlaying chemopreventive activities of anti-inflammatory phytochemicals: down-regulation of COX-2 and iNOS through suppression of NF-κB activation. *Mutat Res* 480–481:243–68.

Surh, YJ, SS Han, YS Keum, HJ Seo, SS Lee. 2000. Inhibitory effect of curcumin and capsaicin on phorbol ester-induced activation of eukaryotic transcription factors, NF-kappaB and AP-1. *Biofactors* 12(1-4)107–12.

Tang, FY, M Meydani. 2001. Green tea catechins and vitamin E inhibit angiogenesis of human microvascular endothelial cells through suppression of IL-8 production. *Nutr Cancer* 41(1–2):119–25.

Tatman, D, H Mo. 2002. Volatile isoprenoids of fruits, vegetables and herbs cumulatively suppress the proliferation of murine B16 melanoma and human HL-60 leukemia cells. *Cancer Lett* 175(2):129–39.

Thatte, U, S Bagadez, S Dahanukar. 2000. Modulation of programmed cell death by medicinal plants. *Cell Mol Biol* 46(1):199–214.

Usia, T, AH Banskota, Y Tezuka. 2002. Constituents of Chinese propolis and their antiproliferative activities. *J Nat Prod* 65(5):673–6.

Valerio, LG, JK Kepa, GV Pickwell, LC Quattrochi. 2001. Induction of human NADPH: quinone reductase (NQO1) gene expression by the flavonol quercetin. *Toxicol Lett* 119:49–57.

Wargovich, MJ, C Woods, DM Hollis, ME Zander. 2001. Herbals, cancer and health. *J Nutr* 131(11S):3034S–6S.

Wasser, SP, AL Weis. 1999. Therapeutic effects of substances occurring in higher Basidiomycetes mushrooms. *Crit Rev Immunol* 19(11):65–96.

13

Phytoestrogens and Cancer

Ruth S. MacDonald,
Ju-yuan Guo,
Mary Sharl Sakla,
Nader Shenouda, and
Dennis B. Lubahn

Several families of compounds found in plants are structurally related to the mammalian hormone estrogen. The most common phytoestrogens in the human diet are shown in Table 13.1. The primary dietary forms of phytoestrogens are derived from the isoflavones, coumestins, lignans, and flavonoids. Additional compounds such as curcumin, resveratrol, and epigallocatechin gallate (EGCG) may also be considered phytoestrogens.

Isoflavones are diphenolic phytoestrogens present in high concentrations in legumes and clover, with soybeans being the main dietary source. In plants, the primary isoflavones genistin, daidzin, and glycetin, are present primarily in the glucoside form and undergo deglycosylation prior to absorption (aglycones are genistein, daidzein, and glycetein).

Coumestins are structurally similar to the isoflavones and are consumed by humans in refried and pinto beans and in alfalfa and soybean sprouts. The most abundant source of coumestins is animal fodder such as alfalfa. Lignans are polyphenols that are widely distributed in fruits, vegetables, and grains, with flaxseed and oil seeds providing the most abundant dietary sources. The lignan precursors matairesinol and secoisolariciresinol are metabolized by intestinal microflora to the weak estrogens enterolactone and enterodiol. Flavonoids, including quercetin, kaempferol, and apigenin, are present in fruits and vegetables, and black and green tea. Berries are also a dietary source of the flavonoid myricetin. Curcumin is present in the spice turmeric, resveratrol is found in grapes and red wine, and EGCG is primarily consumed in tea. In the 1980s phytoestrogens derived from lignans were detected and identified in human urine (Adlercreutz et al. 1982). It was quickly recognized that these compounds were excreted in higher concentrations by vegetarians than omnivores (Adlercreutz et al. 1986) and may be among the factors responsible for the lower incidence of cancer in vegetarian populations (Setchell et al. 1981).

Phytoestrogens may influence cancer via their estrogenic properties. The estrogenic activity of the phytoestrogens is derived from the ability of these compounds to bind to the estrogen receptor (ER). In general, the phytoestrogens bind to ER with a low affinity compared to 17β-estradiol. However, due to the high concentration of phytoestrogens in foods, significant biological responses to these compounds may be achieved. The binding affinity of many phytoestrogens to the rat uterine cytosolic ER has recently been reported

213

Table 13.1.   Phytoestrogen Families, Dietary Sources, and Estrogen Receptor Interaction

Phytoestrogens	Common dietary source	Estrogen receptor binding
Flavones		
Apigenin	Fruits, vegetables	Low[1]
Kaempferol	Green tea	Low[1,2]
Myricetin	Berries, green tea	Moderate[1]
Baicalein	*Sutellaria baicalensis*	Moderate[1]
Quercetin	Green tea, onions	Very low[1,2]
Isoflavones		
Genistein	Soy, peas, and lentils	High[1,2]
Daidzein	Soy, peas, and lentils	Moderate[1,2]
Biochanin A	Soy, peas, and lentils	Moderate[1,2]
Coumarins		
Coumestrol	Refried beans, pinto beans, sprouts	High[1,2]
Lignans		
Matairesinol[6]	Grains, fruits, vegetables	Moderate[5]
Secoisolariciresinol[6]	Grains, fruits, vegetables	Moderate[5]
Curcuminoids		
Curcumin	Tumeric	Moderate[3,4]
Stilbenes		
Resveratrol	Grapes, red wine	Very low[3]
Catechins		
Epigallocatechin gallate	Green tea	Low[3]

[1] Branham et al. 2002.
[2] Kuiper et al. 1998.
[3] Shenouda, N., unpublished data.
[4] Miksicek 1994.
[5] Adlercreutz et al. 2002.
[6] These compounds are metabolized in humans to enterolactone and enterodiol. The estrogen binding potential refers to these metabolites.

(Branham et al. 2002) and the relative binding ability of some are listed in Table 13.1. It has been proposed that the most critical structural feature for estrogenic activity is the diaryl ring structure that is common to all flavonoids and a minimum of one hydroxyl group on each of the aromatic rings (Miksicek 1994). Currently, two types of estrogen receptors have been identified, alpha (ERα) and beta (ERβ). Most tissues express both forms of the estrogen receptor, including the rat prostate, breast, and colon (Kuiper et al. 1998). However, based on the observation that ERβ knockout female mice developed mammary glands with normal ductal structures that were indistinguishable from those of age-matched wild-type females (Couse et al. 2000), ERβ does not seem to have an important role in the mammary gland. Most phytoestrogens were found to have a higher affinity for ERβ than ERα with coumestrol demonstrating a higher binding affinity than 17β-estradiol for ERβ (Kuiper et al. 1998). Genistein, apigenin, naringenin, and kaempferol were also found to compete more strongly for ERβ than ERα binding. The cellular response of phytoestrogen binding to either ERα or ERβ has not been well defined, and there is evidence for both agonist and antagonist activity. It has been demonstrated that the response to phytoestrogens is tissue and cell specific and dependent upon concentration of the phytoestrogen. An example of the concentration effect is shown in human breast cancer cell lines, in which genistein produced a biphasic effect on cell proliferation (Dampier et al. 2001)—stimulatory at low concentrations and inhibitory at high concentrations.

In addition to having estrogenic activity, phytoestrogens influence other aspects of cellular metabolism, which may also contribute to cancer prevention. Some potential mechanisms are shown in Figure 13.1. Genistein, for example, is a potent inhibitor of tyrosine

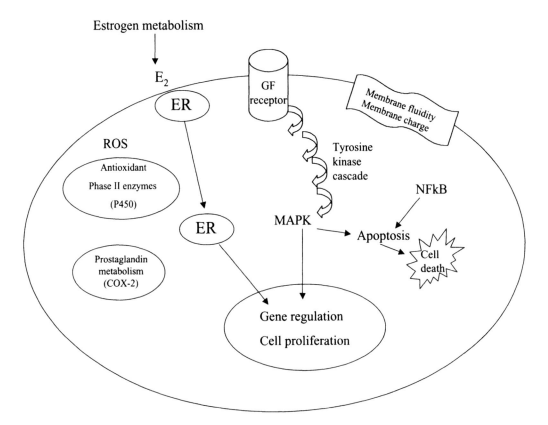

Figure 13.1.   Proposed cellular mechanisms of action of phytoestrogens in hormone-responsive cancers. These pathways are influenced by phytoestrogenic compounds. Taking part in the mechanism are E$_2$, estradiol; ER, estrogen receptor; ROS, reactive oxygen species; GF, growth factor; MAPK, mitogen activated protein kinase; NF-κB, necrosis factor kappa beta; COX-2, cyclooxygenase-2.

kinases both in vitro (Akiyama et al. 1987) and in vivo (Dalu et al. 1998). Genistein induces DNA damage, supposedly through inhibition of topoisomerase II activity (Okura et al. 1988). Such DNA damage may lead to activation of apoptosis through a number of mechanisms, such as increased p53 activation (Fields and Jang, 1990). Many flavonoids are also potent inhibitors of aromatase, 17β-hydroxysteroid dehydrogenase, and other steroid hormone metabolizing enzymes (Kirk et al. 2001). Coumestrol and apigenin are the most potent inhibitors of 17β-hydroxysteroid dehydrogenase, which converts estradiol to the less-active form estrone. Furthermore, many of the phytoestrogens inhibit phenol sulphotransferase, which acts as a secondary enzyme system for estrogen sulphation. And as shown in Figure 13.1, phytoestrogens affect intracellular signaling systems that mediate cell proliferation and apoptosis. These systems include growth factors that activate tyrosine kinases including MAPK. Activated MAPK regulates gene transcription and apoptosis. The estrogen receptor pathway is induced by phytoestrogens, leading to regulation of gene expression. Because many phytoestrogens are also antioxidants, they influence the development of reactive oxygen species (ROS) and the phase II enzymes. There is also evidence that phytoestrogens affect prostaglandin metabolism, including cycolooxygenases (e.g. COX-2), and membrane characteristics. These aspects are discussed in further detail in the following paragraphs.

Hormone-responsive cancers, including breast and prostate, are highly influenced by estrogens. The risk of breast cancer is associated with lifelong estrogen exposure (Kampert et al. 1988), and reducing estrogen is a primary chemotherapeutic approach to breast cancer management. Similarly, prostate cancer management involves suppression of androgens and estrogens (Steiner et al. 2001; Bosland 2000). Recent evidence suggests that colon cancer is also an estrogen-dependent cancer, however, estrogens appear to reduce colon cancer risk. Postmenopausal women using hormone replacement therapy had lower incidence of colon cancer than untreated women (Calle et al. 1995). This observation has been confirmed through a meta-analysis (Grodstein et al. 1999) and in the Women's Health Initiative (Writing Group for the Women's Health Initiative Investigators, 2002). In this review, the role of dietary phytoestrogens on these three hormone-related cancers will be discussed.

COLON CANCER

Colon cancer incidence is significantly lower in populations consuming plant-based diets compared to Western diets (Willett 2001). Early evidence suggested that the higher intake of dietary fiber provided the protective effect in these populations (Reddy 1999). Dietary fiber influences aspects of colon physiology, chemistry, and microbiology—any or all of which may be responsible for the observed protective response. The abundance of phytoestrogens in plant foods suggests another mechanism through which plant-based diets may reduce colon cancer risk. Colon cancer has not been considered to be hormonally responsive until recently. The rate of colon cancer tends to be lower in postmenopausal women than men of similar age, whereas the rate is similar in men and women less than 50 years of age (Potter et al. 1993). This suggests postmenopausal reduction in estrogen would be protective for colon cancer. A review of the literature found five studies in which estrogen replacement therapy (HRT) in postmenopausal women was correlated with colon cancer risk (Potter et al. 1993). Three of the studies showed a reduced risk of colon cancer with hormone use, and none reported an increased risk. More recently, Kampman et al. (1997) reported an inverse association between HRT and colon cancer in older women. Hence, these results suggest replacement of estrogen reduces colon cancer risk, in opposition to the initial finding of reduced risk associated with loss of estrogen post menopause. It has been proposed that estradiol, the naturally occurring form of estrogen in premenopausal women, exerts a promotive effect on colon cancer, whereas estrone, a common estrogen used in HRT, has a protective effect (English et al. 1999). Normal colonic mucosal tissue actively converts estradiol to estrone, and a decrease in that activity occurs in colonic tumors. Estrone has a lower affinity for estrogen receptor binding than does estradiol, although it induces an estrogenic effect. These studies overall suggest that estrogen is a factor in colon cancer risk.

Normal human colon was found to express more ERβ than ERα mRNA (Campbell-Thompson et al. 2001; Foley et al. 2000). A significant loss of ERβ mRNA expression was observed in cancer tissue compared to normal. Similarly, ERβ mRNA was detected in many human colon cancer cell lines (Arai et al. 2000; Fiorelli et al. 1999b). Most of the cell lines were negative for ERα, except for the SW1116 cells that had low levels of ERα. Because of the higher affinity of phytoestrogens for ERβ than ERα, the higher expression of ERβ in the colon may provide a specific target tissue for these compounds.

Soy Isoflavones in Colon Cancer

The effect of soy isoflavones on colon cancer has been examined in animal models, but the results are not consistent. To examine if genistin or a mixture of genistin, daidzin, and glycitin (the three major isoflavone glucosides in soy) would inhibit colon tumor formation, rats were fed (a) defatted soy flour (containing isoflavones), (b) soy flakes (containing isoflavones), (c) soy concentrate (devoid of isoflavones), or (d) soy concentrate plus 150 mg genistein/kg (Thiagarajan et al. 1998). The rats were treated with azoxymethane and aberrant crypts were examined. Aberrant crypt foci are putative precancerous lesions, which can be observed in whole mounts of rat colon (McLellan and Bird 1991). Rats fed soy flour or flakes had fewer aberrant crypt foci than rats fed the soy concentrate devoid of isoflavones. However, the addition of genistein alone to the soy concentration decreased aberrant crypt foci by 50% compared to the soy concentrate. Using the Fisher F344 azoxymethane-treated animal model, diets containing 150 or 75 mg genistein/kg resulted in fewer aberrant crypt foci compared to the control (Pereira et al. 1994). This is similar to the protective effect of genistein observed by Thiagarajan et al. (1998).

In contrast, Fisher F344 rats fed diets containing 250 mg genistein/kg were found to have more colon tumors in response to the colon carcinogen azoxymethane than rats fed the control diet lacking isoflavones (Rao et al. 1997a). A lower activity of 15-prostaglandin dehydrogenase was observed in both normal and tumor tissue from the rats fed genistein. The authors speculate that inhibition of prostaglandin inactivating enzymes could contribute to the tumor-enhancing effect of genistein. Hence, in two studies (Thiagarajan et al. 1998; Pereira et al. 1994), diets containing 150 mg genistein/kg or less appeared to be protective of colon cancer in the same animal model where 250 mg genistein/kg increased colon tumors (Rao et al. 1997a). The studies demonstrating a protective effect measured only precancerous markers, which may not predict tumor outcome, however.

Davies et al. (1999) reported soy isoflavones did not reduce azoxymethane-induced aberrant crypt foci formation in the colon of male rats, nor the formation of colon tumors. In this study, rats were fed high fat (42% of energy) diets containing soy protein with or without isoflavones beginning at 6 weeks of age. An increase in the number of aberrant crypt foci occurred 12 weeks after azoxymethane treatment when the diet contained soy protein with 566 mg isoflavones/kg compared to a low isoflavone soy protein diet. After 31 weeks, rats fed the isoflavone-rich diet had a similar number of tumors as those fed the isoflavone-free control diet. In the same study, however, diets containing 30% rye, as a source of lignans, had significantly fewer colon tumors. The authors speculate that the protective response to rye lignans was due to a nonhormonal mechanism because of the lack or protection by the soy isoflavones.

The Apc^{min} mouse spontaneously develops intestinal tumors due to a nonsense mutation in the Apc gene, which is homologous to the defect commonly observed in human familial adenomatous polyposis coli (Sorensen et al. 1998). To examine the effect of soy isoflavones, Apc^{min} mice were fed from conception a high-risk diet with 20% of energy in animal fat and low in fiber and calcium containing soy protein isolates with either high (280 mg genistein/kg) or low (11.5 mg genistein/kg) levels of isoflavones. When the mice were terminated at 107 days of age, no difference in tumor incidence due to the isoflavone content of the diet was observed.

The evidence that phytoestrogens reduce colon tumor cell growth is much stronger in vitro. The growth of several intestinal cancer cell lines was inhibited by genistein and biochanin A, but diadzein was much less effective (Yanagihara et al. 1993). Genistein and biochanin A induced apoptosis in the cell lines as demonstrated by DNA laddering. Similar inhibition of cell proliferation and induction of apoptosis by genistein was observed in SW620 and HT-29 human colon tumor cells (Booth et al. 1999), but biochanin A was less effective in these cells. The growth of Caco-2 and HT-29 cells was significantly inhibited by genistein, daidzein, kaempferol, naringenin, biochanin A and quercetin (Kuo 1996). The effective concentrations of the compounds ranged from 30 to 90 µM. These compounds also inhibited growth of IEC-6 (Kuo 1996; Booth et al. 1999) and IEC-18 (Booth et al. 1999) cells, which are considered to be nontransformed cells derived from fetal rat intestine. The author was unable to assign specific chemical characteristics of the compounds to explain the antiproliferative effects. Inhibition of HT-29 cell growth with G2/M arrest and induction of apoptosis was also observed with 60–100 µM genistein (Salti et al. 2000). However, when incubated at low concentrations (1–2 µM) genistein induced cell proliferation. This observation was not corroborated however by Arai et al. (2000), who observed no change in cell proliferation of five colon cancer cell lines when incubated with 1 µM genistein. The higher concentrations of genistein induced DNA damage, which suggested the target for genistein was inhibition of topoisomerase IIβ (Salti et al. 2000). Similarly, genistein and genistin (glycoside form) directly induced DNA strand breaks in HT-29 cells, whereas daidzein did not (Plewa et al. 2001).

HCT (human colon tumor) cells demonstrated reduced membrane fluidity when incubated with genistein, and both genistein and daidzein reduced the charge density of the cell surface (Yu et al. 1999). Membrane fluidity and surface charge are usually higher in tumor than in normal cells, hence the isoflavones rendered the membranes more "normal." Altered membrane mechanics in response to dietary factors may affect tumor cell growth and metastases and is a relatively unexplored area.

Cyclooxygenase catalyzes the oxygenation of arachidonic acid, which is the precursor of prostaglandins (Mutoh et al. 2000). One isoform of this enzyme, COX-2 is upregulated in colon cancer and inhibition of COX-2 is an effective therapy for colon cancer. Using a reporter assay for the COX-2 promoter in DLD-1 cells, Mutoh et al. (2000) investigated the ability of a variety of isoflavones to regulate this promoter. The most potent inhibitors were curcumin (10 µM) and quercetin (20 µM), followed by genistein and kaempferol (both 40 µM) and resveratrol (100 µM). Daidzein and epigallocatechin were poor inhibitors (500 µM) of the promoter. The authors speculate that the presence of a resorcin moiety in the effective compounds may be a determining factor in their ability to regulate the COX-2 promoter.

Genistein is a known tyrosine kinase inhibitor, and therefore may influence cell proliferation via alteration of signal transduction cascades. The focal adhesion kinase (FAK) is phosphorylated after integrin activation producing an SH-2 site for binding of intracellular signaling molecules (Weyant et al. 2000). This sequence of events leads to activation of the mitogen-activated protein kinase (MAPK) signaling pathway that regulates cell proliferation. In DLD-1 and HT-29 human colon cancer cells, genistein (100 µM) inhibited FAK phosphorylation (Weyant et al. 2000). Although these data suggest a potential mechanism through which genistein may influence colon cancer cell growth it is unlikely that this dose is physiologically achievable systemically in vivo. However, exposure of colon cells to lumenal contents containing high concentrations of phytoestrogens is possible, as is the accumulation of specific compounds within the intestinal mucosa.

The ability of colon cancer cells to synthesize estrogen was demonstrated in HCT8 and HCT116 cells (Fiorelli et al. 1999a). These cells expressed aromatase cytochrome P450 mRNA and converted androgens to estrogens in vitro. Quercetin (1 µM) inhibited aromatase activity in the cells, but a similar concentration of genistein has a slight stimulatory effect. The presence of estrogen receptors and aromatase activity in colon cancer cells suggests a potential autocrine mechanism for tumor cells.

Other Flavonoids in Colon Cancer

In a thorough study of the effect of 30 flavonoids on colon cell proliferation, Kuntz et al. (1999) reported all of the flavonoids had antiproliferative effects, but no obvious structural features predicted the effectiveness of the compounds. Baicalein was one of the most potent (40 µM) in inhibiting the growth of HT-29 and Caco-2 cells. Apigenin was found to induce G2/M arrest in SW480, HT-29, and Caco-2 cells, which correlated with reduced accumulation of cyclin B1 proteins (Wang and Kurzer 1997). Quercetin induced growth inhibition in HT-29, WiDr, Colo 201, and LS-174T human colon cancer cell lines by blocking cells in the G0/G1 phase (Ranelletti et al. 1992; Hosokawa et al. 1990). Expression of p21-Ras was found to be significantly reduced by 10 μM quercetin in human colon cancer cell lines and primary colorectal tumors (Ranelletti et al. 2000). Quercetin transiently inhibited the epidermal growth factor receptor phosphorylation and reduced the response of colon tumor cells to epidermal growth factor (Richter et al. 1999). The ability of quercetin to inhibit colon tumor cell growth was found to be due to cyto-toxicity of actively proliferating cells (Agullo et al. 1994).

Curcumin is present in turmeric and has been found to possess anti-inflammatory and antioxidant properties. Fisher F344 rats treated with azoxymethane had fewer colon tumors when fed a diet containing 2000 mg curcumin/kg compared to a control diet (Rao et al. 1995). The colon mucosa from rats fed curcumin exhibited lower activities of phospholi-pase A2, phospholipase Cγ (gamma)1, and prostaglandin E2, which suggests altered arachidonic acid metabolism may have contributed to the protective response. An extract of Curcuma was administered to 15 patients with advanced colorectal cancer that had proven to be refractory to standard treatment (Sharma et al. 2001). The patients received doses between 36 and 180 mg curcumin per day. After 29 days, patients on the lowest dose had reduced lymphocytic glutathione S-transferase activity although this effect was not present with the higher doses. In five patients, the cancer was stabilized within 2 to 4 months of treatment. In cultured human colon cancer cells, curcumin is a potent inhibitor of cell pro-liferation. Curcumin inhibited the growth of Lovo cells, produced G2/M arrest, and induced apoptosis (Chen et al. 2001). G2/M arrest and induction of apoptosis was also observed in HCT-116 cells incubated with curcumin (Moragoda et al. 2001). And curcumin inhibited HT-29 cell growth and COX-2 expression in HT-29 cells (Goel et al. 2001).

Administration of black or green tea polyphenols in drinking water (3600 ppm tea polyphenols, 1800 ppm EGCG or 1800 ppm tea polyphenols) to Fisher F344 rats treated with azoxymethane had no effect on tumor development (Weisburger et al. 1998). In con-trast, the number of aberrant crypt foci in rats treated with azoxymethane was significant-ly lower when the animals received EGCG, and EGCG with sulindac resulted in a further reduction in aberrant crypt foci (Ohishi et al. 2002). EGCG and related tea polyphenols inhibited COX and lipoxygenase (LOX) dependent arachidonic acid metabolism in human colon mucosa and colon tumor tissues, which implies a protective effect of these com-pounds on colon cancer (Hong et al. 2001). EGCG may also provide protection through inhibition of topoisomerase I (Berger et al. 2001).

BREAST CANCER

Soy Isoflavones and Breast Cancer

A high dietary intake of soy products, which is common in Asian cultures, has been asso-ciated with reduced incidence of breast cancer (Wu et al. 1998). In a recent review, Messina and Loprinzi (2001) discuss the role of soy isoflavones in breast cancer. A poten-tial mechanism through which soy intake may affect breast cancer risk is by reducing circulating concentrations of estradiol. Lower estradiol levels were reported in pre-menopausal women who consumed a soy-containing diet for one menstrual cycle, although no effect on cycle length was observed (Lu et al. 2000). However, other reports found no significant effect of soy isoflavones on steroid hormone levels in women (Martini et al. 1999; Duncan et al. 1999). Soy isoflavones may act directly on mammary cells. The ability of dietary soy to alter cell proliferation rate in human breast tissue has been report-ed. Women with benign or malignant breast disease were asked to consume breads con-taining 45 mg soy isoflavones per day for 14 days (McMichael-Phillips et al. 1998). Biopsies of mammary tissue were obtained and markers of cell proliferation examined. Increased rates of cell proliferation were observed in the mammary glands of women who had consumed soy isoflavones compared to controls. Hence, soy isoflavones produced an estrogenic response on mammary cell proliferation.

Several animal models of mammary cancer have been used to examine the role of soy isoflavones. Fisher F344 rats were fed diets containing soy protein with or without isoflavones starting from 43 days of age and treated with the carcinogen N-nitroso-N-methylurea (NMU) to induce mammary tumors (Cohen et al. 2000). Overall, no affect of soy isoflavones (about 200 mg/kg diet) on tumor incidence occurred. Compared to the casein control diet, a nonsignificant trend for increased tumor latency occurred in rats fed soy protein (with or without isoflavones). Hilakivi-Clarke et al. (1999b) demonstrated that the mammary epithelial structures of female offspring from mice subcutaneously injected with 20 μg genistein daily during days 15 and 20 of gestation (last third of pregnancy) closely resembled those of mice exposed to 2 μg estradiol. In utero exposure to genistein or estradiol increased the number of terminal end buds present in the offspring at 4–5 weeks of age, thereby increasing the number of epithelial targets for malignant transfor-mation (Russo and Russo 1978). The authors conclude that in utero exposure to genistein, similarly to estradiol, results in increased mammary cancer risk. In contrast, a protective effect of genistein on carcinogen-induced mammary tumors in female offspring of rats fed genistein during pregnancy has been reported (Fritz et al. 1998; Lamartiniere et al. 1995). Diets containing 25 or 250 mg genistein/kg were fed to dams 2 weeks before breeding through weaning of the pups. Thereafter, female pups were fed the basal diet without genistein and DMBA was administered to induce mammary tumors at 50 days postpar-tum. The rats exposed to genistein in utero developed significantly fewer mammary tumors than rats from dams not fed genistein. Similarly, Badger et al (2001) reported rats bred and raised on diets containing soy protein isolate or genistein had reduced incidence of chemically induced mammary cancer than rats fed casein or whey protein. These results conflict with the findings of Hilakivi-Clarke et al. (1999a). The major differences in these studies are that 20 μg genistein was injected (increased tumorigenesis), or 250 mg genis-tein was fed (reduced tumorigenesis). It is possible the concentration or form of genistein provided to the fetus was different in these studies, leading to opposite outcomes. The epi-demiological data would suggest that oral consumption of soy containing isoflavones by mothers may reduce mammary tumorigenesis in their daughters, as first-generation Asian women are protected against breast cancer after migrating to the United States and adopt-ing a Western diet (Ziegler et al. 1993).

There is, however, more consistent evidence for a protective effect of soy isoflavones on mammary cancer when provided during the perinatal and prepubertal periods. Recently, an epidemiological study using the Shanghai Cancer Registry, found an inverse relationship (50%) between adolescent (13–15 yr old) soy food intake and breast cancer incidence later in life (Shu et al. 2001). Injecting genistein into newborn rats protected them from DMBA-induced tumor development as adults (Lamartiniere et al. 1998). A similar reduction in mammary tumor development was observed in rats fed genistein during the prepubertal period (Murrill et al. 1996; Hilakivi-Clarke et al. 1999b; Lamartiniere et al. 1995). A possible explanation for this reduced tumor development may be increased mammary gland maturation. Indeed, a 48% reduction of the terminal end buds and 92% increase in the number of lobules II were observed after prepubertal treatment with 5 mg genistein per rat (Lamartiniere et al. 1995). Furthermore, it has been hypothesized that early exposure to genistein exerts an imprinting effect on the epidermal growth factor (EGF) signaling pathway that plays a significant role in cell proliferation and cancer ontogeny (Brown et al. 1998). Imprinting is considered to set the pattern of gene expression early in development from which the adult responds. The pattern includes regulation of steroid receptor mechanisms and signal transduction. Prepubertal genistein treatment upregulated the expression of the EGF receptor messenger RNA and protein in mammary glands of 21-day-old female rats (Brown et al. 1998). In 50-day-old rats treated prepubertally with genistein, EGF receptor expression was specifically reduced in the epithelial cells of the terminal end buds in comparison with the rest of the mammary gland (Lamartiniere et al. 1998). Targeting genistein to mammary tumors using an EGF-genistein conjugate caused significant shrinkage and even disappearance of implanted tumors in SCID mice (Uckun et al. 1998). The response was thought to occur due to the inhibitory effect of genistein on the EGF receptor tyrosine kinase activity. Hence, reduced EGF receptor mass in the target tissue of adult animals treated with genistein, an effect that could alter signal transduction, mammary gland differentiation, and cell proliferation, may provide protection from mammary tumorigenesis. Another proposed mechanism through which isoflavones may affect mammary tumor development is via activation of phase II enzymes. Sprague-Dawley rats treated with dimethylbenz[a]anthracene (DMBA) to induce mammary tumors had lower tumor incidence when fed soy isoflavones (Appelt and Reicks 1999). This was correlated with higher levels of glutathione reductase, glutathione peroxidase, glutathione S-transferase, and quinone reductase.

Because soy isoflavones have estrogenic effects on the mammary gland, potential promotion of tumor cell growth may occur. Using ovariectomized, athymic mice injected with MCF-7 human breast cancer cells, Ju et al. (2001) observed increased tumor cell proliferation when the mice were fed diets containing 250–1000 mg genistein/kg. Hence, dietary genistein provided in a physiologically relevant concentration range stimulated the growth of estrogen-responsive breast cancer cells. In another study using this model, genistein was observed to decrease the inhibitory effect of tamoxifen on MCF-7 cell proliferation (Ju et al. 2002). A promontory effect of genistein was also observed in a DMBA-induced mouse tumor model (Day et al. 2001). More advanced mammary tumors were observed in mice fed diets containing 1000 mg genistein/kg compared to the controls.

Transgenic mice that overexpress the neu-ErbB2 oncogene spontaneously develop mammary tumors. Neu-ErbB2, which is homologous to HER-2, is a member of the EGF receptor family, and is associated with 30–40% of human breast cancers (Slamon et al. 1987). Using this animal model, a casein-based semipurified diet was compared to two open-formula commercial animal Chow diets (NTP-2000 and NIH-07; Rao et al. 1997b). The open-formula diets contained grains, fish meal, yeast, and molasses but differed slightly in composition. NTP-2000 had lower protein, higher fiber, and higher fat than the NIH-07 diet. Mice fed the casein or NIH-07 diet developed more tumors than mice fed the NTP-2000 diet. The authors speculate that the higher concentration of dietary fiber in the NTP-2000 diet may have contributed to the protective effect by influencing estrogen metabolism. Another explanation for these results may be the presence of phytoestrogens in the nonpurified diets. Jin and MacDonald (2002) recently reported a significant delay in mammary tumor latency in MMTV-neu mice fed diets containing genistein (250 ppm), daidzein (250 ppm), or an isoflavone extract (250 ppm genistein equivalents) compared to a casein control diet. No differences in total tumor burden were observed, however, due to the dietary treatments. Furthermore, there was no difference in tumor development with the three isoflavone diets, suggesting the response was estrogen related.

Genistein has a biphasic effect on cell proliferation in human breast cancer cell lines (Cappelletti et al. 2000). At low concentrations (0.1–2.0 μM), genistein stimulated cell proliferation, and at higher concentrations (6–20 μM), it blocked cell proliferation in the G2/M phase. In humans, serum genistein concentration is estimated to reach 3–4 μM with consumption of a high soy diet (Barnes et al. 1995). However, it is possible that local accumulation of genistein may occur within breast tissues, similar to what occurs with estrogens (Zava and Duwe 1997). Using chimeric proteins for the hormone binding domains of ERα and ERβ, it was clearly demonstrated that at low concentrations (1 μM) both genistein and quercetin are agonists for these receptors (Maggiolini et al. 2001). At higher concentrations (10 μM) however, both compounds were cytotoxic. The cytotoxic effects, but not the proliferative effects, of these compounds were observed in ER-negative and estrogen-independent cells suggesting the inhibitory effects on proliferation are mediated by an ER-independent mechanism. A similar conclusion was reached using ER-positive and ER-negative breast cancer cell lines (Shao et al. 1998, Dampier et al. 2001).

Other Flavonoids and Breast Cancer

Thirteen flavonoids were examined for their effects on ER-dependent and ER-independent breast cancer cell lines (Wang and Kurzer 1997). At concentrations between 20–80 μM the compounds inhibited cell proliferation in both cell lines, but at lower concentrations (0.1–10 μM), stimulation of cell proliferation occurred only in the ER-dependent cell line. Quercetin is a potent inhibitor of cultured mammary tumor cell growth (Choi et al. 2001; Balabhadrapathruni et al. 2000; Rodgers and Grant, 1998; Hansen et al. 1997; Singhal et al. 1995; Avila et al. 1994; Scambia et al. 1993; Scambia et al. 1991; Maggiolini et al. 2001). This effect may be mediated by induction of apoptosis, inhibition of the phosphatidlyinositol kinase, regulation of p53 expression or heat shock proteins.

Curcumin has been found to compete with aryl hydrocarbons for binding the aryl hydrocarbon receptor and cytochrome P450 1A1 (Ciolino et al. 1998). Breast cancer cell lines were arrested in G2/M by curcumin (Mehta et al. 1997) and underwent apoptosis (Ramachandran and You, 1999; Choudhuri et al. 2002). The antiproliferative effects of curcumin were mediated by the ER in ER-dependent cells, but curcumin exerted anti-invasive effects in ER-independent cells also (Shao et al. 2002).

In human breast cancer patients, consumption of green tea was positively associated with decreased numbers of axillary lymph node metastases and decreased recurrence of stage I or II breast cancer (Nakachi et al. 1998). Sprague-Dawley rats treated with DMBA demonstrated a significant delay in mean tumor latency and reduced tumor burden when given green tea compared to controls (Kavanagh et al. 2001). Treatment of mammary tumor cells overexpressing Her-2/neu with EGCG reduced proliferation rate, presumably by inhibiting the PI 3 kinase → Akt kinase → NF-kappa B pathway (Pianetti et al. 2002).

PROSTATE CANCER

SOY ISOFLAVONES IN PROSTATE CANCER

The incidence of prostate cancer is lower in Asia and in vegetarians than in populations consuming a more Western diet (Blumenfeld et al. 2000). Components of the Western diet most often cited as playing a role in the increased prostate cancer risk include animal products (Michaud et al. 2001). However, the most consistent correlation for prostate cancer prevention is consumption of fruits, vegetables, and grains—potential sources of phytoestrogens (Denis et al. 1999). The effects of estrogens on prostate cancer were recently reviewed by Lieberman et al. 2001) and previously by Cox and Crawford (1995). Estrogen therapy, principally the use of DES, is a suggested practice in prostate tumor treatment. Its primary mode of action is through feedback on the anterior pituitary with suppression of gonadotropin secretion and subsequent decrease in testosterone production by Leydig cells of the testis. This would in turn cause a decrease in androgens required for hormone-dependent cancer. However, direct effects of DES are also possible. Whether DES works through a classical ERα pathway, through ERβ or another estrogen-dependent mechanism has not been fully determined. It is possible that genistein, daidzein, and other phytoestrogens affect prostate cancer through similar mechanisms. When male rats were fed diets containing genistein from conception, down-regulation of androgen and estrogen receptors was observed in the dorsolateral prostate in a dose-dependent manner (Fritz et al. 2002). With a high genistein intake, 1000 mg/kg diet, ERα levels were reduced in the prostate compared to rats not fed genistein. Similarly, male Sprague-Dawley rats fed diets containing 600 ppm isoflavones for 20 days had lower circulating levels of testosterone and smaller prostates than rats fed an isoflavone-free diet (Weber et al. 2001). The decreased testosterone was not due to lower 5-α-reductase activity.

The dietary history of newly diagnosed prostate cancer patients was evaluated for phytoestrogen intake (Strom et al. 1999). An inverse relationship between prostate cancer risk and intake of coumestrol, genistein, and daidzein was observed. Furthermore, coumestrol, genistein, and daidzein stimulated the transcriptional activity of the human estrogen receptor in an in vitro model (Miksicek 1994).

Lobund-Wistar rats develop prostate tumors due to overproduction of testosterone. When these rats were fed a diet containing natural products including soy meal, fewer animals developed tumors compared to rats fed a casein-based diet (Pollard and Wolter 2000). The rats fed the soy diet had lower levels of circulating testosterone, which may have contributed to the protective effect. Using subcutaneous injections of 3,2'-dimethyl-4-aminobiphenyl (DMAB) to induce prostate tumors in rats, Kato et al. (2000) observed both dietary genistin and daidzin (1000 mg/kg diet) reduced the number of tumors formed in the ventral prostate. Using a similar carcinogen-induced model, fewer rats developed tumors when they were fed diets containing 100 or 400 ppm isoflavones compared to an isoflavone-free diet (Onozawa et al. 1999).

An animal model of spontaneous prostate cancer has recently been developed. The TRansgenic Adenocarcinoma of the Mouse Prostate (TRAMP) mouse was developed by placing the SV40 large T-antigen gene under the control of the rat probasin promoter, which has been shown to be highly and specifically expressed in the mouse prostate (Gingrich et al. 1996) and no other tissues. The probasin (PB) promoter is androgen and zinc regulated, with two androgen-response elements located in this region. It is localized in the ducts and nucleus of prostate epithelial cells, yet the function for PB has yet to be identified. The transgene, known as PBTag, which is highly expressed in the dorsal and ventral prostate lobes, produces in abundance the T-antigen. This oncoprotein is known to bind tumor suppresser products of p53 and retinoblastoma (Rb). Nearly 100% of TRAMP mice develop prostate cancer spontaneously.

Using this model, the effect of genistein on prostate tumor development was observed. TRAMP mice were fed diets containing varying amounts of genistein (0, 100, 250, or 500 mg/kg diet) from weaning (Mentor-Marcel et al. 2001). The percentage of mice that developed poorly differentiated adenocarcinoma was reduced in a dose-dependent manner by dietary genistein.

When nude mice were injected with the androgen-dependent LNCaP cells, tumor cell growth was reduced by diets containing rye or soy compared to control (Adlercreutz et al. 2000). Rye was more effective than soy in inhibiting the cell growth. Human prostate cancer cells were implanted subcutaneously into severe combined immune-deficient mice (SCID) fed casein or soy protein diets with three levels of soy phytoestrogens (Zhou et al. 1999). Consumption of isoflavones by the mice ranged between 0 and 4.88 mg/day. Tumor cell growth was significantly reduced in vivo in a dose-dependent manner by soy phytoestrogens, which corroborated in vitro assays that showed inhibitory effects of isoflavones on prostate tumor cell proliferation, induced G2/M arrest, and enhanced apoptosis. Using a similar model, SCID mice implanted with LNCaP cells were fed diets containing casein or soy diets (plus isoflavones) with either high or low fat content (Aronson et al. 1999). The tumor cell growth was significantly less in mice fed the low fat soy diet compared to the other diets.

As observed in the mammary gland, dietary genistein inhibited EGF receptor expression and phosphorylation in rat prostate (Dalu et al. 1998). The prostates from rats fed genistein also had reduced tyrosine phosphorylated proteins, specifically between 85 and 170,000 kDa, and reduced ErbB2/neu receptor concentration.

Genistein, daidzein, and coumestrol inhibited the proliferation of androgen receptor negative (PC-3) and androgen receptor positive (LNCaP) cells within a concentration range of 1–10 µM (Mitchell et al. 2000). Genistein induced DNA strand breakage in both cell lines, whereas coumestrol did so only in the PC-3 cells and daidzein did not induce DNA damage. In VeCaP cells, which express the prostate specific antigen (PSA), genistein inhibited cell growth and decreased PSA mRNA, protein expression, and secretion (Davis et al. 2000). A potential mechanism through which genistein may affect cell proliferation in the prostate is by inhibition of phosphorylation of the inhibitory protein I kappa B alpha, which leads to activation of apoptosis (Davis et al. 1999).

Other Flavonoids in Prostate Cancer

Curcumin induced apoptosis in DU145 and LNCaP cells which correlated with decreased activity of NF-kB (Mukhopadhyay et al. 2001). Similarly, Curcumin induced apoptosis in PC-3 and LNCaP cells and was a potent inhibitor of EGF-R signaling (Dorai et al. 2000). When LNCaP cells were injected into nude mice, addition of 2% curcumin to the diet reduced tumor cell growth significantly (Dorai et al. 2001).

Both androgen responsive and independent prostate tumor cells underwent G1 arrest in response to EGCG, with induced apoptosis (Paschka et al. 1998; Lyn-Cook et al. 1999; Gupta et al. 2000). The induction of apoptosis in DU145 cells was found to coincide with an increase in reactive oxygen species and mitochondrial depolarization (Chung et al. 2001). EGCG inhibited proliferation of LNCaP cells, which correlated with suppression of the androgen receptor mRNA (Ren et al. 2000). Genistein and EGCG were found to alter cell cycle regulators, including cyclin-dependent kinase, ERK 1/2, and Cip 1/p21, which led to growth inhibition (Bhatia and Agarwal 2001). The growth of PC-3 and LNCaP cells in nude mice was significantly reduced by intraperitoneal injection of EGCG (Liao et al. 1995).

Resveratrol inhibited growth of hormone-sensitive and insensitive prostate cancer cell lines (Hsieh and Wu 2000). Similarly, baicalein was effective in inhibiting cell proliferation in prostate tumor cells, regardless of androgen sensitivity (Ikezoe et al. 2001; Chen et al. 2001; Chan et al. 2000). Catechin, epicatechin, quercetin, and resveratrol were potent inhibitors of prostate tumor cell lines, LNCaP, DU145, and PC-3 (Kampa et al. 2000). Apigenin also demonstrated inhibitory effects on cell proliferation in prostate tumor cells (Gupta et al. 2002; Gupta et al. 2001). In LNCaP cells, apigenin induced cyclin-dependent kinase inhibitor p21, which plays a role in regulation of cell proliferation (Kobayashi et al. 2002). In the androgen-independent prostate tumor cell line (PC-3), quercetin, kaempferol, and luteolin suppressed growth completely, whereas genistein, apigenin, and myricetin were somewhat less effective (Knowles et al. 2000).

CONCLUSIONS

Dietary phytoestrogens have profound effects on tumor cell growth both in vivo and in vitro. Substantial evidence suggests that colon, breast, and prostate cancer development is reduced in animal models of these diseases by dietary administration of phytoestrogens.

Cell culture evidence suggests multiple mechanisms through which these compounds affect cell growth, through both estrogen-dependent and estrogen-independent systems. Translation of the animal and cell culture data to human cancer prevention is warranted; however, care must be exercised. Whereas the majority of the data suggests dietary phytoestrogens would reduce cancer risk, there remains the possibility that estrogen-responsive tumor cell growth may be promoted by these compounds. The concern for such exacerbating effects is greatest for breast cancer. Consumption of phytoestrogens as they naturally occur in foods is unlikely to increase cancer risk and most probably will provide protection. The safety and efficacy of consuming isolated plant extracts or specific phytoestrogen compounds in concentrations much greater than found in the diet, however, requires addition research.

REFERENCES

Adlercreutz, H., Fotsis, T., Bannwart, C., Wahala, K., Makela, T., Brunow, G., and Hase, T. (1986) Determination of urinary lignans and phytoestrogen metabolites, potential antiestrogens and anticarcinogens, in urine of women on various habitual diets. Journal of Steroid Biochemistry 25: 791–797.

Adlercreutz, H., Fotsis, T., Heikkinen, R., Dwyer, J. T., Woods, M., Goldin, B. R., and Gorbach, S. L. (1982) Excretion of the lignans enterolactone and enterodiol and of equol in omnivorous and vegetarian postmenopausal women and in women with breast cancer. Lancet 2: 1295–1299.

Adlercreutz, H., Mazur, W., Bartels, P., Elomaa, V., Watanabe, S., Wahala, K., Landstrom, M., Lundin, E., Bergh, A., Damber, J. E., Aman, P., Widmark, A., Johansson, A., Zhang, J. X., and Hallmans, G. (2000) Phytoestrogens and prostate disease. Journal of Nutrition 130: 658S–659S.

Agullo, G., Gamet, L., Besson, C., Demigne, C., and Remesy, C. (1994) Quercetin exerts a preferential cytotoxic effect on active dividing colon carcinoma HT29 and Caco-2 cells. Cancer Letters 87: 55–63.

Akiyama, T., Ishida, J., Nakagawa, S., Ogawara, H., Watanabe, S., Itoh, N., Shibuya, M., and Fukami, Y. (1987) Genistein, a specific inhibitor of tyrosine-specific protein kinases. Journal of Biological Chemistry 262: 5592–5595.

Appelt, L. C. and Reicks, M. M. (1999) Soy induces phase II enzymes but does not inhibit dimethylbenz[a]anthracene-induced carcinogenesis in female rats. Journal of Nutrition 129: 1820–1826.

Arai, N., Strom, A., Rafter, J. J., and Gustafsson, J. A. (2000) Estrogen receptor beta mRNA in colon cancer cells: growth effects of estrogen and genistein. Biochemical and Biophysical Research Communications 270: 425–431.

Aronson, W. J., Tymchuk, C. N., Elashoff, R. M., McBride, W. H., McLean, C., Wang, H., and Heber, D. (1999) Decreased growth of human prostate LNCaP tumors in SCID mice fed a low-fat, soy protein diet with isoflavones. Nutrition and Cancer 35: 130–136.

Avila, M. A., Velasco, J. A., Cansado, J., and Notario, V. (1994) Quercetin mediates the down-regulation of mutant p53 in the human breast cancer cell line MDA-MB468. Cancer Research 54: 2424–2428.

Badger, T. M., Ronis, M. J., and Hakkak, R. (2001) Developmental effects and health aspects of soy protein isolate, casein, and whey in male and female rats. International Journal of Toxicology 20: 165–174.

Balabhadrapathruni, S., Thomas, T. J., Yurkow, E. J., Amenta, P. S., and Thomas, T. (2000) Effects of genistein and structurally related phytoestrogens on cell cycle kinetics and apoptosis in MDA-MB-468 human breast cancer cells. Oncology Reports 7: 3–12.

Barnes, S., Peterson, T. G., and Coward, L. (1995) Rationale for the use of genistein-containing soy matrices in chemoprevention trials for breast and prostate cancer. Journal of Cellular Biochemistry, Supplement 22: 181–187.

Berger, S. J., Gupta, S., Belfi, C. A., Gosky, D. M., and Mukhtar, H. (2001) Green tea constituent (—)-epigallocatechin-3-gallate inhibits topoisomerase I activity in human colon carcinoma cells. Biochemical and Biophysical Research Communications 288: 101–105.

Bhatia, N. and Agarwal, R. (2001) Detrimental effect of cancer preventive phytochemicals silymarin, genistein and epigallocatechin 3-gallate on epigenetic events in human prostate carcinoma DU145 cells. Prostate 46: 98–107.

Blumenfeld, A. J., Fleshner, N., Casselman, B., and Trachtenberg, J. (2000) Nutritional aspects of prostate cancer: a review. Canadian Journal of Urology 7: 927–935.

Booth, C., Hargreaves, D. F., Hadfield, J. A., McGown, A. T., and Potten, C. S. (1999) Isoflavones inhibit intestinal epithelial cell proliferation and induce apoptosis in vitro. British Journal of Cancer 80: 1550–1557.

Bosland, M. C. (2000) The role of steroid hormones in prostate carcinogenesis. Journal of the National Cancer Institute Monographs: 39–66.

Branham, W. S., Dial, S. L., Moland, C. L., Hass, B. S., Blair, R. M., Fang, H., Shi, L., Tong, W., Perkins, R. G., and Sheehan, D. M. (2002) Phytoestrogens and mycoestrogens bind to the rat uterine estrogen receptor. Journal of Nutrition 132: 658–664.

Brown, N. M., Wang, J., Cotroneo, M. S., Zhao, Y. X., and Lamartiniere, C. A. (1998) Prepubertal genistein treatment modulates TGF-alpha, EGF and EGF-receptor mRNAs and proteins in the rat mammary gland. Molecular and Cellular Endocrinology 144: 149–165.

Calle, E. E., Miracle-McMahill, H. L., Thun, M. J., and Heath, C. W., Jr. (1995) Estrogen replacement therapy and risk of fatal colon cancer in a prospective cohort of postmenopausal women. Journal of the National Cancer Institute 87: 517–523.

Campbell-Thompson, M., Lynch, I. J., and Bhardwaj, B. (2001) Expression of estrogen receptor (ER) subtypes and ERbeta isoforms in colon cancer. Cancer Research 61: 632–640.

Cappelletti, V., Fioravanti, L., Miodini, P., and Di Fronzo, G. (2000) Genistein blocks breast cancer cells in the G(2)M phase of the cell cycle. Journal of Cellular Biochemistry 79: 594–600.

Chan, F. L., Choi, H. L., Chen, Z. Y., Chan, P. S., and Huang, Y. (2000) Induction of apoptosis in prostate cancer cell lines by a flavonoid, baicalin. Cancer Letters 160: 219–228.

Chen, S., Ruan, Q., Bedner, E., Deptala, A., Wang, X., Hsieh, T. C., Traganos, F., and Darzynkiewicz, Z. (2001) Effects of the flavonoid baicalin and its metabolite baicalein on androgen receptor expression, cell cycle progression and apoptosis of prostate cancer cell lines. Cell Proliferation 34: 293–304.

Choi, J. A., Kim, J. Y., Lee, J. Y., Kang, C. M., Kwon, H. J., Yoo, Y. D., Kim, T. W., Lee, Y. S., and Lee, S. J. (2001) Induction of cell cycle arrest and apoptosis in human breast cancer cells by quercetin. International Journal of Oncology 19: 837–844.

Choudhuri, T., Pal, S., Agwarwal, M. L., Das, T., and Sa, G. (2002) Curcumin induces apoptosis in human breast cancer cells through p53-dependent Bax induction. FEBS Letters 512: 334–340.

Chung, L. Y., Cheung, T. C., Kong, S. K., Fung, K. P., Choy, Y. M., Chan, Z. Y., and Kwok, T. T. (2001) Induction of apoptosis by green tea catechins in human prostate cancer DU145 cells. Life Sciences 68: 1207–1214.

Ciolino, H. P., Daschner, P. J., Wang, T. T., and Yeh, G. C. (1998) Effect of curcumin on the aryl hydrocarbon receptor and cytochrome P450 1A1 in MCF-7 human breast carcinoma cells. Biochemical Pharmacology 56: 197–206.

Cohen, L. A., Zhao, Z., Pittman, B., and Scimeca, J. A. (2000) Effect of intact and isoflavone-depleted soy protein on NMU-induced rat mammary tumorigenesis. Carcinogenesis 21: 929–935.

Couse, J. F., Curtis, H. S., and Korach, K. S. (2000) Receptor null mice reveal contrasting roles for estrogen receptor alpha and beta in reproductive tissues. Journal of Steroid Biochemistry and Molecular Biology 74: 287–296.

Cox, R. L., and Crawford, E. D. (1995) Estrogens in the treatment of prostate cancer. [Review] [96 refs]. Journal of Urology 154: 1991–1998.

Dalu, A., Haskell, J. F., Coward, L., and Lamartiniere, C. A. (1998) Genistein, a component of soy, inhibits the expression of the EGF and ErbB2/Neu receptors in the rat dorsolateral prostate. Prostate 37: 36–43.

Dampier, K., Hudson, E. A., Howells, L. M., Manson, M. M., Walker, R. A., and Gescher, A. (2001) Differences between human breast cell lines in susceptibility towards growth inhibition by genistein. British Journal of Cancer 85: 618–624.

Davies, M. J., Bowey, E. A., Adlercreutz, H., Rowland, I. R., and Rumsby, P. C. (1999) Effects of soy or rye supplementation of high-fat diets on colon tumour development in azoxymethane-treated rats. Carcinogenesis 20: 927–931.

Davis, J. N., Kucuk, O., and Sarkar, F. H. (1999) Genistein inhibits NF-kappa B activation in prostate cancer cells. Nutrition and Cancer 35: 167–174.

Davis, J. N., Muqim, N., Bhuiyan, M., Kucuk, O., Pienta, K. J., and Sarkar, F. H. (2000) Inhibition of prostate specific antigen expression by genistein in prostate cancer cells. International Journal of Oncology 16: 1091–1097.

Day, J. K., Besch-Williford, C., McMann, T. R., Hufford, M. G., Lubahn, D. B., and MacDonald, R. S. (2001) Dietary genistein increased DMBA-induced mammary adenocarcinoma in wild-type, but not ER alpha KO, mice. Nutrition and Cancer 39: 226–232.

Denis, L., Morton, M. S., and Griffiths, K. (1999) Diet and its preventive role in prostatic disease. European Urology 35: 377–387.

Dorai, T., Gehani, N., and Katz, A. (2000) Therapeutic potential of curcumin in human prostate cancer. II. Curcumin inhibits tyrosine kinase activity of epidermal growth factor receptor and depletes the protein. Molecular Urology 4: 1–6.

Duncan, A. M., Merz, B. E., Xu, X., Nagel, T. C., Phipps, W. R., and Kurzer, M. S. (1999) Soy isoflavones exert modest hormonal effects in premenopausal women. Journal of Clinical Endocrinology and Metabolism 84: 192–197.

English, M. A., Kane, K. F., Cruickshank, N., Langman, M. J., Stewart, P. M., and Hewison, M. (1999) Loss of estrogen inactivation in colonic cancer. Journal of Clinical Endocrinology and Metabolism 84: 2080–2085.

Fields, S., and Jang, S. K. (1990) Presence of a potent transcription activating sequence in the p53 protein. Science 249: 1046–1049.

Fiorelli, G., Picariello, L., Martineti, V., Tonelli, F., and Brandi, M. L. (1999a) Estrogen synthesis in human colon cancer epithelial cells. Journal of Steroid Biochemistry and Molecular Biology 71: 223–230.

Fiorelli, G., Picariello, L., Martineti, V., Tonelli, F., and Brandi, M. L. (1999b) Functional estrogen receptor beta in colon cancer cells. Biochemical and Biophysical Research Communications 261: 521–527.

Foley, E. F., Jazaeri, A. A., Shupnik, M. A., Jazaeri, O., and Rice, L. W. (2000) Selective loss of estrogen receptor beta in malignant human colon. Cancer Research 60: 245–248.

Fritz, W. A., Coward, L., Wang, J., and Lamartiniere, C. A. (1998) Dietary genistein: perinatal mammary cancer prevention, bioavailability and toxicity testing in the rat. Carcinogenesis 19: 2151–2158.

Fritz, W. A., Wang, J., Eltoum, I. E., and Lamartiniere, C. A. (2002) Dietary genistein down-regulates androgen and estrogen receptor expression in the rat prostate. Molecular and Cellular Endocrinology 186: 89–99.

Gingrich, J. R., Barrios, R. J., Morton, R. A., Boyce, B. F., DeMayo, F. J., Finegold, M. J., Angelopoulou, R., Rosen, J. M., and Greenberg, N. M. (1996) Metastatic prostate cancer in a transgenic mouse. Cancer Research 56: 4096–4102.

Goel, A., Boland, C. R., and Chauhan, D. P. (2001) Specific inhibition of cyclooxygenase-2 (COX-2) expression by dietary curcumin in HT-29 human colon cancer cells. Cancer Letters 172: 111–118.

Grodstein, F., Newcomb, P. A., and Stampfer, M. J. (1999) Postmenopausal hormone therapy and the risk of colorectal cancer: a review and meta-analysis. American Journal of Medicine 106: 574–582.

Gupta, S., Ahmad, N., Nieminen, A. L., and Mukhtar, H. (2000) Growth inhibition, cell cycle dysregulation, and induction of apoptosis by green tea constituent (-)-epigallocatechin-3-gallate. Toxicology and Applied Pharmacology 164: 82–90.

Gupta, S., Afaq, F., and Mukhtar, H. (2001) Selective growth-inhibitory, cell-cycle deregulatory and apoptotic response of apigenin in normal versus human prostate carcinoma cells. Biochemical and Biophysical Research Communications 287: 914–920.

Gupta, S., Afaq, F., and Mukhtar, H. (2002) Involvement of nuclear factor-kappa B, Bax and Bcl-2 in induction of cell cycle arrest and apoptosis by apigenin in human prostate carcinoma cells. Oncogene 21: 3727–3738.

Hansen, R. K., Oesterreich, S., Lemieux, P., Sarge, K. D., and Fuqua, S. A. (1997) Quercetin inhibits heat shock protein induction but not heat shock factor DNA-binding in human breast carcinoma cells. Biochemical and Biophysical Research Communications 239: 851–856.

Hilakivi-Clarke, L., Cho, E., Onojafe, I., Raygada, M., and Clarke, R. (1999a) Maternal exposure to genistein during pregnancy increases carcinogen-induced mammary tumorigenesis in female rat offspring. Oncology Reports 6: 1089–1095.

Hilakivi-Clarke, L., Onojafe, I., Raygada, M., Cho, E., Skaar, T., Russo, I., and Clarke, R. (1999b) Prepubertal exposure to zearalenone or genistein reduces mammary tumorigenesis. British Journal of Cancer 80: 1682–1688.

Hong, J., Smith, T. J., Ho, C. T., August, D. A., and Yang, C. S. (2001) Effects of purified green and black tea polyphenols on cyclooxygenase- and lipoxygenase-dependent metabolism of arachidonic acid in human colon mucosa and colon tumor tissues. Biochemical Pharmacology 62: 1175–1183.

Hosokawa, N., Hosokawa, Y., Sakai, T., Yoshida, M., Marui, N., Nishino, H., Kawai, K., and Aoike, A. (1990) Inhibitory effect of quercetin on the synthesis of a possibly cell-cycle-related 17-kDa protein, in human colon cancer cells. International Journal of Cancer 45: 1119–1124.

Hsieh, T. C. and Wu, J. M. (2000) Grape-derived chemopreventive agent resveratrol decreases prostate-specific antigen (PSA) expression in LNCaP cells by an androgen receptor (AR)-independent mechanism. Anticancer Research 20: 225–228.

Ikezoe, T., Chen, S. S., Heber, D., Taguchi, H., and Koeffler, H. P. (2001) Baicalin is a major component of PC-SPES which inhibits the proliferation of human cancer cells via apoptosis and cell cycle arrest. Prostate 49: 285–292.

Jin, Z., MacDonald, R. S. 2002. Soy isoflavones increase latency of spontaneous mammary tumors in mice. Journal of Nutrition 132(10): 3186–3190.

Ju, Y. H., Allred, C. D., Allred, K. F., Karko, K. L., Doerge, D. R., and Helferich, W. G. (2001) Physiological concentrations of dietary genistein dose-dependently stimulate growth of estrogen-dependent human breast cancer (MCF-7) tumors implanted in athymic nude mice. Journal of Nutrition 131: 2957–2962.

Ju, Y. H., Doerge, D. R., Allred, K. F., Allred, C. D., and Helferich, W. G. (2002) Dietary genistein negates the inhibitory effect of tamoxifen on growth of estrogen-dependent human breast cancer (MCF-7) cells implanted in athymic mice. Cancer Research 62: 2474–2477.

Kampa, M., Hatzoglou, A., Notas, G., Damianaki, A., Bakogeorgou, E., Gemetzi, C., Kouroumalis, E., Martin, P. M., and Castanas, E. (2000) Wine antioxidant polyphenols inhibit the proliferation of human prostate cancer cell lines. Nutrition and Cancer 37: 223–233.

Kampert, J. B., Whittemore, A. S., and Paffenbarger, R. S., Jr. (1988) Combined effect of child-bearing, menstrual events, and body size on age-specific breast cancer risk. American Journal of Epidemiology 128: 962–979.

Kampman, E., Potter, J. D., Slattery, M. L., Caan, B. J., and Edwards, S. (1997) Hormone replacement therapy, reproductive history, and colon cancer: a multicenter, case-control study in the United States. Cancer Causes and Control 8: 146–158.

Kato, K., Takahashi, S., Cui, L., Toda, T., Suzuki, S., Futakuchi, M., Sugiura, S., and Shirai, T. (2000) Suppressive effects of dietary genistin and daidzin on rat prostate carcinogenesis. Japanese Journal of Cancer Research 91: 786–791.

Kavanagh, K. T., Hafer, L. J., Kim, D. W., Mann, K. K., Sherr, D. H., Rogers, A. E., and Sonenshein, G. E. (2001) Green tea extracts decrease carcinogen-induced mammary tumor burden in rats and rate of breast cancer cell proliferation in culture. Journal of Cellular Biochemistry 82: 387–398.

Kirk, C. J., Harris, R. M., Wood, D. M., Waring, R. H., and Hughes, P. J. (2001) Do dietary phytoestrogens influence susceptibility to hormone-dependent cancer by disrupting the metabolism of endogenous oestrogens? Biochemical Society Transactions 29: 209–216.

Knowles, L. M., Zigrossi, D. A., Tauber, R. A., Hightower, C., and Milner, J. A. (2000) Flavonoids suppress androgen-independent human prostate tumor proliferation. Nutrition and Cancer 38: 116–122.

Kobayashi, T., Nakata, T., and Kuzumaki, T. (2002) Effect of flavonoids on cell cycle progression in prostate cancer cells. Cancer Letters 176: 17–23.

Kuiper, G. G., Lemmen, J. G., Carlsson, B., Corton, J. C., Safe, S. H., van der Saag, P. T., van der, B. B., and Gustafsson, J. A. (1998) Interaction of estrogenic chemicals and phytoestrogens with estrogen receptor beta. Endocrinology 139: 4252–4263.

Kuntz, S., Wenzel, U., and Daniel, H. (1999) Comparative analysis of the effects of flavonoids on proliferation, cytotoxicity, and apoptosis in human colon cancer cell lines. European Journal of Nutrition 38: 133–142.

Kuo, S. M. (1996) Antiproliferative potency of structurally distinct dietary flavonoids on human colon cancer cells. Cancer Letters 110: 41–48.

Lamartiniere, C. A., Moore, J., Holland, M., and Barnes, S. (1995) Neonatal genistein chemo prevents mammary cancer. Proceedings of the Society for Experimental Biology and Medicine 208: 120–123.

Lamartiniere, C. A., Murrill, W. B., Manzolillo, P. A., Zhang, J. X., Barnes, S., Zhang, X., Wei, H., and Brown, N. M. (1998) Genistein alters the ontogeny of mammary gland development and protects against chemically-induced mammary cancer in rats. Proceedings of the Society for Experimental Biology and Medicine 217: 358–364.

Liao, S., Umekita, Y., Guo, J., Kokontis, J. M., and Hiipakka, R. A. (1995) Growth inhibition and regression of human prostate and breast tumors in athymic mice by tea epigallocatechin gallate. Cancer Letters 96: 239–243.

Lieberman, R., Bermejo, C., Akaza, H., Greenwald, P., Fair, W., and Thompson, I. (2001) Progress in prostate cancer chemoprevention: modulators of promotion and progression. [Review] [29 refs]. Urology 58: 835–842.

Lu, L. J., Anderson, K. E., Grady, J. J., Kohen, F., and Nagamani, M. (2000) Decreased ovarian hormones during a soya diet: implications for breast cancer prevention. Cancer Research 60: 4112–4121.

Lyn-Cook, B. D., Rogers, T., Yan, Y., Blann, E. B., Kadlubar, F. F., and Hammons, G. J. (1999) Chemopreventive effects of tea extracts and various components on human pancreatic and prostate tumor cells in vitro. Nutrition and Cancer 35: 80–86.

Maggiolini, M., Bonofiglio, D., Marsico, S., Panno, M. L., Cenni, B., Picard, D., and Ando, S. (2001) Estrogen receptor alpha mediates the proliferative but not the cytotoxic dose-dependent effects of two major phytoestrogens on human breast cancer cells. Molecular Pharmacology 60: 595–602.

Martini, M. C., Dancisak, B. B., Haggans, C. J., Thomas, W., and Slavin, J. L. (1999) Effects of soy intake on sex hormone metabolism in premenopausal women. Nutrition and Cancer 34: 133–139.

McLellan, E. and Bird, R. P. (1991) Effect of disulfiram on 1,2-dimethylhydrazine- and azoxymethane-induced aberrant crypt foci. Carcinogenesis 12: 969–972.

McMichael-Phillips, D. F., Harding, C., Morton, M., Roberts, S. A., Howell, A., Potten, C. S., and Bundred, N. J. (1998) Effects of soy-protein supplementation on epithelial proliferation in the histologically normal human breast. American Journal of Clinical Nutrition 68: 1431S–1435S.

Mehta, K., Pantazis, P., McQueen, T., and Aggarwal, B. B. (1997) Antiproliferative effect of curcumin (diferuloylmethane) against human breast tumor cell lines. Anti-Cancer Drugs 8: 470–481.

Mentor-Marcel, R., Lamartiniere, C. A., Eltoum, I. E., Greenberg, N. M., and Elgavish, A. (2001) Genistein in the diet reduces the incidence of poorly differentiated prostatic adenocarcinoma in transgenic mice (TRAMP). Cancer Research 61: 6777–6782.

Messina, M. J., and Loprinzi, C. L. (2001) Soy for breast cancer survivors: a critical review of the literature. Journal of Nutrition 131: 3095S–3108S.

Michaud, D. S., Augustsson, K., Rimm, E. B., Stampfer, M. J., Willet, W. C., and Giovannucci, E. (2001) A prospective study on intake of animal products and risk of prostate cancer. Cancer Causes and Control 12: 557–567.

Miksicek, R. J. (1994) Interaction of naturally occurring nonsteroidal estrogens with expressed recombinant human estrogen receptor. Journal of Steroid Biochemistry and Molecular Biology 49: 153–160.

Mitchell, J. H., Duthie, S. J., and Collins, A. R. (2000) Effects of phytoestrogens on growth and DNA integrity in human prostate tumor cell lines: PC-3 and LNCaP. Nutrition and Cancer 38: 223–228.

Moragoda, L., Jaszewski, R., and Majumdar, A. P. (2001) Curcumin induced modulation of cell cycle and apoptosis in gastric and colon cancer cells. Anticancer Research 21: 873–878.

Mukhopadhyay, A., Bueso-Ramos, C., Chatterjee, D., Pantazis, P., and Aggarwal, B. B. (2001) Curcumin downregulates cell survival mechanisms in human prostate cancer cell lines. Oncogene 20: 7597–7609.

Murrill, W. B., Brown, N. M., Zhang, J. X., Manzolillo, P. A., Barnes, S., and Lamartiniere, C. A. (1996) Prepubertal genistein exposure suppresses mammary cancer and enhances gland differentiation in rats. Carcinogenesis 17: 1451–1457.

Mutoh, M., Takahashi, M., Fukuda, K., Matsushima-Hibiya, Y., Mutoh, H., Sugimura, T., and Wakabayashi, K. (2000) Suppression of cyclooxygenase-2 promoter-dependent transcriptional activity in colon cancer cells by chemopreventive agents with a resorcin-type structure. Carcinogenesis 21: 959–963.

Nakachi, K., Suemasu, K., Suga, K., Takeo, T., Imai, K., and Higashi, Y. (1998) Influence of drinking green tea on breast cancer malignancy among Japanese patients. Japanese Journal of Cancer Research 89: 254–261.

Ohishi, T., Kishimoto, Y., Miura, N., Shiota, G., Kohri, T., Hara, Y., Hasegawa, J., and Isemura, M. (2002) Synergistic effects of (-)-epigallocatechin gallate with sulindac against colon carcinogenesis of rats treated with azoxymethane. Cancer Letters 177: 49–56.

Okura, A., Arakawa, H., Oka, H., Yoshinari, T., and Monden, Y. (1988) Effect of genistein on topoisomerase activity and on the growth of [Val 12]Ha-ras-transformed NIH 3T3 cells. Biochemical and Biophysical Research Communications 157: 183–189.

Onozawa, M., Kawamori, T., Baba, M., Fukuda, K., Toda, T., Sato, H., Ohtani, M., Akaza, H., Sugimura, T., and Wakabayashi, K. (1999) Effects of a soybean isoflavone mixture on carcinogenesis in prostate and seminal vesicles of F344 rats. Japanese Journal of Cancer Research 90: 393–398.

Paschka, A. G., Butler, R., and Young, C.Y. (1998) Induction of apoptosis in prostate cancer cell lines by the green tea component, (-)-epigallocatechin-3-gallate. Cancer Letter 130: 1–7.

Pereira, M. A., Barnes, L. H., Rassman, V. L., Kelloff, G. V., and Steele, V. E. (1994) Use of azoxymethane-induced foci of aberrant crypts in rat colon to identify potential cancer chemopreventive agents. Carcinogenesis 15: 1049–1054.

Pianetti, S., Guo, S., Kavanagh, K. T., and Sonenshein, G. E. (2002) Green tea polyphenol epigallocatechin-3 gallate inhibits Her-2/neu signaling, proliferation, and transformed phenotype of breast cancer cells. Cancer Research 62: 652–655.

Plewa, M. J., Berhow, M. A., Vaughn, S. F., Woods, E. J., Rundell, M., Naschansky, K., Bartolini, S., and Wagner, E. D. (2001) Isolating antigenotoxic components and cancer cell growth suppressors from agricultural by-products. Mutation Research 480–481: 109–120.

Pollard, M., and Wolter, W. (2000) Prevention of spontaneous prostate-related cancer in Lobund-Wistar rats by a soy protein isolate/isoflavone diet. Prostate 45: 101–105.

Potter, J. D., Slattery, M. L., Bostick, R. M., and Gapstur, S. M. (1993) Colon cancer: a review of the epidemiology. Epidemiologic Reviews 15: 499–545.

Ramachandran, C., and You, W. (1999) Differential sensitivity of human mammary epithelial and breast carcinoma cell lines to curcumin. Breast Cancer Research and Treatment 54: 269–278.

Ranelletti, F. O., Maggiano, N., Serra, F. G., Ricci, R., Larocca, L. M., Lanza, P., Scambia, G., Fattorossi, A., Capelli, A., and Piantelli, M. (2000) Quercetin inhibits p21-RAS expression in human colon cancer cell lines and in primary colorectal tumors. International Journal of Cancer 85: 438–445.

Ranelletti, F. O., Ricci, R., Larocca, L. M., Maggiano, N., Capelli, A., Scambia, G., Benedetti-Panici, P., Mancuso, S., Rumi, C., and Piantelli, M. (1992) Growth-inhibitory effect of quercetin and presence of type-II estrogen-binding sites in human colon-cancer cell lines and primary colorectal tumors. International Journal of Cancer 50: 486–492.

Rao, C. V., Rivenson, A., Simi, B., and Reddy, B. S. (1995) Chemoprevention of colon carcinogenesis by dietary curcumin, a naturally occurring plant phenolic compound. Cancer Research 55: 259–266.

Rao, C. V., Wang, C. X., Simi, B., Lubet, R., Kelloff, G., Steele, V., and Reddy, B. S. (1997a) Enhancement of experimental colon cancer by genistein. Cancer Research 57: 3717–3722.

Rao, G. N., Ney, E., and Herbert, R. A. (1997b) Influence of diet on mammary cancer in transgenic mice bearing an oncogene expressed in mammary tissue. Breast Cancer Research and Treatment 45: 149–158.

Reddy, B. S. (1999) Role of dietary fiber in colon cancer: an overview. American Journal of Medicine 106: 16S–19S.

Ren, F., Zhang, S., Mitchell, S. H., Butler, R., and Young, C. Y. (2000) Tea polyphenols down-regulate the expression of the androgen receptor in LNCaP prostate cancer cells. Oncogene 19: 1924–1932.

Richter, M., Ebermann, R., and Marian, B. (1999) Quercetin-induced apoptosis in colorectal tumor cells: possible role of EGF receptor signaling. Nutrition and Cancer 34: 88–99.

Rodgers, E. H., and Grant, M. H. (1998) The effect of the flavonoids, quercetin, myricetin and epicatechin on the growth and enzyme activities of MCF7 human breast cancer cells. Chemico-Biological Interactions 116: 213–228.

Russo, I. H., and Russo, J. (1978) Developmental stage of the rat mammary gland as determinant of its susceptibility to 7,12-dimethylbenz[a]anthracene. Journal of the National Cancer Institute 61: 1439–1449.

Salti, G. I., Grewal, S., Mehta, R. R., Das Gupta, T. K., Boddie, A. W., Jr., and Constantinou, A. I. (2000) Genistein induces apoptosis and topoisomerase II-mediated DNA breakage in colon cancer cells. European Journal of Cancer 36: 796–802.

Scambia, G., Ranelletti, F. O., Benedetti, P. P., Piantelli, M., Bonanno, G., De Vincenzo, R., Ferrandina, G., Pierelli, L., Capelli, A., and Mancuso, S. (1991) Quercetin inhibits the growth of a multidrug-resistant estrogen-receptor-negative MCF-7 human breast-cancer cell line expressing type II estrogen-binding sites. Cancer Chemotherapy and Pharmacology 28: 255–258.

Scambia, G., Ranelletti, F. O., Panici, P. B., Piantelli, M., De Vincenzo, R., Ferrandina, G., Bonanno, G., Capelli, A., and Mancuso, S. (1993) Quercetin induces type-II estrogen-binding sites in estrogen-receptor-negative (MDA-MB231) and estrogen-receptor-positive (MCF-7) human breast-cancer cell lines. International Journal of Cancer 54: 462–466.

Setchell, K. D., Lawson, A. M., Borriello, S. P., Harkness, R., Gordon, H., Morgan, D. M., Kirk, D. N., Adlercreatz, H., Anderson, L. C., and Axelson, M. (1981) Lignan formation in man-microbial involvement and possible roles in relation to cancer. Lancet 2: 4–7.

Shao, Z. M., Alpaugh, M. L., Fontana, J. A., and Barsky, S. H. (1998) Genistein inhibits proliferation similarly in estrogen receptor-positive and negative human breast carcinoma cell lines characterized by P21WAF1/CIP1 induction, G2/M arrest, and apoptosis. Journal of Cellular Biochemistry 69: 44–54.

Shao, Z. M., Shen, Z. Z., Liu, C. H., Sartippour, M. R., Go, V. L., Heber, D., and Nguyen, M. (2002) Curcumin exerts multiple suppressive effects on human breast carcinoma cells. International Journal of Cancer 98: 234–240.

Sharma, R. A., McLelland, H. R., Hill, K. A., Ireson, C. R., Euden, S. A., Manson, M. M., Pirmohamed, M., Marnett, L. J., Gescher, A. J., and Steward, W. P. (2001) Pharmacodynamic and pharmacokinetic study of oral Curcuma extract in patients with colorectal cancer. Clinical Cancer Research 7: 1894–1900.

Shu, X. O., Jin, F., Dai, Q., Wen, W., Potter, J. D., Kushi, L. H., Ruan, Z., Gao, Y. T., and Zheng, W. (2001) Soyfood intake during adolescence and subsequent risk of breast cancer among Chinese women. Cancer Epidemiology, Biomarkers and Prevention 10: 483–488.

Singhal, R. L., Yeh, Y. A., Praja, N., Olah, E., Sledge, G. W., Jr., and Weber, G. (1995) Quercetin down-regulates signal transduction in human breast carcinoma cells. Biochemical and Biophysical Research Communications 208: 425–431.

Slamon, D. J., Clark, G. M., Wong, S. G., Levin, W. J., Ullrich, A., and McGuire, W. L. (1987) Human breast cancer: correlation of relapse and survival with amplification of the HER-2/neu oncogene. Science 235: 177–182.

Sorensen, I. K., Kristiansen, E., Mortensen, A., Nicolaisen, G. M., Wijnands, J. A., van Kranen, H. J., and van Kreijl, C. F. (1998) The effect of soy isoflavones on the development of intestinal neoplasia in ApcMin mouse. Cancer Letters 130: 217–225.

Steiner, M. S., Raghow, S., and Neubauer, B. L. (2001) Selective estrogen receptor modulators for the chemoprevention of prostate cancer. Urology 57: 68–72.

Strom, S. S., Yamamura, Y., Duphorne, C. M., Spitz, M. R., Babaian, R. J., Pillow, P. C., and Hursting, S. D. (1999) Phytoestrogen intake and prostate cancer: a case-control study using a new database. Nutrition and Cancer 33: 20–25.

Thiagarajan, D. G., Bennink, M. R., Bourquin, L. D., and Kavas, F. A. (1998) Prevention of precancerous colonic lesions in rats by soy flakes, soy flour, genistein, and calcium. American Journal of Clinical Nutrition 68: 1394S–1399S.

Uckun, F. M., Narla, R. K., Zeren, T., Yanishevski, Y., Myers, D. E., Waurzyniak, B., Ek, O., Schneider, E., Messinger, Y., Chelstrom, L. M., Gunther, R., and Evans, W. (1998) In vivo toxicity, pharmacokinetics, and anticancer activity of Genistein linked to recombinant human epidermal growth factor. Clinical Cancer Research 4: 1125–1134.

Wang, C., and Kurzer, M. S. (1997) Phytoestrogen concentration determines effects on DNA synthesis in human breast cancer cells. Nutrition and Cancer 28: 236–247.

Weber, K. S., Setchell, K. D., Stocco, D. M., and Lephart, E. D. (2001) Dietary soy-phytoestrogens decrease testosterone levels and prostate weight without altering LH, prostate 5alpha-reductase or testicular steroidogenic acute regulatory peptide levels in adult male Sprague-Dawley rats. Journal of Endocrinology 170: 591–599.

Weisburger, J. H., Rivenson, A., Aliaga, C., Reinhardt, J., Kelloff, G. J., Boone, C. W., Steele, V. E., Balentine, D. A., Pittman, B., and Zang, E. (1998) Effect of tea extracts, polyphenols, and epigallocatechin gallate on azoxymethane-induced colon cancer. Proceedings of the Society for Experimental Biology and Medicine 217: 104–108.

Weyant, M. J., Carothers, A. M., Bertagnolli, M. E., and Bertagnolli, M. M. (2000) Colon cancer chemopreventive drugs modulate integrin-mediated signaling pathways. Clinical Cancer Research 6: 949–956.

Willett, W. C. (2001) Diet and cancer: one view at the start of the millennium. Cancer Epidemiology, Biomarkers and Prevention 10: 3–8.

Writing Group for the Women's Health Initiative Investigators. (2002) Risks and benefits of estrogen plus progestin in healthy postmenopausal women: principal results from the Women's Health Initiative randomized controlled trial. JAMA 288: 321–333.

Wu, A. H., Ziegler, R. G., Nomura, A. M., West, D. W., Kolonel, L. N., Horn-Ross, P. L., Hoover, R. N., and .Pike, M. C. (1998) Soy intake and risk of breast cancer in Asians and Asian Americans. American Journal of Clinical Nutrition 68: 1437S–1443S.

Yanagihara, K., Ito, A., Toge, T., and Numoto, M. (1993) Antiproliferative effects of isoflavones on human cancer cell lines established from the gastrointestinal tract. Cancer Research 53: 5815–5821.

Yu, J., Cheng, Y., Xie, L., and Zhang, R. (1999) Effects of genistein and daidzein on membrane characteristics of HCT cells. Nutrition and Cancer 33: 100–104.

Zava, D. T. and Duwe, G. (1997) Estrogenic and antiproliferative properties of genistein and other flavonoids in human breast cancer cells in vitro. Nutrition and Cancer 27: 31–40.

Zhou, J. R., Gugger, E. T., Tanaka, T., Guo, Y., Blackburn, G. L., and Clinton, S. K. (1999) Soybean phytochemicals inhibit the growth of transplantable human prostate carcinoma and tumor angiogenesis in mice. Journal of Nutrition 129: 1628–1635.

Ziegler, R. G., Hoover, R. N., Pike, M. C., Hildesheim, A., Nomura, A. M., West, D. W., Wu-Williams, A. H., Kolonel, L. N., Horn-Ross, P. L., and Rosenthal, J. F. (1993) Migration patterns and breast cancer risk in Asian-American women. Journal of the National Cancer Institute 85: 1819–1827.

14

Herbals and Cancer Prevention

Michael J. Wargovich,
Destiny M. Hollis,
and Mary E. S. Zander

INTRODUCTION

Over the last decade the use of dietary supplements (including botanicals) has risen in prevalence to one in three Americans. Botanical supplements include whole leaf, stems and roots of plants, and prepared extracts from plant components. Most human cultures have a tradition of botanical medicine. Plants, especially herbs, have been valued by indigenous cultures for health care and a large percentage of the world relies on plants and extracts of plants for sources of medicine. Today, there is a resurgence of interest, especially among the well-read population, in herbal medicine. The most commonly cited reasons for the use of botanical supplements are similar to those for use of other "alternative" medicine modalities. These include the beliefs that (1) there are limitations to conventional medicine, (2) conventional medications are artificial and alternative medicine is natural, (3) conventional medicine treats the disease while alternative medicine treats the person, (4) alternative medicines provide hope of help with chronic disease while offering a sense of self-control. In several recent studies the prevalence of supplement use was studied among cancer patients. It was found that use was higher than the general public (50–80% were users) and, while cancer patients share the same motivations as the general public, they do so with greater intensity (Bernstein and Grasso 2001).

Botanicals have a long history of use in the treatment of cancer. Many cancer chemotherapeutic drugs are derived from plants including the alkaloids of the Vinca species (vincristine and vinblastine), the Pacific yew, *Taxus brevifolia* (Taxol), and *Campotheca acuminata* (Irinotecan) to name a few. More recently, there is speculation that herbal products and constituents may be useful in the prevention of cancer. Use of botanicals for cancer prevention is consonant with public health advice offered by governmental and other health agencies to modify diet and lifestyle. This review explores the use of herbal products for the prevention of cancer.

HISTORICAL USE OF HERBS FOR CANCER

Ancient cultures throughout the world have used a plethora of techniques to treat and prevent diseases, and to maintain health. One subset of these techniques is herbals. It is often found that the same or similar plants are used in a number of cultures for the same symptoms or diseases, signifying that it is probably medicinally quite effective for those types of ailments (Borchers et al. 2000). Despite modern medical advances, cancer remains a worldwide health problem. A number of herbs have been traditionally used for treating and preventing cancer. An example is the herb ginseng, which has been used for more than two thousand years beginning in ancient China. It was noted during China's Liang Dynasty that the habitual use of ginseng not only helped cure acute problems, but also showed life-prolongation effects, leading to the hypothesis that ginseng may have chemo-preventive properties (Bruss et al. 2000; Yun and Choi 1998).

As we progress in the scientific understanding of the mechanisms of herbs that have been used for centuries, we may discover new uses for ancient sources of medicine.

HERBAL MARKET AND CANCER

The use of herbs as medicines has played an important role in nearly every culture on earth. Recent surveys suggest that one in three Americans use dietary supplements daily and the rate of usage is much higher in cancer patients. A study of one hundred cancer patients in a South Florida hospital reported that 57% of cancer patients take herbal products (Bernstein and Grasso 2001). Among the many reasons cited by the general public for use of herbal medicines is the belief that botanicals will provide some benefit over and above traditional allopathic medical approaches. There is also the sense that taking supplements allows some measure of self-choice in medical care. Table 14.1 outlines some of the more commonly consumed herbals and their medicinal claims.

As a result of the increased interest in herbal use for medicinal purposes, sales of herbal supplements have increased substantially over the past decade. Herbal sales in the United States alone are over $4 billion annually. Some of the top herbs sold in the United States include *Ginkgo biloba*, St. John's wort, ginseng, garlic, echinacea, and saw palmetto (Brevoort 1998). In an attempt to scientifically validate the historical claims or observational analyses associated with many of these herbs, scientists have begun rigorously testing these products, or their active ingredients, in cell culture, animal models, and humans in a variety of disease intervention strategies.

In 1994, the U.S. Congress passed the Dietary Supplement Health and Education Act (DSHEA) to govern the manufacturing, classification, and distribution of these herbal supplements. Under DSHEA, botanicals can be sold as foods, or as dietary supplements with claims as to their effect on the structure and function of the human body, providing the company has adequate documentation for the claim. The product must also display the disclaimer, "This statement has not been evaluated by the Food and Drug Administration. This product is not intended to diagnose, treat, cure or prevent any disease." Herbals can also be sold as over-the-counter medication after receiving approval from the Food and Drug Administration (FDA). These medications can carry more specific therapeutic claims. Herbals also can be submitted to the FDA as an Investigational New Drug/New Drug Application (IND/NDA). Herbal IND applications may be treated differently from pharmaceutical drug trials, that is, they may require little or no chemistry or toxicology data (Temple 2002).

Table 14.1.   Commonly Consumed Herbals for Cancer Prevention

Herbal supplement	Components	Mechanism of action
Aged garlic extract	S-allylcysteine, allyl sulfides	Reduces cholesterol, reduces cancer risk, boosts immune function
Black tea extract	Proanthocyanidins, bisflavanols, theaflavins, and thearubigin	Antioxidant
EGb 761	Standardized *Gingko biloba* leaf extract	Stabilizes or improves dementia, anti-inflammatory
Flaxseed	Omega-3-fatty acids and lignan	Anti-angiogenic, anti-inflammatory
Ginger	6-Gingerol	Antioxidant
Ginseng	Ginsenosides	Antioxidant, anti-inflammatory
Grape seed extract	Range of proanthocyanidins	Antioxidant
Green tea extract	EGCG and related catechins theogallin	Antioxidant
Milk thistle	Silymarin	Anti-angiogenic, anti-inflammatory
Rosemary	Carnosol, carnosic acid, ursolic acid, rosmarinic acid, caffeic acid	Antioxidant, inhibits carcinogen activation, anti-inflammatory
Saw palmetto	Extract of saw palmetto berries	Inhibitor of 5alpha-reductase, anti-inflammatory
Soy isoflavones	Predominantly genistein and daidzein	Alternative to hormone replacement therapy
Turmeric	Curcumin	Antioxidant, anti-inflammatory

HERBALS AND CANCER PREVENTION

Antioxidants

Oxidative damage to DNA contributes to a variety of diseases, including cancer (Sharma et al. 2001) and antioxidant depletion in circulation is a characteristic finding in malignant transformation (Dreher and Junod 1996). Reactive oxygen species (ROS) are generated endogenously and by chemical carcinogens. These ROS can act as second messengers to stimulate cells to activate transcription factors regulated by the intracellular redox state and promote the development of inflammation, which can lead to cancer. Many chemical carcinogens exert their mutagenic effects by covalently binding to and modifying electron-rich sources in the cells such as DNA, RNA, lipids, and proteins. If modifications are not repaired and apoptosis is not initiated, mutagenesis and cancer could occur.

   One of the most widely studied herbals with respect to chemopreventive efficacy is green tea and its associated polyphenols. Protection against oxidative damage is one of the most widely described attributes of polyphenols and one of the major selling points on which these compounds are marketed as dietary supplements. Tea preparations have been shown to trap reactive oxygen species, such as superoxide radical, singlet oxygen, hydroxy radical, peroxyl radical, nitric oxide, nitrogen dioxide, and peroxynitrite (Yang et al. 2002). The interaction of catechins with intracellular antioxidative species such as glutathione peroxidase may enhance their antioxidant activities (Nagata et al. 1999). In mice, both green and black tea were capable of inducing the free radical scavenger superoxide dismutase (Das et al. 2002).

Garlic has been reported to modulate lipid peroxidation levels and enhance the status of antioxidants (Balasenthil et al. 1999; Balasenthil et al. 2000). Aged garlic extract (AGE) is an antioxidant-rich extract derived from prolonged extraction of fresh garlic at room temperature. AGE consists of water-soluble S-allylcysteine (SAC) and S-allylmercaptocysteine (SAMC), and lipid-soluble diallyl sulfide (DAS), diallyl disulfide (DADS), triallyl sulfide, and diallyl polysulfide. AGE increases cellular glutathione in a variety of cells. As a substrate for the antioxidant enzyme glutathione peroxidase, glutathione protects cells from the damaging effects of peroxides formed in metabolism and through other ROS reactions. Decreased glutathione levels are associated with cell damage and may increase the risk of cancer development (Borek 2001).

[6]-Gingerol, the pharmacologically active component of ginger, possesses substantial antioxidant and antitumor activity. [6]-Gingerol inhibits xanthine oxidase activity, which is responsible for the generation of ROS such as superoxide anion (Chang et al. 1994). Diarylheptanoids, which are phenolic substances from plants of the ginger family, protect against superoxide anion generation in HL-60 skin cancer cells in culture (Lee et al. 1998).

Rosemary and its constituents (carnosol, carnosic acid, ursolic acid, rosmarinic acid, caffeic acid) have been studied extensively for their chemopreventive effects in various cancer models, including breast and skin cancer. Slamenova et al. suggested that the extract of rosemary exhibits a protective effect against oxidative damage to DNA as a consequence of scavenging ROS (Slamenova et al. 2002). Licorice may also be an effective antioxidant for chemoprevention. There is a growing body of evidence to suggest that licorice possesses anticarcinogenic properties because of its content of triterpenoids and polyphenols. Glabridin, a polyphenol found in licorice, inhibited superoxide release from macrophages in response to 12-O-tetradecanoylphorbol-13-acetate (TPA), or to low-density lipoprotein (LDL) when added together with copper ions, by up to 60% (Singletary and MacDonald 2000).

Many studies have demonstrated the antioxidant activities of ginsengs (examples include *Panax ginseng*, or Asian ginseng, and *Panax quinquefolius*, or American ginseng) (Bucci 2000; Keum et al. 2000; Surh et al. 2001a). They have been found to protect against fatty acid peroxidation as well as free radical-induced injury (Keum et al. 2000). Additionally, they were found to induce the expression of superoxide dismutase (Keum et al. 2000; Shin et al. 2000a), attenuate lipid peroxidation (Keum et al. 2000; Surh et al. 2001b), and suppress cytochrome P450 IIE1 (CYP2E1) (Keum et al. 2000), all of which demonstrate ginseng's antioxidant activities. Furthermore, at least one study has found that this herbal's antioxidant activities are dose dependent (Keum et al. 2000). In addition, certain ginseng fractions have been shown to scavenge reactive oxygen intermediates, including both superoxide and hydroxyl (Keum et al. 2000; Kitts et al. 2000; Surh et al.

2001b). Ginseng has been found to reduce the activity and expression of ornithine decarboxylase (ODC), which plays an important role in tumor promotion (Surh et al. 2001b). These activities have been found to inhibit virtually all stages of cancer. In addition, it increased glutathione content (Bucci 2000) and stimulated nitric oxide production (Bucci 2000; Shin et al. 2000b). Finally, in a comparison of a large number of medicinal plants, ginseng showed some of the highest antioxidant activities of over 40 herbs tested (Mantle et al. 2000).

Quercetin is the most common biologically active plant flavonoid, and it is often found in the outer layers of fruits and vegetables, as well as in tea leaves and wine (Mahmoud et al. 2000; Yang et al. 2000). Though many antioxidants and flavonoids are usually found in plant materials, quercetin is often the most abundant and/or the most active antioxidant in the plant (Bedir et al. 2002; Myhrstad et al. 2002; Pedrielli et al. 2001; Tanaka 1994). The average human intake of quercetin has been estimated to be from 20 to 500 mg per day, though most sources agree that it is just under 100 mg per day (Myhrstad et al. 2002; Tanaka 1994; Yang et al. 2000). Nevertheless, its high consumption makes it an important flavonoid and antioxidant to study. Quercetin has demonstrated antioxidant activities through a wide variety of mechanisms. Included in this list is inhibition of cytochrome c (P450) reductase (Tanaka 1994), reduction of lipid peroxidation (Pedrielli et al. 2001), direct reduction of oxidative stress by scavenging reactive oxygen species, and indirect protection of cells through phase II detoxification and antioxidant enzymes such as glutathione (GSH) and gamma-glutamylcysteine synthetase (GCS) (Myhrstad et al. 2002). In fact, it was determined that quercetin significantly increased GSH and GCS levels in a dose-dependent manner without cytotoxic effects in an in vitro model (Myhrstad et al. 2002). However, it should be noted that antioxidants have also been shown to induce DNA damage, especially at high concentrations, though these effects were neither statistically significant nor in physiological conditions (Szeto et al. 2002).

Flavonoids often exist in plants as sugar conjugates. Quercetin is no exception: Rutin is the glycosidic form of quercetin, and it is hydrolyzed to quercetin by the colonic microflora through beta-glucosidase activity (Mahmoud et al. 2000; Myhrstad et al. 2002; Yang et al. 2000). This glucosidase activity may enhance the bioavailability of the antioxidant activity (Mahmoud et al. 2000), but before this product conversion, rutin may not be an effective antioxidant (Myhrstad et al. 2002).

Carcinogen Activation and Detoxification

Phase I and phase II enzymes represent activation and detoxification pathways, respectively, for environmental and chemical carcinogens. The mechanism of action of many herbals includes their ability to decrease phase I and/or increase phase II enzyme activity.

Organosulfur compounds present in garlic represent some of the more efficient phase I/II modulators. DAS, which has been shown to inhibit chemically induced cancers of the colon and esophagus, is a potent inhibitor of CYP2E1. CYP2E1 is involved in the metabolic activation of several carcinogens, including dimethylhydrazine and several nitrosamines (Brady et al. 1988; Hollis et al. 2002). DADS, also an inhibitor of experimentally induced cancers in various animal models (Wargovich 1997), significantly increased several phase II enzymes, including GST, quinone reductase (QR), and UDP-glucuronosyltransferase (UGT), in the liver of male SPF Wistar rats. These enzymes catalyze the detoxification of carcinogens through reduction, hydrolysis, or conjugation with endogenous compounds, thereby blocking the ability of these carcinogens to bind to DNA (Guyonnet et al. 1999).

Cytochrome P450 1A (CYP1A) is involved in the metabolic activation of 2-amino-1-methyl-6-phenylimidazo[4,5-b]pyridine (PhIP), which is one of the most prevalent carcinogenic heterocyclic amines in the environment. PhIP targets the colon, prostate, pancreas, and mammary gland in rodents and humans (Hirose et al. 2002; Sinha et al. 2000). Rosemary inhibited CYP1A1 activity by 70–90% in a mouse mammary tumor model. Additionally, carnosol from rosemary induced GST and QR expression (Offord et al. 1997).

Resveratrol (trans-3,5,4'-trihydroxystilbene) is a polyphenolic phytoalexin present in several plants, and is especially abundant in the skin of grapes, as well as in peanuts (Wolter et al. 2001). The anti-initiating activity of resveratrol is linked to the suppression of metabolic activation of carcinogens and/or enhancement of their detoxification. Resveratrol inhibits hepatic cytochrome P450-linked alkoxyresorufin O-dealkylase activities responsible for oxidative metabolism of a wide array of carcinogenic aromatic hydrocarbons (Teel and Huynh 1998). Additionally, resveratrol has been reported to inhibit transcription of CYP1A1 (Plouzek et al. 1999).

Steroid Metabolism

Endogenous and exogenous steroid hormones are involved in the development of breast, prostate, and other cancers. Hormonal activity is associated with increased cell turnover, which might be expected to increase genomic instability. The estrogenic phytochemicals appear to primarily function by binding to and activating the estrogen receptor (ER), but at concentrations one hundred to one thousand times higher than 17β-estradiol (Collins et al. 1997; Gehm et al. 1997; Miksicek 1993; Miksicek 1994). Some of the most potent ER-binding herbals are soy, licorice, and red clover (Zava et al. 1998).

Soy phytochemicals genistein and daidzein can function as estradiol agonists, but the ability of these compounds to inhibit chemically induced mammary carcinogenesis suggests that they have antiestrogenic qualities as well. Genistein acts as an antiestrogen by binding to estrogen receptors and by stimulating sex hormone-binding globulin production to decrease the free and active hormone in the blood (Messina et al. 1994). It has been postulated that soy isoflavones exert antiestrogenic effects when placed in high-estrogen environments and estrogenic effects when placed in low-estrogen environments. This hypothesis could explain the epidemiological evidence that suggests soy shows a protective effect against breast cancer predominantly in premenopausal women.

Genistein is also effective in the inhibition of both androgen-dependent and androgen-independent prostate cancer cells in vitro and in vivo. Although the precise role of estrogen in prostate cancer is not well defined, the potential estrogenic effects of isoflavones from soy may be protective because estrogens have been used successfully as a form of hormone therapy for metastatic prostate cancer (Messina 1999).

The enzyme steroid 5α-reductase catalyzes the conversion of testosterone to 5α-dihydrotestosterone. In humans, 5α-reductase activity may be involved in the development of prostate cancer and may be responsible for differences in prostate cancer mortality among different racial groups (Ross et al. 1992). Several compounds derived from plant sources are inhibitors of 5α-reductase activity, including myricetin, quercetin, daidzein, genistein, kaempferol, and green tea catechins (Hiipakka et al. 2002). However, a recent report suggests that dihydrotestosterone suppresses tumor growth in androgen-independent tumors. Therefore, a decrease in 5α-reductase activity may actually potentiate tumor development in androgen-independent cancers (Liao 2001).

Signal Transduction Regulation

In addition to their direct effects on carcinogen activation and function, several herbals also maintain the ability to modify signal transduction events in a cell such that the basic patterns of cell growth and function are manipulated. Such modifications can contribute to the progression or regression of a malignant phenotype.

The *ras* family of protooncogenes encodes 21-kDa proteins (p21^{ras}), which play an important role in the transduction of extracellular signals to the cell nucleus. Oncogenic *ras* has been identified in 30–50% of human cancers, and plasma membrane association of p21^{ras} is necessary for its cell transformation activity. Farnesylation, catalyzed by farnesyl transferase, is required for plasma membrane association (Kato et al. 1992). Mevalonate is a precursor to farnesyl pyrophosphate and is synthesized from 3-hydroxy-3-methylglutaryl coenzyme A (HMG-CoA), a reaction catalyzed by HMG-CoA reductase (Goldstein and Brown 1990). Oral administration of DADS from garlic significantly inhibits the growth of H-*ras* oncogene transformed tumors in nude mice by inhibiting p21^{ras} farnesylation. This inhibition occurs via depletion of the farnesyl pyrophosphate pool due to inhibition by DADS of HMG-CoA reductase activity (Singh 2001).

Isoprenoids are a large group of anticarcinogenic phytochemicals present in a variety of herbs, including basil, marjoram, peppermint, and thyme, which are secondary products of plant mevalonate metabolism. The potency with which an isoprenoid suppresses hepatic HMG-CoA reductase activity predicts its potency as an antitumor agent (Mo and Elson 1999). The breakdown of lamin B processing subsequent to isoprenoid-mediated HMG-CoA reductase inhibition interferes with the assembly of daughter nuclei and renders DNA available to the p53-independent apoptotic endonuclease activities (Mo and Elson 1999).

Ornithine decarboxylase (ODC) catalyzes the rate-limiting step in the biosynthesis of polyamines and is closely linked to cellular proliferation and carcinogenesis. Inhibitors of ODC have been used for many years in the prevention and treatment of various cancers. Polyphenols present in green tea are effective inhibitors of ODC activity (Bachrach and Wang 2002). Glycyrrhetinic acid from licorice extract and diarylheptanoids present in *Alpinia oxyphylla Miquel* (Zingiberaceae) inhibit TPA-induced ODC activity (Surh 1999; Wang et al. 1991).

The induction of apoptosis in different cancer cell lines and in tumors is a common mechanism of cancer prevention by dietary agents. DAS from garlic induced apoptosis in human non-small-cell lung cancer cell lines as evidenced by an increase in the proapoptotic protein Bax and a decrease in anti-apoptotic protein Bcl-2 (Hong et al. 2000). Bcl-2 inhibits apoptosis and Bax counteracts the effects of Bcl-2 by forming a heterodimer with Bcl-2 (Kobayashi et al. 1998). Carnosol from rosemary induced apoptosis accompanied by a disruption of the mitochondrial membrane potential and downregulation of Bcl-2 (Dorrie et al. 2001). Licochalcone A isolated from licorice decreased Bcl-2 and altered the Bcl-2 to Bax ratio in favor of apoptosis (Rafi et al. 2000). S-allylmercaptocysteine, a water-soluble garlic OSC, induced apoptosis in erythroleukemia cell lines (Sigounas et al. 1997). There is also evidence to suggest that these allylic sulfur compounds, possibly due to their inactivation of sulfhydryl enzymes within rapidly dividing cancer cells, preferentially suppress neoplastic over non-neoplastic cells (Dorrie et al. 2001). Because tumor tissues have a higher concentration of sulfhydryl enzymes than normal tissues, a decrease in the availability of sulfhydryl enzymes could result in inhibition of tumor growth (Moon et al. 2000).

Apoptosis can be mediated by oxidative stress, which is in turn mediated by the generation of reactive oxygen intermediates (Buttke and Sandstrom 1994). Oxidative stress activates caspases, a family of cysteine proteases that are involved in the induction of cell death by apoptosis (Grimm et al. 1996; Polverino and Patterson 1997). DADS can induce apoptosis in human leukemia HL-60 cells by the generation of hydrogen peroxide with subsequent induction of caspase-3 (Kwon et al. 2002). Similar results were obtained by treatment of human chondrosarcoma HTB-94 cells by catechins from green tea (Islam et al. 2000).

The Her-2/neu oncogene is a second messenger of the EGFR family that promotes cell proliferation, survival, and transformed phenotype. Overexpression of Her-2/neu, which has been seen in approximately 30% of breast cancer patients, is associated with poor overall survival possibly due to increased metastatic potential and resistance to chemotherapeutic agents (Guy et al. 1992). A recent study demonstrated that epigallocatechin gallate from green tea can ablate the Her-2/neu signaling cascade in breast cancer cells by reducing basal Her-2/neu receptor phosphorylation (Pianetti et al. 2002).

Anti-inflammatory Mechanisms

An important manner in which herbals aid in cancer prevention is through anti-inflammatory mechanisms. The use of anti-inflammatory drugs has proven to be effective in reducing the incidence of several cancers, most notably colon cancer (Tosetti et al. 2002). A potential problem with using traditional NSAIDs (nonsteroidal anti-inflammatory drugs) such as aspirin or ibuprofen is that there are numerous side effects associated with their habitual use. Thus, safe and effective natural herbals with strong anti-inflammatory activities could greatly help reduce cancer rates without the adverse side effects commonly associated with habitual NSAID use.

Curcumin, or diferuloylmethane, is a constituent of the plant turmeric (*Curcuma longa*), and is a low molecular weight polyphenol. Its characteristic yellow color has made it an ideal coloring agent for many foods, and it is used to flavor mustards, curry powders, and other spice mixtures (Goel et al. 2001; Huang et al. 1997; Surh et al. 2001a). In addition to its practical uses, this herbal has a wide variety of medicinally beneficial activities, including anti-inflammatory activities. In fact, its traditional uses include treating inflammatory disorders (Churchill et al. 2000; Cipriani et al. 2001; Hanif et al. 1997). It has been shown to inhibit the activity of cyclooxygenase (COX) and lipoxygenase (LOX), both of which are strongly believed to be involved in inflammatory and carcinogenic processes (Churchill et al. 2000; Goel et al. 2001; Plummer et al. 1999; Surh et al. 2001a; Tanaka 1994). Furthermore, it has been found to suppress the expression of COX at the protein and mRNA levels (Churchill et al. 2000; Plummer et al. 1999; Surh et al. 2001a). Goel et al. determined that the COX inhibitory effects of curcumin were specific for only one isoform of this enzyme: COX-2, the isoform responsible for the inflammatory effects in the cell (Goel et al. 2001). Curcumin inhibits COX directly and indirectly. Plummer et al. demonstrated that curcumin inhibits activation of nuclear factor kappa B (NF-κB), which in turn inhibits expression of the COX-2 gene (Plummer et al. 1999). This effect has been confirmed in several different models (Cipriani et al. 2001; Li and Lin-Shia 2001; Surh et al. 2001a). Furthermore, curcumin blocked the degradation of the inhibitory protein IκBα, and the subsequent nuclear translocation of NF-κB. IκBα normally binds to NF-κB, keeping it in the inactive form and preventing it from translocating to the nucleus. In addition, curcumin inhibited nitric oxide (NO) production and mRNA and protein expression of iNOS (inducible nitric oxide synthase). iNOS catalyzes the production of NO, a potent inflammatory mediator believed to activate COX-2. The decrease of iNOS was attributed to c-Jun and AP-1 suppression. Additionally, c-fos has been found to be strongly inhibited by curcumin, as has jun N-terminal kinase (JNK) activation (Surh et al. 2001a). These transcription factors are all part of the MAPK (mitogen activated protein kinase) pathway, which is among the most extensively studied signaling cascades involved in inflammatory responses. It is believed that activation of this pathway leads to COX-2 and iNOS induction (Surh et al. 2001a). Curcumin also significantly lowered levels of inflammatory cytokines involved in what is thought to be the damaging steps leading to Alzheimer's disease (Lim et al. 2001). Finally, topical application of curcumin has strongly inhibited chemically induced inflammation, as well as the formation of tumors on the skin of mice (Churchill et al. 2000; Huang et al. 1997; Surh et al. 2001a). All of these examples show that curcumin has very strong anti-inflammatory activities; since cancer is thought to be prevented with NSAIDs, curcumin seems a great candidate for a chemopreventive agent. See Figure 14.1.

Green tea is one of the most widely consumed beverages worldwide, and it has been reported to have a number of medicinally beneficial properties, including chemopreventive properties. However, the experimental and epidemiological data have not always been in agreement (Metz et al. 2000). Nevertheless, there have been a number of studies that have shown chemopreventive effects through green tea, and it was suggested that it worked via an anti-inflammatory pathway. It has been shown to dramatically reduce COX-2 levels and activity in multiple animal models, without affecting COX-1 (Haqqi et al. 1999; Metz et al. 2000). It also lowered the amounts of TNF-alpha (tumor necrosis factor-

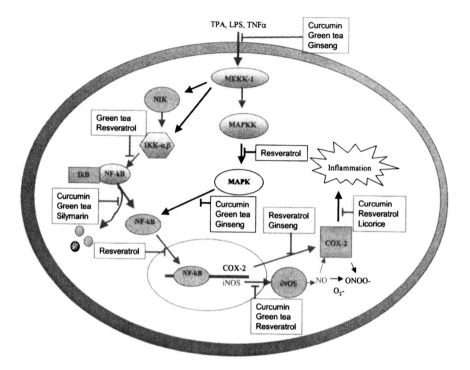

Figure 14.1.   Several herbals inhibit inflammation by blocking activation of COX-2. Some of these herbals can inhibit COX-2 by blocking the activation of NF-κB by blocking IKK-mediated phosphorylation of the inhibitory protein IκB (green tea, resveratrol), preventing the degradation of IκB (curcumin, green tea, silymarin), or blocking the translocation of NF-κB to the nucleus (resveratrol). These herbals can also inhibit the phosphorylation and subsequent nuclear translocation of NF-κB by inhibiting MAPK or MAPKK (resveratrol, curcumin, green tea, ginseng). Curcumin, ginseng, green tea, and resveratrol can also block inflammation by directly inhibiting translation of the COX-2 gene, by blocking the iNOS-mediated activation of COX-2, or by inhibiting the activity of the COX-2 protein.

alpha) and IFN-gamma (interferon-gamma), which are inflammatory cytokines, as well as the number of TNF-alpha and IFN-gamma expressing cells in a mouse model (Haqqi et al. 1999).

The polyphenol content of green tea accounts for up to 30% of its dry weight; with the average consumption of three-100 mL servings a day, approximately 240–320 mg of polyphenols are consumed (Haqqi et al. 1999). One of the most abundant and most effective of these polyphenols is epigallocatechin gallate (EGCG), which accounts for over 40% of the total polyphenolic content (Yang et al. 1998). This substance has anti-inflammatory properties. It dramatically inhibits TNF-alpha expression in a dose dependent manner (Levites et al. 2002; Surh et al. 2001a; Yang et al. 1998). It has been shown to inhibit NO production and iNOS gene expression through the decreased activation of NF-κB (Levites et al. 2002; Surh 1999; Surh et al. 2001a; Yang et al. 1998). Furthermore, it was found to abolish the activation of NF-κB in an in vitro model, as well as inhibit its translocation to the nucleus. Several NSAIDs inhibit IKK activity, and it has been found that EGCG is also a very effective inhibitor of this kinase. IκB kinases (IKK) phospoho-rylate IκB, which causes it to dissociate from NF-κB, become degraded, and allow NF-κB to stimulate cytokines in the inflammatory pathway. EGCG demonstrated decreased IκBα phosphorylation in a dose-dependent manner (Surh et al. 2001a; Yang et al. 2001) and decreased the NF-κB activity through the down-regulation of IκB kinase activity (Levites et al. 2002). Finally, EGCG has been found to decrease the expression of sever-al MAPK transcription factors, including c-jun, c-myc, JNK, ERK, and p38 MAPK (Surh et al. 2001a).

The phytoalexin resveratrol is especially abundant in the skin of grapes (Wolter et al. 2001). The chemopreventive properties of resveratrol have been associated with anti-inflammatory effects because of the epidemiological studies that defined the "French par-adox," which showed reduced mortality from heart disease and cancers with increased consumption of red wine (Holmes-McNary and Baldwin, Jr. 2000). Since this correlation was shown, several mechanisms through which resveratrol exerts its anti-inflammatory effects have been elucidated. Included in this list is the inhibition of COX transcription and activity, which subsequently causes suppression of prostaglandin biosynthesis (Baek et al. 2002; Gao et al. 2001; Holmes-McNary and Baldwin, Jr. 2000; Manna et al. 2000; Surh 1999; Surh et al. 2001a; Tou and Urbizo 2001; Wolter et al. 2001). This compound has also been found to inhibit LOX (Tou and Urbizo 2001). Additionally, resveratrol repressed the activation of AP-1 (Manna et al. 2000; Surh 1999; Surh et al. 2001a). One of the strongest mechanisms through which this compound may exert its anti-inflamma-tory effects is by suppressing the NF-κB activation pathway. It was found to completely inhibit NF-κB activation in a dose and time-dependent manner (Holmes-McNary and Baldwin, Jr. 2000; Manna et al. 2000). It is proposed that it works through this manner by inhibiting the nuclear translocation of NF-κB not through the degradation of IκBα, but by blocking the phosphorylation of the p65 subunit of NF-κB (Manna et al. 2000). Another hypothesis for how it blocks NF-κB activity is through the inhibition of IKK activity (Holmes-McNary and Baldwin, Jr. 2000). Furthermore, it has been shown to inhibit the activation of MAPK and its pathways (Surh et al. 2001a; Tou and Urbizo 2001): it was found to inhibit JNK and MEK in a dose-dependent manner (Manna et al. 2000) decrease the expression of c-fos (Manna et al. 2000; Surh 1999; Surh et al. 2001a), as well as reduce the phosphorylation of ERK-1/2 and p38 MAPK (Surh et al. 2001a). Finally, resveratrol suppresses the induction of iNOS and NO production (Gao et al. 2001; Holmes-McNary and Baldwin, Jr. 2000; Surh et al. 2001a).

There are several other herbals that appear to be chemopreventive through anti-inflam-matory mechanisms. Ginseng, including Asian ginseng (*Panax ginseng*) and American ginseng (*Panax quinquefolius*), is one of the most widely consumed herbals worldwide. The pharmacologically active constituents of ginseng are a series of saponin glycosides collectively known as the ginsenosides. Several case-control and cohort studies in Korea support experimental evidence that shows an inverse correlation with intake of ginseng and cancer risk at several sites. Included in its list of chemopreventive properties is an anti-inflammatory effect. Keum et al. showed that it dramatically lowered TNF-alpha pro-duction (Keum et al. 2000). Furthermore, Surh et al. found that all of the ginsenosides tested inhibited the effects of NF-κB. They also found that multiple ginsenosides inhibited several of the transcription factors in the MAPK pathway, including p38 MAPK, and ERK. Finally, they determined that one ginsenoside in particular, Rg3, suppressed COX-2 expression (Surh et al. 2001b). Several other groups also support the idea that ginseng suppresses COX (Ang-Lee et al. 2001; Borchers et al. 2000; Kimura et al. 1988; Park et al. 1996; Teng et al. 1989).

Other herbals with potential chemopreventive effects through an anti-inflammatory mechanism are milk thistle (*Silybum marianum*) and licorice. Silymarin, a polyphenolic flavonoid, is one of the main and most active ingredients in milk thistle. Silymarin has been found to inhibit COX and LOX (Luper 1998). Furthermore, it has been demonstrated to inhibit Kuppfer cells, inhibit neutrophil migration, and stabilize mast cells, which are components of the inflammatory response (Luper 1998). Manna et al. showed that this compound could inhibit NF-κB activation in a dose and time-dependent manner. Furthermore, it was determined that the effects on NF-κβ were due to silymarin's inhibition of the phosphorylation and degradation of Iκβα. Though they found that silymarin did not inhibit AP-1 activation, it did inhibit the activation of JNK and MEK (Manna et al. 1999). Licorice root has been used in Chinese medicine since at least 2100 B.C. One of its constituents, the triterpenoid GL, exerts a hydrocortisone-like anti-inflammatory effect. Finally, multiple constituents of licorice have demonstrated an inhibitory effect on LOX and COX (Wang and Nixon 2001). Thus, there are quite a number of herbals that can exert chemopreventive effects through anti-inflammatory mechanisms.

Antiangiogenic Mechanisms

Another mechanism through which several herbals have expressed chemopreventive properties is through inhibition of angiogenesis. Angiogenesis is the process of forming new blood vessels from preexisting ones (Berbari et al. 1999; Tosetti et al. 2002). This process is very important in cancer because a tumor cannot grow more than about 1 mm^3 without vasculature. The endothelial cell represents a preferential target for therapy, as it is a cell type common to all solid tumors (Ferrara 2000). Therefore, if an herbal supplement can aid in preventing or slowing angiogenesis, tumor progression can be prevented. There are several ways in which antiangiogenic compounds could work. One is by inhibiting matrix metalloproteinases (MMPs), which would then block the breakdown of the matrix surrounding the cells. Another is by directly inhibiting endothelial cells. A third mechanism is by blocking the activation of angiogenesis, for example blocking fibroblast growth factor (FGF), platelet-derived growth factor (PDGF), or vascular endothelial growth factor (VEGF) signaling. The last defined mechanism by which they could work is through the inhibition of endothelial-specific integrin signaling, or survival signaling (Unpublished data 2001).

One of the strongest herbals that has shown potential antiangiogenic capabilities is green tea (Bertolini et al. 2000; Jung et al. 2001; Yang et al. 2002). EGCG, the main polyphenol in green tea, has been demonstrated to inhibit MMP2 and MMP9 (Garbisa et al. 2001; Tosetti et al. 2002). It has also been shown to block the induction of VEGF, and

VEGF-receptor activity (Jung et al. 2001; L'Allemain 1999; Lamy et al. 2002; Tosetti et al. 2002). Furthermore, it has elevated the levels of IL-12, which is capable of activating an antiangiogenic process. It has also shown to inhibit EGF-R and PDGF-R beta (Tosetti et al. 2002).

Another herbal that has shown antiangiogenic activities is curcumin. This herbal has demonstrated these capabilities through the inhibition of MMP-2, and the upregulation of tissue inhibitor of metalloproteinase (TIMP)-1 (Shao et al. 2002). It has been shown to strongly decrease VEGF production (Pollmann et al. 2001). Dorai et al. demonstrated in an in vivo model that it significantly decreased the size and number of blood vessels in the animals' tumors (Dorai et al. 2001). Other studies have found similar results, and showed that curcumin targets FGF-2 and MMPs in the process (Arbiser et al. 1998; Mohan et al. 2000; Thaloor et al. 1998).

The isoflavone genistein inhibited the invasion of MCF-7 and MDA-MB-231 breast carcinoma cells by inhibiting MMP-9 and upregulating the tissue inhibitor of matrix met-alloproteinase-1 (TIMP-1), and inhibited angiogenesis by decreasing vessel density and levels of VEGF and TGF-β1 (Shao et al. 1998). The high excretion of genistein in urine of vegetarians suggests that genistein may contribute to the chemopreventive effects of a plant-based diet on tumor formation by inhibiting neovascularization (Fotsis et al. 1993).

Other herbals have also been demonstrated to have antiangiogenic properties. Resveratrol is included in this list, demonstrated through the inhibition of VEGF (Igura et al. 2001; Kimura and Okuda 2001). Silymarin is another, and it has also been shown to inhibit VEGF, along with MMP-2 (Jiang et al. 2000; Tosetti et al. 2002). Other herbals that have shown antiangiogenic properties through in vivo and in vitro data include ginseng, quercetin, and licorice (Igura et al. 2001; Kobayashi et al. 1995; Mochizuki et al. 1995; Morrow et al. 2001; Sato et al. 1994; Shibata 2001).

Other Mechanisms

Other mechanisms of cancer prevention by herbals have been explored. While some herbals can prevent the activation of carcinogens in an organism, others can actually inhib-it the formation of the carcinogen prior to ingestion. Heterocyclic aromatic amines com-prise a group of highly potent carcinogens that are formed during the cooking of meat and fish. The levels of the heterocyclic aromatic amines PhIP and 2-amino-3,8-dimethylimi-dazo[4,5-f]quinoxaline (MeIQx) that are formed in the cooking of beef can be signifi-cantly decreased by marinating with turmeric and garlic (Nerurkar et al. 1999), or with polyphenolic extracts from green tea (Weisburger et al. 2002).

Multidrug resistance (MDR), the cross-resistance of tumor cells to a variety of struc-turally and functionally unrelated anticancer drugs, is a major obstacle in treating cancer (Lehnert 1998). One mechanism of MDR involves the overexpression of the 170kDa plas-ma membrane-associated glycoprotein (Pgp). Pgp acts as an energy-dependent drug efflux pump that decreases intracellular drug accumulation, thereby decreasing the effectiveness of many chemotherapeutic agents (Gottesman et al. 1996). In drug-resistant MCF-7 breast cancer cells, rosemary extract inhibits the efflux of the common chemotherapeutic drugs doxorubicin and vinblastine, which are known substrates of Pgp, but does not affect accumulation of doxorubicin in wild-type MCF-7 cells, which lack Pgp (Plouzek et al. 1999). Similar results were observed using green tea polyphenols in the multidrug resistant cell line CH^{R}C5 (Jodoin et al. 2002).

Topoisomerase enzymes are DNA-associated enzymes that cleave and then reseal either one (topo I) or two (topo II) strands of DNA during processes such as replication or transcription. A number of compounds interfere in these processes by inhibiting the relegation of DNA double-strand breaks and enhancing the formation of cleavable DNA-enzyme complexes (Ferguson and Baguley 1994). Several chemotherapeutic agents, such as the antileukemic drug amsacrine, work by this mechanism (Finlay et al. 1994). It is possible that some of the observed anticancer effects of plant polyphenols may actually relate to their action as topo II poisons, making them potential antitumor agents. Topo II inhibition may be responsible for several of the known effects of genistein, including antiproliferative activity (Fotsis et al. 1993), apoptosis induction (McCabe, Jr. and Orrenius 1993), and effects on differentiation (Kondo et al. 1991; Watanabe et al. 1991).

Herbal Mixtures

Prostate cancer is a significant health problem in U.S. men, ranking first in incidence and second in the cause of cancer deaths (Jemal et al. 2002). In addition to surgery, the most common medical treatment for prostate cancer is androgen ablation therapy since prostate cells, at least in the initial stages of tumor formation, are androgen dependent for survival and proliferation. However, with time, it is the androgen independent tumor cells that become clinically aggressive and result in cancer deaths. A number of herbal products are used by men with prostate cancer in the hopes of modulating their disease, and it is possible that some of these herbal products work through androgen dependent or androgen independent pathways.

For practical purposes the most common herbal supplements taken for prostate cancer are saw palmetto, PC-SPES, pygeum, and flaxseed. Other less-common herbal supplements include lycopene and pumpkin seed oil. Saw palmetto is derived from the ripened fruits of *Serenoa repens,* an evergreen palm growing commonly in the southeastern United States. Saw palmetto was widely used as a food and tonic among the Seminole Indians and was considered to be useful in relieving irritation of the respiratory, digestive, and urinary tracts (Tyler 1993). An array of fatty acids and sterols have been identified in saw palmetto including phytosterols (β sitosterol and its glucoside) and free fatty acids (Fan and Wang 1995). Saw palmetto has been used to relieve the symptoms caused by a swollen prostate gland. It became widely used in the treatment of lower urinary tract symptoms, particulary secondary to benign prostatic hyperplasia (BPH) (U.S. Pharmacopeia 2002). Over 30 published studies have been conducted with saw palmetto but these studies have rarely had sufficient size, power, duration, or clinical study design quality to conclusively establish the efficacy of saw palmetto in BPH. In many of these studies a liposterolic extract of saw palmetto was used. The U.S. Pharmacopeia has evaluated the scientific literature relevant to saw palmetto and BPH. Seven trials were placebo controlled, one compared saw palmetto to finesteride, and one was a meta-analysis of 18 published studies, which did include saw palmetto in combination with other herbal products. Dosage of extract most commonly used was 160 mg taken twice per day. At this dose or higher, the report concluded that use of saw palmetto is more effective than placebo in relieving lower urinary tract symptoms (frequency, urgency, nocturia, and urine flow) (Wilt et al. 1998).

Another common herbal preparation used by men for treatment of their prostate cancer is PC-SPES. It consists of a blend of eight plants: baikal skullcap root, rabdosia root, saw palmetto, ginseng root, licorice root, dyer's woad root, reishi fungus, and chrysanthemum (Tiwari et al. 1999). PC-SPES inhibits proliferation and induces apoptosis in prostate cells in culture and inhibits tumorigenesis in rats implanted with prostate tumors (DiPaola et al. 1998). In the clinical arena, PC-SPES treatment has been shown to reduce blood PSA levels with concomitant reports of breast tenderness, indicating that PC-SPES may have estrogenic activity (Hsieh et al. 1997). Another recent study confirmed that PC-SPES has potent estrogenic activity in yeast, mice, and humans with side effects reported to be similar to pharmacologic doses of estrogen. PSA levels in eight patients treated with PC-SPES declined while on treatment (Oh et al. 2002). Studies on prostate cancer cells and studies on xenografted human prostate cancer in mice suggest that PC-SPES inhibits cell proliferation and tumor growth (Chenn 2001). Grave concerns have recently been raised by the FDA over accidental or intentional adulteration of PC-SPES with known pharmaceuticals. The recent discovery of traces of warfarin and alprazolam in samples of PC-SPES have led to a removal of this herbal mixture from the market pending investigation.

Pygeum, the extracted bark of the African prune tree (*Pygeum africanum*), has been used widely in Europe over the last two decades to treat mild to moderate symptoms of BPH (Longo and Tira 1983). A systematic scientific review of 31 studies was subjected to a meta-analysis and 18 studies met inclusion criteria; only one was not double blinded (Chatelain et al. 1999). Most of the studies compared a commercial pygeum extract (Tadenan) to placebo, while others compared pygeum to other herbals. While suffering from the same problems facing saw palmetto trials (short duration, inefficient study design, concurrent phytotherapies), the evidence is suggestive that pygeum significantly improves urological symptoms and urine flow in men with BPH (Chatelain et al. 1999). Its mechanism of action is not known.

Another dietary supplement widely used by men with symptoms of BPH or prostate cancer is flaxseed. Flaxseed contains omega-3 fatty acids and lignan and animal studies have supported the hypothesis that its consumption is preventive for certain cancers (Thompson 1994). In a clinical study, 25 men awaiting prostatectomy were placed on a low-fat diet supplemented with 30 g of flaxseed for an average of 34 days. Men taking the flaxseed experienced decreased testosterone levels, inhibition of tumor cell proliferation, and increases in apoptotic rates in tumor samples compared with men who did not receive flaxseed (Demark-Wahnefried et al. 2001).

Green tea drinking has been associated in a limited number of epidemiologic studies with a lower risk for prostate cancer (Heilbrun et al. 1986). Japanese and Chinese men have a prostate cancer incidence that ranks among the world's lowest. However, other factors in the Asian diet could also provide a level of protection not observed in Western nations. In vitro studies strongly suggest that the polyphenols in green tea impart growth inhibition of prostate cancer cells in culture and induce apoptosis (Gupta et al. 1999a; Gupta et al. 1999b). In possibly the most noteworthy study to date, a green tea polyphenol infusion at a dose equivalent to six cups of green tea a day inhibited prostate cancer development and extended survival in TRAMP mice, a strain of mouse that has been engineered with a transgene to develop metastatic prostate cancer (Gupta et al. 2001). Of interest in this study was the decreased activity of IGF-1 binding protein, a protein that has been shown to be elevated in several common forms of cancer.

CONCLUSION

Plant-based medicines were used by indigenous cultures to treat disease or alleviate its symptoms. In modern times, epidemiological investigations have strongly implicated a plant-based diet as the foundation for good health and linked its practice to prevention of chronic debilitating diseases such as heart disease and cancer. In the field of cancer prevention, the term "chemoprevention" has been adopted to include the discipline of cancer research that investigates the use of natural products or pharmaceuticals as possible modulators of the cancer process. It is clear that chemoprevention research is at a place where it now intersects ethnobotanical research. Indeed, many phytochemicals show promise as inhibitors of cancer. One of the limitations of chemoprevention in humans is the underlying toxicity of certain classes of chemopreventive drugs as illustrated by the use of retinoids in patients with recurrent head and neck cancer (Kurie et al. 1996). The next frontier of this research may well be to incorporate herbal compounds in cancer prevention clinical trials to reduce the potential toxicity of pharmaceuticals when given to at-risk populations over a long course of time. If herbal products with similar mechanisms of action can be employed with a far greater range of safety, long-term cancer prevention may become a reality.

REFERENCES

Ang-Lee, M. K., J. Moss, and C. S. Yuan. 2001. "Herbal medicines and perioperative care." *JAMA.* 286:208–216.

Arbiser, J. L., N. Klauber, R. Rohan, R. van Leeuwen, M. T. Huang, C. Fisher, E. Flynn, and H. R. Byers. 1998. "Curcumin is an in vivo inhibitor of angiogenesis." *Mol. Med.* 4:376–383.

Bachrach, U., and Y. C. Wang. 2002. "Cancer therapy and prevention by green tea: role of ornithine decarboxylase." *Amino. Acids.* 22:1–13.

Baek, S. J., L. C. Wilson, and TrE. Eling. 2002. "Resveratrol enhances the expression of nonsteroidal anti-inflammatory drug-activated gene (NAG-1) by increasing the expression of p53." *Carcinogenesis.* 23:425–434.

Balasenthil, S., S. Arivazhagan, and S. Nagini. 2000. "Garlic enhances circulatory antioxidants during 7, 12- dimethylbenz[a]anthracene-induced hamster buccal pouch carcinogenesis." *J Ethnopharmacol.* 72:429–433.

Balasenthil, S., S. Arivazhagan, C. R. Ramachandran, and S. Nagini. 1999. "Effects of garlic on 7,12-Dimethylbenz[a]anthracene-induced hamster buccal pouch carcinogenesis." *Cancer Detect. Prev.* 23:534–538.

Bedir, E., I. I. Tatli, R. A. Khan, J. Zhao, S. Takamatsu, L. A. Walker, P. Goldman, and I. A. Khan. 2002. "Biologically Active Secondary Metabolites from Ginkgo biloba." *J. Agric. Food Chem.* 50:3150–3155.

Berbari, P., A. Thibodeau, L. Germain, M. Saint-Cyr, P. Gaudreau, S. Elkhouri, E. Dupont, D. R. Garrel, S. Elkouri, and S. El Khouri. 1999. "Antiangiogenic effects of the oral administration of liquid cartilage extract in humans." *J. Surg. Res.* 87:108–113.

Bernstein, B. J., and T. Grasso. 2001. "Prevalence of complementary and alternative medicine use in cancer patients." *Oncology (Huntingt).* 15:1267–1272.

Bertolini, F., L. Fusetti, C. Rabascio, S. Cinieri, G. Martinelli, and G. Pruneri. 2000. "Inhibition of angiogenesis and induction of endothelial and tumor cell apoptosis by green tea in animal models of human high-grade non- Hodgkin's lymphoma." *Leukemia.* 14:1477–1482.

Borchers, A. T., C. L. Keen, J. S. Stern, and M. E. Gershwin. 2000. "Inflammation and Native American medicine: the role of botanicals." *Am. J. Clin. Nutr.* 72:339–347.

Borek, C. 2001. "Antioxidant health effects of aged garlic extract." *J Nutr.* 131:1010S–1015S.

Brady, J. F., D. C. Li, H. Ishizaki, and C. S. Yang. 1988. "Effect of diallyl sulfide on rat liver microsomal nitrosamine metabolism and other monooxygenase activities." *Cancer Res.* 48:5937–5940.

Brevoort, P. 1998. "The Booming U.S. Botanical Market: A New Overview." *HerbalGram.* 44:33–46.

Bruss, K., E. Galán and C. Salter, ed. 2000. American Cancer Society's Guide to Complementary and Alternative Cancer Methods. American Cancer Society.

Bucci, L. R. 2000. "Selected herbals and human exercise performance." *Am. J. Clin. Nutr.* 72:624S–636S.

Buttke, T. M., and P. A. Sandstrom. 1994. "Oxidative stress as a mediator of apoptosis." *Immunol Today.* 15:7–10.

Chang, W. S., Y. H. Chang, F. J. Lu, and H. C. Chiang. 1994. "Inhibitory effects of phenolics on xanthine oxidase." *Anticancer Res.* 14:501–506.

Chatelain, C., W. Autet, and F. Brackman. 1999. "Comparison of once and twice daily dosage forms of Pygeum africanum extract in patients with benign prostatic hyperplasia: a randomized, double-blind study, with long-term open label extension." *Urology.* 54:473–478.

Chenn, S. 2001. "In vitro mechanism of PC SPES." *Urology.* 58:28–35.

Churchill, M., A. Chadburn, R. T. Bilinski, and M. M. Bertagnolli. 2000. "Inhibition of intestinal tumors by curcumin is associated with changes in the intestinal immune cell profile." *J. Surg. Res.* 89:169–175.

Cipriani, B., G. Borsellino, H. Knowles, D. Tramonti, F. Cavaliere, G. Bernardi, L. Battistini, and C. F. Brosnan. 2001. "Curcumin inhibits activation of Vgamma9Vdelta2 T cells by phosphoantigens and induces apoptosis involving apoptosis-inducing factor and large scale DNA fragmentation." *J. Immunol.* 167:3454–3462.

Collins, B. M., J. A. McLachlan, and S. F. Arnold. 1997. "The estrogenic and antiestrogenic activities of phytochemicals with the human estrogen receptor expressed in yeast." *Steroids.* 62:365–372.

Das, M., P. Sur, A. Gomes, J. R. Vedasiromoni, and D. K. Ganguly. 2002. "Inhibition of tumour growth and inflammation by consumption of tea." *Phytother. Res.* 16 Suppl 1:S40–S44.

Demark-Wahnefried, W., D. T. Price, T. J. Polascik, C. N. Robertson, E. E. Anderson, D. F. Paulson, P. J. Walther, M. Gannon, and R. T. Vollmer. 2001. "Pilot study of dietary fat restriction and flaxseed supplementation in men with prostate cancer before surgery: exploring the effects on hormonal levels, prostate-specific antigen, and histopathologic features." *Urology.* 58:47–52.

DiPaola, R. S., H. Zhang, G. H. Lambert, R. Meeker, E. Licitra, M. M. Rafi, B. T. Zhu, H. Spaulding, S. Goodin, M. B. Toledano, W. N. Hait, and M. A. Gallo. 1998. "Clinical and biologic activity of an estrogenic herbal combination (PC-SPES) in prostate cancer." *N. Engl. J Med.* 339:785–791.

Dorai, T., Y. C. Cao, B. Dorai, R. Buttyan, and A. E. Katz. 2001. "Therapeutic potential of curcumin in human prostate cancer. III. Curcumin inhibits proliferation, induces apoptosis, and inhibits angiogenesis of LNCaP prostate cancer cells in vivo." *Prostate.* 47:293–303.

Dorrie, J., K. Sapala, and S. J. Zunino. 2001. "Carnosol-induced apoptosis and downregulation of Bcl-2 in B-lineage leukemia cells." *Cancer Lett.* 170:33–39.

Dreher, D. and A. F. Junod. 1996. "Role of oxygen free radicals in cancer development." *Eur. J Cancer.* 32A:30–38.

Fan, D. and X. Wang. PC-SPES Composition of Herbal Extracts. [Patent no. 5,417,979]. Patent report, 1995.

Ferguson, L. R., and B. C. Baguley. 1994. "Topoisomerase II enzymes and mutagenicity." *Environ. Mol. Mutagen.* 24:245–261.

Ferrara, N. 2000. "VEGF: an update on biological and therapeutic aspects." *Curr. Opin. Biotechnol.* 11:617–624.

Finlay, G. J., K. M. Holdaway, and B. C. Baguley. 1994. "Comparison of the effects of genistein and amsacrine on leukemia cell proliferation." *Oncol. Res.* 6:33–37.

Fotsis, T., M. Pepper, H. Adlercreutz, G. Fleischmann, T. Hase, R. Montesano, and L. Schweigerer. 1993. "Genistein, a dietary-derived inhibitor of in vitro angiogenesis." *Proc. Natl. Acad. Sci. U.S.A.* 90:2690–2694.

Gao, X., Y. X. Xu, N. Janakiraman, R. A. Chapman, and S. C. Gautam. 2001. "Immunomodulatory activity of resveratrol: suppression of lymphocyte proliferation, development of cell-mediated cytotoxicity, and cytokine production." *Biochem. Pharmacol.* 62:1299–1308.

Garbisa, S., L. Sartor, S. Biggin, B. Salvato, R. Benelli, and A. Albini. 2001. "Tumor gelatinases and invasion inhibited by the green tea flavanol epigallocatechin-3-gallate." *Cancer.* 91:822–832.

Gehm, B. D., J. M. McAndrews, P. Y. Chien, and J. L. Jameson. 1997. "Resveratrol, a polyphenolic compound found in grapes and wine, is an agonist for the estrogen receptor." *Proc. Natl. Acad. Sci. U.S.A.* 94:14138–14143.

Goel, A., C. R. Boland, and D. P. Chauhan. 2001. "Specific inhibition of cyclooxygenase-2 (COX-2) expression by dietary curcumin in HT-29 human colon cancer cells." *Cancer Lett.* 172:111–118.

Goldstein, J. L., and M. S. Brown. 1990. "Regulation of the mevalonate pathway." *Nature.* 343:425–430.

Gottesman, M. M., I. Pastan, and S. V. Ambudkar. 1996. "P-glycoprotein and multidrug resistance." *Curr. Opin. Genet. Dev.* 6:610–617.

Grimm, S., M. K. Bauer, P. A. Baeuerle, and K. Schulze-Osthoff. 1996. "Bcl-2 down-regulates the activity of transcription factor NF-kappa B induced upon apoptosis." *J Cell Biol.* 134:13–23.

Gupta, S., N. Ahmad, R. R. Mohan, M. M. Husain, and H. Mukhtar. 1999a. "Prostate cancer chemoprevention by green tea: in vitro and in vivo inhibition of testosterone-mediated induction of ornithine decarboxylase." *Cancer Res.* 59:2115–2120.

Gupta, S., N. Ahmad, and H. Mukhtar. 1999b. "Prostate cancer chemoprevention by green tea." *Semin. Urol. Oncol.* 17:70–76.

Gupta, S., K. Hastak, N. Ahmad, J. S. Lewin, and H. Mukhtar. 2001. "Inhibition of prostate carcinogenesis in TRAMP mice by oral infusion of green tea polyphenols." *Proc Natl. Acad. Sci. U.S.A.* 98:10350–10355.

Guy, C. T., M. A. Webster, M. Schaller, T. J. Parsons, R. D. Cardiff, and W. J. Muller. 1992. "Expression of the neu protooncogene in the mammary epithelium of transgenic mice induces metastatic disease." *Proc. Natl. Acad. Sci. U.S.A.* 89:10578–10582.

Guyonnet, D., M. H. Siess, A. M. Le Bon, and M. Suschetet. 1999. "Modulation of phase II enzymes by organosulfur compounds from allium vegetables in rat tissues." *Toxicol. Appl. Pharmacol.* 154:50–58.

Hanif, R., L. Qiao, S. J. Shiff, and B. Rigas. 1997. "Curcumin, a natural plant phenolic food additive, inhibits cell proliferation and induces cell cycle changes in colon adenocarcinoma cell lines by a prostaglandin-independent pathway." *J Lab Clin. Med.* 130:576–584.

Haqqi, T. M., D. D. Anthony, S. Gupta, N. Ahmad, M. S. Lee, G. K. Kumar, and H. Mukhtar. 1999. "Prevention of collagen-induced arthritis in mice by a polyphenolic fraction from green tea." *Proc. Natl. Acad. Sci. U.S.A.* 96:4524–4529.

Heilbrun, L. K., A. Nomura, and G. N. Stemmermann. 1986. "Black tea consumption and cancer risk: a prospective study." *Br J Cancer.* 54:677–683.

Hiipakka, R. A., H. Z. Zhang, W. Dai, Q. Dai, and S. Liao. 2002. "Structure-activity relationships for inhibition of human 5 alpha-reductases by polyphenols." *Biochem. Pharmacol.* 63:1165–1176.

Hirose, M., A. Nishikawa, M. Shibutani, T. Imai, and T. Shirai. 2002. "Chemoprevention of heterocyclic amine-induced mammary carcinogenesis in rats." *Environ. Mol. Mutagen.* 39:271–278.

Hollis, D. M., S. J. Muga, and M. J. Wargovich. Structure-activity relationships of garlic compounds and the inhibition of hepatic CYP2E1. Proc. Amer. Assoc. Cancer Res. [42], 661. 2002.

Holmes-McNary, M., and A. S. Baldwin, Jr. 2000. "Chemopreventive properties of trans-resveratrol are associated with inhibition of activation of the I kappa B kinase." *Cancer Res.* 60:3477–3483.

Hong, Y. S., Y. A. Ham, J. H. Choi, and J. Kim. 2000. "Effects of allyl sulfur compounds and garlic extract on the expression of Bcl-2, Bax, and p53 in non small cell lung cancer cell lines." *Exp. Mol. Med.* 32:127–134.

Hsieh, T., S. S. Chen, X. Wang, and J. M. Wu. 1997. "Regulation of androgen receptor (AR) and prostate specific antigen (PSA) expression in the androgen-responsive human prostate LNCaP cells by ethanolic extracts of the Chinese herbal preparation, PC-SPES." *Biochem. Mol. Biol. Int.* 42:535–544.

Huang, M. T., H. L. Newmark, and K. Frenkel. 1997. "Inhibitory effects of curcumin on tumorigenesis in mice." *J. Cell Biochem. Suppl.* 27:26–34.

Igura, K., T. Ohta, Y. Kuroda, and K. Kaji. 2001. "Resveratrol and quercetin inhibit angiogenesis in vitro." *Cancer Lett.* 171:11–16.

Islam, S., N. Islam, T. Kermode, B. Johnstone, H. Mukhtar, R. W. Moskowitz, V. M. Goldberg, C. J. Malemud, and T. M. Haqqi. 2000. "Involvement of caspase-3 in epigallocatechin-3-gallate-mediated apoptosis of human chondrosarcoma cells." *Biochem. Biophys. Res. Commun.* 270:793–797.

Jemal, A., A. Thomas, T. Murray, and M. Thun. 2002. "Cancer statistics, 2002." *CA Cancer J Clin.* 52:23–47.

Jiang, C., R. Agarwal, and J. Lu. 2000. "Anti-angiogenic potential of a cancer chemopreventive flavonoid antioxidant, silymarin: inhibition of key attributes of vascular endothelial cells and angiogenic cytokine secretion by cancer epithelial cells." *Biochem. Biophys. Res. Commun.* 276:371–378.

Jodoin, J., M. Demeule, and R. Beliveau. 2002. "Inhibition of the multidrug resistance P-glycoprotein activity by green tea polyphenols." *Biochim. Biophys. Acta.* 1542:149–159.

Jung, Y. D., M. S. Kim, B. A. Shin, K. O. Chay, B. W. Ahn, W. Liu, C. D. Bucana, G. E. Gallick, and L. M. Ellis. 2001. "EGCG, a major component of green tea, inhibits tumour growth by inhibiting VEGF induction in human colon carcinoma cells." *Br. J Cancer.* 84:844–850.

Kato, K., A. D. Cox, M. M. Hisaka, S. M. Graham, J. E. Buss, and C. J. Der. 1992. "Isoprenoid addition to Ras protein is the critical modification for its membrane association and transforming activity." *Proc. Natl. Acad. Sci. U.S.A.* 89:6403–6407.

Keum, Y. S., K. K. Park, J. M. Lee, K. S. Chun, J. H. Park, S. K. Lee, H. Kwon, and Y. J. Surh. 2000. "Antioxidant and anti-tumor promoting activities of the methanol extract of heat-processed ginseng." *Cancer Lett.* 150:41–48.

Kimura, Y. and H. Okuda. 2001. "Resveratrol isolated from Polygonum cuspidatum root prevents tumor growth and metastasis to lung and tumor-induced neovascularization in Lewis lung carcinoma-bearing mice." *J. Nutr.* 131:1844–1849.

Kimura, Y., H. Okuda, and S. Arichi. 1988. "Effects of various ginseng saponins on 5-hydroxytryptamine release and aggregation in human platelets." *J. Pharm. Pharmacol.* 40:838–843.

Kitts, D. D., A. N. Wijewickreme, and C. Hu. 2000. "Antioxidant properties of a North American ginseng extract." *Mol. Cell Biochem.* 203:1–10.

Kobayashi, S., T. Miyamoto, I. Kimura, and M. Kimura. 1995. "Inhibitory effect of isoliquiritin, a compound in licorice root, on angiogenesis in vivo and tube formation in vitro." *Biol. Pharm. Bull.* 18:1382–1386.

Kobayashi, T., S. Ruan, K. Clodi, K. O. Kliche, H. Shiku, M. Andreeff, and W. Zhang. 1998. "Overexpression of Bax gene sensitizes K562 erythroleukemia cells to apoptosis induced by selective chemotherapeutic agents." *Oncogene.* 16:1587–1591.

Kondo, K., K. Tsuneizumi, T. Watanabe, and M. Oishi. 1991. "Induction of in vitro differentiation of mouse embryonal carcinoma (F9) cells by inhibitors of topoisomerases." *Cancer Res.* 51:5398–5404.

Kurie, J. M., J. S. Lee, T. Griffin, S. M. Lippman, P. Drum, M. P. Thomas, C. Weber, M. Bader, G. Massimini, and W. K. Hong. 1996. "Phase I trial of 9-cis retinoic acid in adults with solid tumors." *Clin. Cancer Res.* 2:287–293.

Kwon, K. B., S. J. Yoo, D. G. Ryu, J. Y. Yang, H. W. Rho, J. S. Kim, J. W. Park, H. R. Kim, and B. H. Park. 2002. "Induction of apoptosis by diallyl disulfide through activation of caspase-3 in human leukemia HL-60 cells." *Biochem. Pharmacol.* 63:41–47.

L'Allemain, G. 1999. "[Multiple actions of EGCG, the main component of green tea]." *Bull. Cancer.* 86:721–724.

Lamy, S., D. Gingras, and R. Beliveau. 2002. "Green tea catechins inhibit vascular endothelial growth factor receptor phosphorylation." *Cancer Res.* 62:381–385.

Lee, E., K. K. Park, J. M. Lee, K. S. Chun, J. Y. Kang, S. S. Lee, and Y. J. Surh. 1998. "Suppression of mouse skin tumor promotion and induction of apoptosis in HL-60 cells by Alpinia oxyphylla Miquel (Zingiberaceae)." *Carcinogenesis.* 19:1377–1381.

Lehnert, M. 1998. "Chemotherapy resistance in breast cancer." *Anticancer Res.* 18:2225–2226.

Levites, Y., M. B. Youdim, G. Maor, and S. Mandel. 2002. "Attenuation of 6-hydroxydopamine (6-OHDA)-induced nuclear factor-kappa B (NF-kappa B) activation and cell death by tea extracts in neuronal cultures." *Biochem. Pharmacol.* 63:21–29.

Li, J. K. and S. Y. Lin-Shia. 2001. "Mechanisms of cancer chemoprevention by curcumin." *Proc. Natl. Sci. Counc. Repub. China B.* 25:59–66.

Liao, S. 2001. "The medicinal action of androgens and green tea epigallocatechin gallate." *Hong. Kong. Med. J.* 7:369–374.

Lim, G. P., T. Chu, F. Yang, W. Beech, S. A. Frautschy, and G. M. Cole. 2001. "The curry spice curcumin reduces oxidative damage and amyloid pathology in an Alzheimer transgenic mouse." *J. Neurosci.* 21:8370–8377.

Longo, R. and S. Tira. 1983. "Steroidal and other components of Pygeum africanum bark." *Farmaco [Prat.].* 38:287–292.

Luper, S. 1998. "A review of plants used in the treatment of liver disease: part 1." *Altern. Med. Rev.* 3:410–421.

Mahmoud, N. N., A. M. Carothers, D. Grunberger, R. T. Bilinski, M. R. Churchill, C. Martucci, H. L. Newmark, and M. M. Bertagnolli. 2000. "Plant phenolics decrease intestinal tumors in an animal model of familial adenomatous polyposis." *Carcinogenesis.* 21:921–927.

Manna, S. K., A. Mukhopadhyay, and B. B. Aggarwal. 2000. "Resveratrol suppresses TNF-induced activation of nuclear transcription factors NF-kappa B, activator protein-1, and apoptosis: potential role of reactive oxygen intermediates and lipid peroxidation." *J. Immunol.* 164:6509–6519.

Manna, S. K., A. Mukhopadhyay, N. T. Van, and B. B. Aggarwal. 1999. "Silymarin suppresses TNF-induced activation of NF-kappa B, c-Jun N-terminal kinase, and apoptosis." *J. Immunol.* 163:6800–6809.

Mantle, D., F. Eddeb, and A. T. Pickering. 2000. "Comparison of relative antioxidant activities of British medicinal plant species in vitro." *J. Ethnopharmacol.* 72:47–51.

McCabe, M. J., Jr., and S. Orrenius. 1993. "Genistein induces apoptosis in immature human thymocytes by inhibiting topoisomerase-II." *Biochem. Biophys. Res. Commun.* 194:944–950.

Messina, M. J. 1999. "Legumes and soybeans: overview of their nutritional profiles and health effects." *Am. J Clin. Nutr.* 70:439S–450S.

Messina, M. J., V. Persky, K. D. Setchell, and S. Barnes. 1994. "Soy intake and cancer risk: a review of the in vitro and in vivo data." *Nutr. Cancer.* 21:113–131.

Metz, N., A. Lobstein, Y. Schneider, F. Gosse, R. Schleiffer, R. Anton, and F. Raul. 2000. "Suppression of azoxymethane-induced preneoplastic lesions and inhibition of cyclooxygenase-2 activity in the colonic mucosa of rats drinking a crude green tea extract." *Nutr. Cancer.* 38:60–64.

Miksicek, R. J. 1993. "Commonly occurring plant flavonoids have estrogenic activity." *Mol. Pharmacol.* 44:37–43.

Miksicek, R. J. 1994. "Interaction of naturally occurring nonsteroidal estrogens with expressed recombinant human estrogen receptor." *J Steroid Biochem. Mol. Biol.* 49:153–160.

Mo, H. and C. E. Elson. 1999. "Apoptosis and cell-cycle arrest in human and murine tumor cells are initiated by isoprenoids." *J Nutr.* 129:804–813.

Mochizuki, M., Y. C. Yoo, K. Matsuzawa, K. Sato, I. Saiki, S. Tono-oka, K. Samukawa, and I. Azuma. 1995. "Inhibitory effect of tumor metastasis in mice by saponins, ginsenoside- Rb2, 20(R)- and 20(S)-ginsenoside-Rg3, of red ginseng." *Biol. Pharm. Bull.* 18:1197–1202.

Mohan, R., J. Sivak, P. Ashton, L. A. Russo, B. Q. Pham, N. Kasahara, M. B. Raizman, and M. E. Fini. 2000. "Curcuminoids inhibit the angiogenic response stimulated by fibroblast growth factor-2, including expression of matrix metalloproteinase gelatinase B." *J. Biol. Chem.* 275:10405–10412.

Moon, D. G., J. Cheon, D. H. Yoon, H. S. Park, H. K. Kim, J. J. Kim, and S. K. Koh. 2000. "Allium sativum potentiates suicide gene therapy for murine transitional cell carcinoma." *Nutr. Cancer.* 38:98–105.

Morrow, D. M., P. E. Fitzsimmons, M. Chopra, and H. McGlynn. 2001. "Dietary supplementation with the anti-tumour promoter quercetin: its effects on matrix metalloproteinase gene regulation." *Mutat. Res.* 480–481:269–276.

Myhrstad, M. C., H. Carlsen, O. Nordstrom, R. Blomhoff, and J. J. Moskaug. 2002. "Flavonoids increase the intracellular glutathione level by transactivation of the gamma-glutamylcysteine synthetase catalytical subunit promoter." *Free Radic. Biol. Med.* 32:386–393.

Nagata, H., S. Takekoshi, T. Takagi, T. Honma, and K. Watanabe. 1999. "Antioxidative action of flavonoids, quercetin and catechin, mediated by the activation of glutathione peroxidase." *Tokai J Exp. Clin. Med.* 24:1–11.

Nerurkar, P. V., L. Le Marchand, and R. V. Cooney. 1999. "Effects of marinating with Asian marinades or western barbecue sauce on PhIP and MeIQx formation in barbecued beef." *Nutr. Cancer.* 34:147–152.

Offord, E. A., K. Mace, O. Avanti, and A. M. Pfeifer. 1997. "Mechanisms involved in the chemoprotective effects of rosemary extract studied in human liver and bronchial cells." *Cancer Lett.* 114:275–281.

Oh, W. K., D. J. George, and P. W. Kantoff. 2002. "Rapid rise of serum prostate specific antigen levels after discontinuation of the herbal therapy PC-SPES in patients with advanced prostate carcinoma: report of four cases." *Cancer.* 94:686–689.

Park, H. J., J. H. Lee, Y. B. Song, and K. H. Park. 1996. "Effects of dietary supplementation of lipophilic fraction from Panax ginseng on cGMP and cAMP in rat platelets and on blood coagulation." *Biol. Pharm. Bull.* 19:1434–1439.

Pedrielli, P., G. F. Pedulli, and L. H. Skibsted. 2001. "Antioxidant mechanism of flavonoids. Solvent effect on rate constant for chain-breaking reaction of quercetin and epicatechin in autoxidation of methyl linoleate." *J. Agric. Food Chem.* 49:3034–3040.

Pianetti, S., S. Guo, K. T. Kavanagh, and G. E. Sonenshein. 2002. "Green tea polyphenol epigallocatechin-3 gallate inhibits Her-2/neu signaling, proliferation, and transformed phenotype of breast cancer cells." *Cancer Res.* 62:652–655.

Plouzek, C. A., H. P. Ciolino, R. Clarke, and G. C. Yeh. 1999. "Inhibition of P-glycoprotein activity and reversal of multidrug resistance in vitro by rosemary extract." *Eur. J Cancer.* 35:1541–1545.

Plummer, S. M., K. A. Holloway, M. M. Manson, R. J. Munks, A. Kaptein, S. Farrow, and L. Howells. 1999. "Inhibition of cyclo-oxygenase 2 expression in colon cells by the chemopreventive agent curcumin involves inhibition of NF-kappaB activation via the NIK/IKK signalling complex." *Oncogene.* 18:6013–6020.

Pollmann, C., X. Huang, J. Mall, D. Bech-Otschir, M. Naumann, and W. Dubiel. 2001. "The constitutive photomorphogenesis 9 signalosome directs vascular endothelial growth factor production in tumor cells." *Cancer Res.* 61:8416–8421.

Polverino, A. J. and S. D. Patterson. 1997. "Selective activation of caspases during apoptotic induction in HL-60 cells. Effects Of a tetrapeptide inhibitor." *J Biol. Chem.* 272:7013–7021.

Rafi, M. M., R. T. Rosen, A. Vassil, C. T. Ho, H. Zhang, G. Ghai, G. Lambert, and R. S. DiPaola. 2000. "Modulation of bcl-2 and cytotoxicity by licochalcone-A, a novel estrogenic flavonoid." *Anticancer Res.* 20:2653–2658.

Ross, R. K., L. Bernstein, R. A. Lobo, H. Shimizu, F. Z. Stanczyk, M. C. Pike, and B. E. Henderson. 1992. "5-alpha-reductase activity and risk of prostate cancer among Japanese and US white and black males." *Lancet.* 339:887–889.

Sato, K., M. Mochizuki, I. Saiki, Y. C. Yoo, K. Samukawa, and I. Azuma. 1994. "Inhibition of tumor angiogenesis and metastasis by a saponin of Panax ginseng, ginsenoside-Rb2." *Biol. Pharm. Bull.* 17:635–639.

Shao, Z. M., J. Wu, Z. Z. Shen, and S. H. Barsky. 1998. "Genistein exerts multiple suppressive effects on human breast carcinoma cells." *Cancer Res.* 58:4851–4857.

Shao, Z. M., Z. Z. Shen, C. H. Liu, M. R. Sartippour, V. L. Go, D. Heber, and M. Nguyen. 2002. "Curcumin exerts multiple suppressive effects on human breast carcinoma cells." *Int. J. Cancer.* 98:234–240.

Sharma, R. A., C. R. Ireson, R. D. Verschoyle, K. A. Hill, M. L. Williams, C. Leuratti, M. M. Manson, L. J. Marnett, W. P. Steward, and A. Gescher. 2001. "Effects of dietary curcumin on glutathione S-transferase and malondialdehyde-DNA adducts in rat liver and colon mucosa: relationship with drug levels." *Clin. Cancer Res.* 7:1452–1458.

Shibata, S. 2001. "Chemistry and cancer preventing activities of ginseng saponins and some related triterpenoid compounds." *J. Korean Med. Sci.* 16 Suppl:S28–S37.

Shin, H. R., J. Y. Kim, T. K. Yun, G. Morgan, and H. Vainio. 2000a. "The cancer-preventive potential of Panax ginseng: a review of human and experimental evidence." *Cancer Causes Control.* 11:565–576.

Shin, H. R., J. Y. Kim, T. K. Yun, G. Morgan, and H. Vainio. 2000b. "The cancer-preventive potential of Panax ginseng: a review of human and experimental evidence." *Cancer Causes Control.* 11:565–576.

Sigounas, G., J. L. Hooker, W. Li, A. Anagnostou, and M. Steiner. 1997. "S-allylmercaptocysteine, a stable thioallyl compound, induces apoptosis in erythroleukemia cell lines." *Nutr. Cancer.* 28:153–159.

Singh, S. V. 2001. "Impact of garlic organosulfides on p21(H-ras) processing." *J Nutr.* 131:1046S–1048S.

Singletary, K. and C. MacDonald. 2000. "Inhibition of benzo[a]pyrene- and 1,6-dinitropyrene-DNA adduct formation in human mammary epithelial cells bydibenzoylmethane and sulforaphane." *Cancer Lett.* 155:47–54.

Sinha, R., D. R. Gustafson, M. Kulldorff, W. Q. Wen, J. R. Cerhan, and W. Zheng. 2000. "2-amino-1-methyl-6-phenylimidazo[4,5-b]pyridine, a carcinogen in high- temperature-cooked meat, and breast cancer risk." *J Natl. Cancer Inst.* 92:1352–1354.

Slamenova, D., K. Kuboskova, E. Horvathova, and S. Robichova. 2002. "Rosemary-stimulated reduction of DNA strand breaks and FPG-sensitive sites in mammalian cells treated with H_2O_2 or visible light-excited Methylene Blue." *Cancer Lett.* 177:145–153.

Surh, Y. 1999. "Molecular mechanisms of chemopreventive effects of selected dietary and medicinal phenolic substances." *Mutat. Res.* 428:305–327.

Surh, Y. J., H. K. Na, J. Y. Lee, and Y. S. Keum. 2001b. "Molecular mechanisms underlying antitumor promoting activities of heat- processed Panax ginseng C. A. Meyer." *J. Korean Med. Sci.* 16 Suppl:S38–S41.

Surh, Y. J., K. S. Chun, H. H. Cha, S. S. Han, Y. S. Keum, K. K. Park, and S. S. Lee. 2001a. "Molecular mechanisms underlying chemopreventive activities of anti- inflammatory phytochemicals: down-regulation of COX-2 and iNOS through suppression of NF-kappa B activation." *Mutat. Res.* 480-481:243–268.

Szeto, Y. T., A. R. Collins, and I. F. Benzie. 2002. "Effects of dietary antioxidants on DNA damage in lysed cells using a modified comet assay procedure." *Mutat. Res.* 500:31–38.

Tanaka, T. Cancer chemoprevention by natural products (Review). Oncology Reports 1, 1139–1155. 1994.

Teel, R. W., and H. Huynh. 1998. "Modulation by phytochemicals of cytochrome P450-linked enzyme activity." *Cancer Lett.* 133:135–141.

Temple, R. FDA Office of Drug Evaluation. DIA Annual Meeting . 2002.

Teng, C. M. , S. C. Kuo, F. N. Ko, J. C. Lee, L. G. Lee, S. C. Chen, and T. F. Huang. 1989. "Antiplatelet actions of panaxynol and ginsenosides isolated from ginseng." *Biochim. Biophys. Acta.* 990:315–320.

Thaloor, D., A. K. Singh, G. S. Sidhu, P. V. Prasad, H. K. Kleinman, and R. K. Maheshwari. 1998. "Inhibition of angiogenic differentiation of human umbilical vein endothelial cells by curcumin." *Cell Growth Differ.* 9:305–312.

Thompson, L. U. 1994. "Antioxidants and hormone-mediated health benefits of whole grains." *Crit Rev. Food Sci. Nutr.* 34:473–497.

Tiwari, R. K., J. Geliebter, V. P. Garikapaty, S. P. Yedavelli, S. Chen, and A. Mittelman. 1999. "Antitumor effects of PC-SPES, an herbal formulation in prostate cancer." *Int. J Oncol.* 14:713–719.

Tosetti, F., N. Ferrari, S. De Flora, and A. Albini. 2002. "Angioprevention': angiogenesis is a common and key target for cancer chemopreventive agents." *FASEB J.* 16:2–14.

Tou, J., and C. Urbizo. 2001. "Resveratrol inhibits the formation of phosphatidic acid and diglyceride in chemotactic peptide- or phorbol ester-stimulated human neutrophils." *Cell Signal.* 13:191–197.

Tyler, V. T. 1993. "The Honest Herbal." *The Honest Herbal.* Pharmaceutical Product Press. Binghamton, MY. 285–287.

Unpublished data. Comprehensive Cancer Care Conference. 2001.

U.S. Pharmacopeia. Saw Palmetto Summary. 2002. US Pharmacopeia. Ref Type: Report. See at http://www.usp.org/cgibin/catalog/SoftCart.exe/catalog/frameset.htm?E+uspstore.

Wang, Z. Y., and D. W. Nixon. 2001. "Licorice and cancer." *Nutr. Cancer.* 39:1–11.

Wang, Z. Y., R. Agarwal, Z. C. Zhou, D. R. Bickers, and H. Mukhtar. 1991. "Inhibition of mutagenicity in Salmonella typhimurium and skin tumor initiating and tumor promoting activities in SENCAR mice by glycyrrhetinic acid: comparison of 18 alpha- and 18 beta-stereoisomers." *Carcinogenesis.* 12:187–192.

Wargovich, M. J. 1997. "Experimental evidence for cancer preventive elements in foods." *Cancer Lett.* 114:11–17.

Watanabe, T., K. Kondo, and M. Oishi. 1991. "Induction of in vitro differentiation of mouse erythroleukemia cells by genistein, an inhibitor of tyrosine protein kinases." *Cancer Res.* 51:764–768.

Weisburger, J. H., E. Veliath, E. Larios, B. Pittman, E. Zang, and Y. Hara. 2002. "Tea polyphenols inhibit the formation of mutagens during the cooking of meat." *Mutat. Res.* 516:19–22.

Wilt, T. J., A. Ishani, G. Stark, R. MacDonald, J. Lau, and C. Mulrow. 1998. "Saw palmetto extracts for treatment of benign prostatic hyperplasia: a systematic review." *JAMA.* 280:1604–1609.

Wolter, F., B. Akoglu, A. Clausnitzer, and J. Stein. 2001. "Downregulation of the cyclin D1/Cdk4 complex occurs during resveratrol- induced cell cycle arrest in colon cancer cell lines." *J. Nutr.* 131:2197–2203.

Yang, C. S., P. Maliakal, and X. Meng. 2002. "Inhibition of carcinogenesis by tea." *Annu. Rev. Pharmacol. Toxicol.* 42:25–54.

Yang, F., H. S. Oz, S. Barve, W. J. de Villiers, C. J. McClain, and G. W. Varilek. 2001. "The green tea polyphenol (-)-epigallocatechin-3-gallate blocks nuclear factor-kappa B activation by inhibiting I kappa B kinase activity in the intestinal epithelial cell line IEC-6." *Mol. Pharmacol.* 60:528–533.

Yang, F., W. J. de Villiers, C. J. McClain, and G. W. Varilek. 1998. "Green tea polyphenols block endotoxin-induced tumor necrosis factor- production and lethality in a murine model." *J. Nutr.* 128:2334–2340.

Yang, K., S. A. Lamprecht, Y. Liu, H. Shinozaki, K. Fan, D. Leung, H. Newmark, V. E. Steele, G. J. Kelloff, and M. Lipkin. 2000. "Chemoprevention studies of the flavonoids quercetin and rutin in normal and azoxymethane-treated mouse colon." *Carcinogenesis.* 21:1655–1660.

Yun, T. K., and S. Y. Choi. 1998. "Non-organ specific cancer prevention of ginseng: a prospective study in Korea." *Int. J. Epidemiol.* 27:359–364.

Zava, D. T., C. M. Dollbaum, and M. Blen. 1998. "Estrogen and progestin bioactivity of foods, herbs, and spices." *Proc. Soc. Exp. Biol. Med.* 217:369–378.

15

Cruciferous Vegetables and Cancer Prevention

Cynthia A. Thomson
and Tina L. Green

INTRODUCTION

The association between vegetable consumption and cancer prevention has been supported by epidemiological studies, particularly for colon and breast cancer (1, 2, 3). Among studies that demonstrated no protective effect there is a generally accepted assumption that intake was either too low or not of sufficient nutrient or phytochemical content to afford protection. Among the vegetables that may be of particular importance in the prevention of breast and colon cancer are the vegetables of the *Brassica oleracea* species. Although there is a general lack of clinical intervention trials in this area, cell culture models, animal studies, and epidemiological research each support a protective role and have offered a number of viable biological mechanisms for a protective effect. This chapter will define and describe cruciferous vegetables, review current data on intake and measurement of metabolites of intake, describe the association between intake and cancer as well as describe the known and postulated biological mechanisms by which constituents of cruciferous vegetables protect against cancer.

INTAKE OF CRUCIFEROUS VEGETABLES

There is some degree of confusion in the current literature as to what constitutes a cruciferous vegetable. The lay understanding is that cruciferous vegetables are the "gas-forming" vegetables that release a distinct, strong odor when cooked. The Cruciferae are also known as Brassicaceae, which constitute a family of plants that include the *Brassica* genus. There are 20 species in the *Brassica* genus with 2000 accessions. Research has focused on the various members of the species *Brassica oleracea*. The most commonly consumed cruciferous vegetables in the United States include broccoli, cauliflower, a number of types of cabbage, kale, kohlrabi, and brussels sprouts. Also included in this species is broccoflower and purple broccoli, designer foods that increase the complexity of accurate measurement of intake. The International community consumes a wide variety of other cruciferous vegetables beyond those consumed commonly in the United States. These include such vegetables as arugula, watercress, daikon root, wasabi, or mustards. Availability of a variety of cruciferous vegetables will impact the overall intake of phytochemicals as well as the ability to determine if an inverse association exists between cancer incidence and cruciferous vegetable intake (4,5). Table 15.1 provides a listing of common and less commonly consumed cruciferous vegetables.

Cruciferous vegetable intake in the United States was recently estimated from the USDA 1994–1996 CSFII data by Johnston and colleagues. They estimated that less than 20% of Americans consumed a cruciferous vegetable during the diet reporting period of two nonconsecutive calendar days. This translated to 0.2 servings/day on average for U.S. adults (7). Nestle has estimated intake of cruciferous vegetables at 5 grams per person per day (8). A recent analysis of cruciferous vegetable intake among U.S. participants in a case-control study assessing the relationship between isothiocyanate intake and lung cancer risk indicated that the mean intake of broccoli among all study participants was approximately 1.1 servings/week, cauliflower and brussels sprouts was   0.39 servings/week, and overall cruciferous vegetable intake was estimated at 2.3 servings per week (9). Significant differences in cruciferous vegetable intake can be seen across cultures and in relation to country of residence. For example, while Americans consume primarily broccoli, cauliflower, and cabbage, residents of Japan favor daikon, Chinese cab-

Table 15.1.   Commonly and Less Commonly Consumed Cruciferous Vegetables

Brassicaceae/ Cruciferae family	Genus	Species	Plant
Brassicaceae	*Brassica*	*oleracea*	Broccoli, brussels sprouts, cabbage, savoy cabbage, red cabbage, cauliflower, collards, kale, Chinese kale, Italian broccoli, asparagus broccoli, sea kale, wild cabbage, kohlrabi
Brassicaceae	*Brassica*	*rapa*	Chinese cabbage, celery, cabbage, spinach mustard, turnip, turnip tops, turnip broccoli, toria
Brassicaceae	*Brassica*	*napus*	Rape, colza, Siberian kale, rutabaga
Brassicaceae	*Brassica*	*japonica*	Wasabi
Brassicaceae	*Brassica*	*juncea*	Chinese mustards, mustard greens, curled mustard, pak choi, bok celery, brown mustard
Brassicaceae/ Cruciferae	*Brassica*	*alba*	White mustard
Brassicaceae	*Brassica*	*negra*	Black mustard oil, black mustard seeds
	Sisymbrium	*officinale*	Hedge mustard
	Nasturtium	*amoracia*	Horseradish
Cruciferae	*Nasturtium*	*officinale*	Watercress
Ranunculaceae	*Anemone*	*acutiloba*	Liverwort
Brassicaceae	*Raphanus*	*naphanistrum*	Wild radish
Brassicaceae	*Raphanus*	*sativus*	Radish

bage, wasabi, watercress, and oriental mustards. Those residing in the United Kingdom prefer cabbage, sauerkraut, and brussels sprouts. Seow and coworkers estimated daily cruciferous vegetable intake among Singapore Chinese men and women (N = 246) participating in the Singapore Cohort Study to be 40.6 grams per day with choi sum, bok choi, and cabbage contributing greater than 50% of daily intake (10).

An assessment of genetic taste markers and preference for or dislike of cruciferous vegetables such as Brussels sprouts, indicated that lower consumption levels of cruciferous vegetables commonly seen in Americans may be related to a genetic sensitivity to the bitter taste of 6-n-propylthiouracil (PROP) (11). This was particularly true for females (12,13) and included breast cancer patients (14). Although the investigator demonstrated a reduction in cruciferous vegetable intake among those with PROP-sensitivity, it is unknown whether those with PROP-sensitivity are at any higher risk of cancer. Also of interest is the fact that this genetic sensitivity is reduced with age while at the same time age remains the primary risk factor for the majority of cancers. If there is an association, increased consumption with advancing age may or may not offer protection (15).

DIETARY METHODS USED IN THE MEASUREMENT OF CRUCIFEROUS VEGETABLE INTAKE

Despite the limitations in quantifying and qualifying the glucosinolate and isothiocyanate content of specific cruciferous vegetables, efforts to quantify human intake continue. Currently, data regarding cruciferous vegetable intake is limited by the fact that food frequency questionnaires are not highly specific in regards to cruciferous vegetable intake. In fact, the most commonly employed food frequency instruments generally include broccoli, cabbage, cauliflower, and kale, thus omitting several other glucosinolate-rich vegetables. These items may be grouped with other vegetables or together on a single line of the food frequency questionnaire making it difficult to estimate the contribution to total cruciferous intake derived from each vegetable. In addition, cruciferous vegetables such as watercress, oriental mustards, or wasabi may not be consumed in large amounts by the predominantly Caucasian participants in dietary studies, but could be eaten in considerable amounts by those of select ethnicities. Finally, the increasing availability of *Brassica* supplements in the form of dehydrated cruciferous vegetables or even sulfurophane-enriched *Brassica* tea further complicates our ability to accurately measure intake.

Other dietary methods, such as food records or dietary recalls, provide more specific data but tend to introduce recall bias as well as participant burden and are less commonly used in epidemiological research particularly longitudinal studies. Although recalls and food records may be more cost-effective in studies with reduced sample size, the power to detect statistically significant differences between "high consumers" and "low consumers" of cruciferous vegetables and disease outcomes may not be demonstrated. One possible approach would be to develop a focused food frequency questionnaire such as has been suggested (16) and employed (17, 18) for other phytochemicals.

Recently, researchers at the University of Arizona developed an abbreviated food frequency questionnaire for application in larger, longitudinal epidemiological studies to quantify intake of cruciferous vegetables cost-effectively and with reduced participant burden. The instrument is currently being validated against biological markers of isothiocyanate intake. Finally, the lack of a well-defined database of the glucosinolate or isothiocyanate content of cruciferous vegetables has also stifled efforts to advance science in this area since the relationship between exposure and disease cannot, at this time, be accurately assessed. The prototype phytochemical database is the carotenoid database established by NCI and USDA (19) and efforts to expand to other disease-preventive phytochemicals such as glucosinolates and isothiocyanates found in cruciferous vegetables are under consideration. The availability of the paired-ion chromatography (20) and cyclo-condensation reaction assays makes the reliable quantification of the phytochemical content of foods now possible (21).

PHYTOCHEMICAL CONTENT OF CRUCIFEROUS VEGETABLES

Role of Metabolism

The metabolism of glucosinolates and other phytochemical constituents in cruciferous vegetables is complex and has not been fully determined. Cruciferous vegetables have several hundred naturally occurring plant chemicals called phytochemicals that contribute to the health-promoting effects. The Brassicaceae family alone contains greater than 350 genera and 3000 species. Table 15.2 lists select phytochemicals isolated from several cruciferous vegetables.

Of greatest importance are the more than 120 identified glucosinolates that are beta-thioglucoside N-hydroximinosulfate esters or the sulfur-containing S-glucopyranosyl thiohydroximates with variable side chains. The bioavailability of health-promoting phytochemicals is largely dependent on their exposure to metabolic enzymes (24). When hydrolyzed through the process of cutting or mastication, glucosinolates yield biologi-

Table 15.2.   Cruciferous Vegetables and Associated Phytochemicals

Cruciferous vegetable	Isothiocyanate	Phytochemical
Broccoli, broccoli sprouts, garden cress, cabbage, horseradish, turnips, brussels sprouts, collard greens, tender greens, water cress, turnips	Glucoraphanin	Sulforaphane (SUL)
	Glucopaeolin	Benzylisothiocyanate (BITC)
	Gluconasturtin	Phenethylisothiocyanate (PEITC)
	Indoles	
Broccoli, brussels sprouts, cabbage, cauliflower, radish		Ascorbigen (ASG)
		Diindolylmethane (DIM)
	Neoglucobrassin	Indolylcarbazole (ICZ)
	Glucobrassin	Indole-3-carbinol (I3C)

cally active isothiocyanate derivatives. This hydrolysis is dependent largely on the enzyme myrosinase and in humans on beta-thioglucosidase present in gut microflora (25). Once hydrolyzed, glucosinolates yield a wide variety of isothiocyanates and indoles. Several have shown promise as potential cancer chemoprevention agents including the isothiocyanates sulforaphane (SUL), benzyl isothiocyanate (BITC), and phenylethyl isothiocyanate (PEITC), the indoles indole-3-carbinol (I3C), ascorbigen (ASG), 3,3'-diindolylmethane (DIM), and indolylcarbazole (ICZ), and the sulfur-containing glucosinolates such as methylthioalkyl. A comprehensive review of glucosinolates and isothiocyanates has been recently published (26) and expands on earlier work published regarding the specific chemical entities of indole glucosinolates (27) and those identified within the Brassicaceae family (28). Most glucosinolate-rich plants are clustered in three families—Brassicaceae, Capparaceae, and Caricaceae (29; see Figs. 15.1 and 15.2). The formation of isothiocyanates and indoles from glucosinolates are illustrated in Figure 15.1 (30).

Measurement of Glucosinolate and Isothiocyanate Content in Foods

Measurement of glucosinolate content of cruciferous vegetables is generally accomplished using high performance liquid chromatography (33). However, this methodology yields incomplete glucosinolate quantification. In addition, the desulfoglucosinolates are not responsive to myrosinase degradation to yield specific isothiocyanates. The isothiocyanates are more relevant to the study of the biological, health-promoting activity of cruciferous vegetables in humans. Ion-pair, reverse-phase chromatography (IPC) has improved upon HPLC methodology by neutralizing the highly charged sulfur groups thus allowing more effective and quantitative measurement of glucosinolate (20). Recently, hydrophilic interaction liquid chromatography (HILIC) was developed as a complement to IPC by Troyer and colleagues at Johns Hopkins School of Medicine (34). HILIC more specifically separates the highly polar glucosinolates. Ideally, methodology that allows for hydrolytic removal of the sulfur group from glucosinolates followed by separation of both polar and nonpolar glucosinolates, the enzymatic conversion of glucosinolates to isothio-

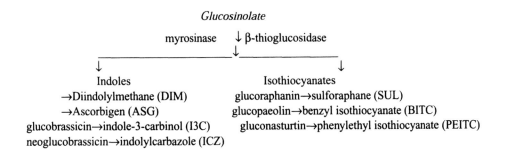

Figure 15.1.   Formation of phytochemicals. (Adapted from P. J. Thornalley 2002 [30])

Indoles

Isothiocyanates

Diindolylmethane

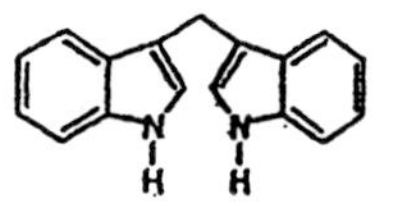

Sulforaphane

DIM

$$CH_3-\overset{\overset{O}{\parallel}}{S}-(CH_2)_4-R^* \longrightarrow H_3C-\overset{\overset{O}{\underset{O}{\parallel}}}{S}-CH_2-CH_2-CH_2-CH_2-N=C=S$$

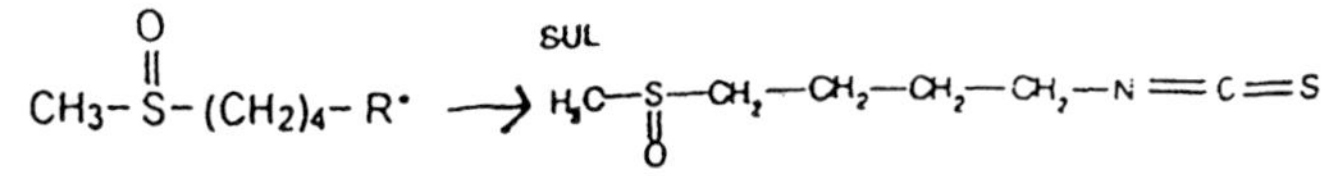

Glucoraphanin
(4-methylsulfinylbutyl glucosinolate)

Ascorbigen

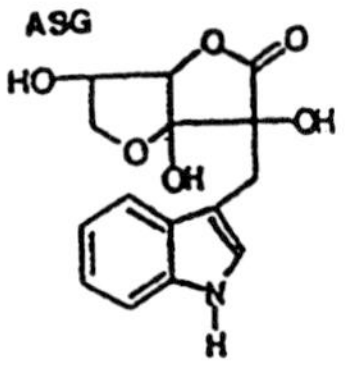

Benzyl isothiocyanate

ASG

BITC

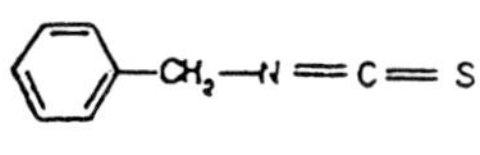

Indole-3-carbinol

Phenylethyl isothiocyanate

I3C

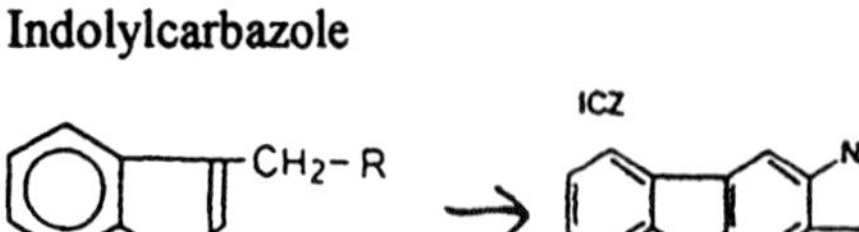

Glucobrassicin
(indole-3-ylmethyl glucosinolate)

PEITC

Indolylcarbazole

ICZ

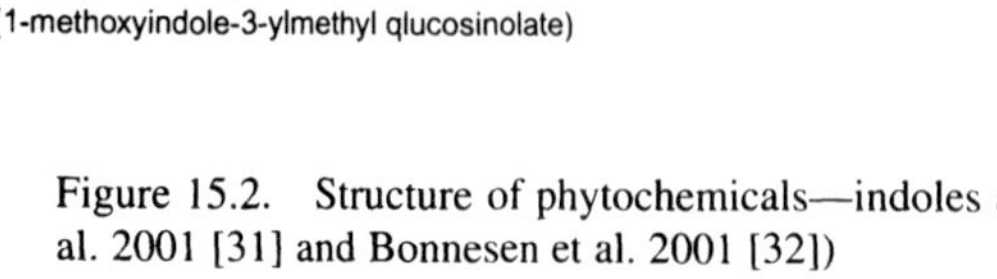

Neoglucobrassicin
(1-methoxyindole-3-ylmethyl glucosinolate)

Figure 15.2. Structure of phytochemicals—indoles and isothiocyanates. (Adapted from Steinkellner et al. 2001 [31] and Bonnesen et al. 2001 [32])

cyanates through exposure to myrosinase, and finally quantification of ITC content using the cyclocondensation assay was developed by Zhang (21).

Determinants of Phytochemical Content

The phytochemical content of cruciferous vegetables can vary considerably, even across the same family and species (35). Seeds or sprouts of young plants tend to have higher concentrations of glucosinolates, at times approaching a 100-fold difference (36, 37). Age has also been shown to influence the quantity of specific glucosinolates in plants, for example, broccoli sprouts are rich in aliphatic glucosinolates while mature broccoli has equal amounts of aliphatic and indole glucosinolates (36). The specific variety of plant is also an important factor in the amount of glucosinolates the plant contains. For example, broccoli of the Peto no.7 accession contains 35.6 micromoles glucosinolates per gram dry weight, while Zeus accession contains only 6.4 micromoles glucosinolates per gram dry weight (35, 38). The accessions with the highest sulfurophane content include Brigadier, Majestic, and Saga (39). Labeling of cruciferous vegetables with information regarding the specific variety is not yet available at point-of-purchase and thus quantifying intake among individuals is extremely difficult.

Preparation, processing, and storage can also impact the available glucosinolates in a given serving of cruciferous vegetables (24, 40). Hydrolysis is a critical step in enhancing the bioavailability of isothiocyanates (41). Breaking the cell membrane and causing cellular disruption through crushing, chopping, or masticating cruciferous vegetables has been shown to release the enzyme myrosinase, converting the glucosinolate to its active forms making the isothiocyanates bioavailable (42, 43). Although cooking has been shown to destroy myrosinase, human feeding studies using cooked cruciferous vegetables have demonstrated cancer-preventive biological activity (44, 45, 46) supporting at least one other existing mechanism for glucosinolate hydrolysis (47, 48). One well-accepted hypothesis is that the enzyme beta-thioglucosidase in the gut microflora is capable of hydrolyzing glucosinolates to their active forms (49, 50). The relationship between glucosinolate bioavailability and cooking methods has not been described. However, hydrophilic glucosinolates are likely to be lost during boiling or steaming where exposure to water is greater than during baking or microwaving (51). In addition, defrosting of frozen vegetables has been postulated to release myrosinase thus enhancing the bioavailability of glucosinolates (27). Glucosinolate hydrolysis is also affected by the species of brassica and the presence of ascorbic acid (40). Glucosinolate content and type can differ related to the brassica species, growing conditions, and the part of the plant.

Evidence suggests that isothiocyanates are not the only chemopreventive phytochemicals found in cruciferous vegetables. Fractionation followed by purification of several whole vegetables has led to the isolation of a few candidate phytochemicals that warrant further study. The phytochemicals that have demonstrated biological activity in terms of upregulation of phase II enzymes include crambene, a stable nitrile, and S-methyl cysteine sulfoxide and dithiolethione. In animal models, crambene has demonstrated synergistic effects with indole-3-carbinol in inducing quinone reductase and glutathione-S-transferase (52).

BIOLOGICAL BIOMARKERS OF CRUCIFEROUS VEGETABLE CONSUMPTION

The identification of accurate, reliable, and valid biomarkers of cruciferous vegetable intake is a pivotal step toward more clearly evaluating the relationship between cruciferous vegetable intake and disease. Characteristics of strong biomarkers include (1) significant correlation between biomarker and exposure (dietary intake), (2) response to significant changes in intake, (3) low variability in populations or within an individual on repeat measurement, (4) readily available biological sample (urine, blood, buccal cells, etc.) for analysis, (5) stable with long-term storage, and (6) cost- and time-efficient. Chung and colleagues have identified a promising urinary biomarker of dietary uptake of isothiocyanates in humans (53). This HPLC-based assay quantifies total ITC and dithiocarbamates in human urine using a cyclocondensation reaction quantifying 1,3-benzodithiole-2-thione. The assay was validated using a controlled diet including 20 grams of brown mustard or watercress and the collection of urine at variable time points throughout a 24-hour period. Variation coefficients were determined to be 1.4% interday and 0.5% intraday and standard deviations supported high reproducibility of the assay. There are, however, limitations to the use of this assay in clinical trials of diet and disease prevention. First, for optimal quantification, 24-hour urines are preferable. Given the fact that the peak excretion for the majority of ITCs is within 8 hours of intake and excretion is 80% complete within 24 hours (25), at minimum, urine should be collected overnight to reflect the timing of highest intake of cruciferous vegetables in humans (lunch and supper). Second, the assay is unable to differentiate the relative contribution of individual ITCs to the total. HPLC is, however, more specific than measurement of ITC mercapturic acid metabolites and assays to quantify phenethyl (54) and allyl isothiocyanate (55) have also been developed.

Application of this assay to stored urine samples from Chinese elderly living in Singapore, indicated that when intake is high (mean intake of cruciferous vegetables of 40.6 grams/day), correlations between reported dietary intake and urinary excretion of total ITCs were significant (10). A study by Shapiro et al. carefully quantified the isothiocyanate content of a controlled cruciferous vegetable diet regime and compared intake to excretion of proportionate amounts of urinary dithiocarbamates by analytical recovery using the cyclocondensation assay. This allows the measurement of the extent of metabolism and kinetics of the excretion of defined quantities of dietary glucosinolates (25). Fowke and colleagues demonstrated the efficacy of the cyclocondensation ITC analysis among free-living subjects who regularly consume approximately 100 grams (one serving) of cruciferous vegetables daily. Interestingly, the biomarker was shown to be less accurate during periods of low or sporadic intake and when intake was greater than 200 grams per day (56). Raw vegetable intake was more strongly associated with urinary ITC than cooked vegetable intake ($r = 0.23$ versus 0.07, respectively), a hypothesis that has been supported by a controlled feeding study using fresh versus cooked broccoli in which a threefold increase in ITC metabolites was demonstrated for raw broccoli (57).

Efforts to employ the cyclocondensation assay to biological samples other than urine, such as plasma, serum, or erythrocytes, have recently been improved by precipitation of sample proteins using polyethylene glycol and introducing a solid phase extraction of the cyclocondensation product. This sensitive and specific method indicates that there is active renal tubular excretion of isothiocyanates and peak levels following controlled feedings with 200 micromoles of broccoli sprouts, which can be measured in plasma and serum one hour after feeding (58). A similar methodology using the cyclocondensation reaction, hexane extraction, and HPLC with UV detection has also been demonstrated to provide reproducible and valid measurement of intake of phenethyl isothiocyanate with only 5.6% variability in multiple-day samples (59).

CRUCIFEROUS VEGETABLES AND CANCER PREVENTION

Evidence from Animal Models

Studies using animals induced with chemical carcinogens have provided strong evidence that cruciferous vegetables can alter the carcinogenesis pathway. A highly publicized study by Talalay and colleagues showed that rats fed broccoli sprouts with high concentrations of sulfurophane and then exposed to a chemical carcinogen demonstrated a significant reduction in both mammary tumor multiplicity and tumor size compared to rats fed either the control diet or a mature broccoli diet (60). A more recent study using a high-selenium broccoli diet fed to Sprague-Dawley rats induced with mammary or colon cancer showed similar chemopreventive effects and demonstrated the synergy among select dietary constituents—nutrient and others—in optimizing these effects (61). Chung also demonstrated a protective role for ITCs in a Fischer rat model of colonic aberrant crypt foci (ACF). In this case, sulfurophane and phenethylisothiocyanate significantly reduced ACF during the initiation and postinitiation phases of carcinogenesis, while the N-acetylcysteine conjugates demonstrated efficacy only postinitiation (62). Research using A/J mice as a model for lung cancer tumorigenesis has also shown a chemopreventive effect of isothiocyanates (63).

Epidemiological Evidence

Epidemiological evidence exists to support a protective role for certain fruits and vegetables in reducing the risk of cancer (2, 3, 64, 65, 66, 67, 68, 69, 70). For the past decade, public health efforts in the form of the 5-a-day for better health program have focused on increasing fruit and vegetable intake among Americans. The 1994–1996 Continuing Survey of Food Intakes by Individuals (CSFII) reported that their sample population consumed 3.6 +/- 2/3 servings of vegetables per day. Only 3% of the sample consumed broccoli during the reporting period. Between 1991 and 1994, fruit and vegetable consumption, combined, increased by 12%. The 1994–1996 CSFII reported that 45% of Americans consumed at least five servings of fruits and vegetables per day (7).

Yet data related to specific types or families of vegetables, including cruciferous vegetables, have not been adequately tested (64, 71). The relationship between cruciferous vegetable intake and cancer prevention has gained increased focus among cancer prevention scientists in recent years. Table 15.3 lists select epidemiologic studies focused on the role of cruciferous vegetables or their biologically active constituents on carcinogenesis. Driven by our advancing understanding of the underlying chemopreventive mechanisms, growing epidemiological evidence, and recent development of analytical assays to quan-

Table 15.3. Epidemiologic Studies Focused on Cruciferous Vegetables

Study	Cancer site	Cruciferous vegetable or biologically active constituent	Relative risk/odds ratio and 95% confidence interval
Brennan 2000 (72) (European multi-center study)		Brassica vegetables	N = RR = 0.5 95% CI = 0.3–0.9
Cohen 2000 (65) (Prostate Cancer)	Prostate	Cruciferous vegetables	N = 1230 OR =0.59 CI = 0.39–0.90
Ewertz 1990 (73)	Breast	Broccoli, green cabbage (spinach)	N = 1474 OR = 0.9 CI = 0.8–1.1
Graham 1978 (74)	Rectum	Cabbage	N = OR = 0.7 (P =0.05)
Jain, 1999 (67)	Prostate	Cruciferous vegetables	N = 1253 OR = 0.69 CI = 0.52–0.91
Katsouyanni 1986 (75) Greece	Breast	Total vegetables	N = 120 Negative association
LeMarchand 1989 (76) Hawaii	Lung	Cruciferous vegetables	Men N = 230 OR = 0.5 CI = (NA) Women N =102 OR = 0.2 CI = (NA)
Levi 1999 (68)	Colorectal	Cruciferous vegetables	N =714 Raw OR = 0.85 CI = 0.74–0.98 Cooked OR = 0.69 CI = 0.57–0.98
Lin 1998 (77)	Colorectal adenomas	Broccoli	N = 1213 OR = 0.47 95% CI = 0.30–0.73
Michaud, 1999 (69) (Health Professionals Follow-up Study) (Bladder)	Bladder	Cruciferous vegetables (broccoli and cabbage statistically significant)	N = 47,909 RR = 0.49 CI = 0.32–0.75
Slattery 1988 (78) USA	Colon	Brassica vegetables	N = 229 OR = 0.3 CI = 0.1–0.8
Slattery 2000 (79)	Breast	Brassica vegetables	N =5482 RR = 0.58 CI = 0.42–0.79

Table 15.3. (*Continued*)

Study	Cancer site	Cruciferous vegetable or biologically active constituent	Relative risk/odds ratio and 95% confidence interval
Smith-Warner 2001 (80)	Breast	Broccoli, brussels sprouts, and cabbage	N = 351, 825 RR = 0.96 CI = 0.87–1.06
Steinmetz 1993 (81)	Lung	Broccoli	N = 41,837 OR = 0.7 CI =0.4–1.3
Steinmetz 1994 (82)	Colon	Cruciferous	N = 41,837 RR = 1.1 CI = 0.7–1.7
Terry 2001 (83) Sweden	Breast	Brassica vegetables	N = 5482 RR = 0.58 CI = 0.42–0.79
Voorrips 2000 (84) (Netherlands Cohort Study)	Distal colon cancer	Brassica and total vegetables	Men (brassica) N = 58,279 RR = 0.68 CI = 0.41–1.15 Women (brassica) N = 62,573 RR = 0.47 CI = 0.25–0.89

tify intake, cancer prevention researchers are expanding investigations into these promising chemopreventive foods and food constituents (23).

Evidence for Breast Cancer

A recent pooled analysis of the protective effect of vegetables against breast cancer indicated that no protective association was demonstrated for cruciferous vegetables (RR = 0.96, CI = 0.87–1.06). However, cruciferous intake was limited to intake of broccoli, brussels sprouts, and cabbage as assessed by a food frequency questionnaire and did not reflect significant differences in intake across quartiles (80). This finding was not supported by Terry and colleagues who reported a significant reduction in breast cancer risk with increasing cruciferous vegetable intake (RR = 0.58, 95% CI, 0.42–0.79) (83). Levi also demonstrated a 60% reduction in risk among participants in a case-control study conducted in Switzerland (68). Several studies from the 1980s demonstrated a 6% reduction in risk associated with broccoli, spinach, and green cabbage consumption (85, 75); and p-for-trend significance for intake of raw cabbage, cooked cabbage, and cauliflower in residents of Greece (75).

Evidence for Other Cancers

Cohen and colleagues reported a protective effect of cruciferous vegetables in relation to risk for prostate cancer (RR = 0.59, 95% CI = 0.39–0.90) (65) that has also been substantiated in other cohorts (67, 86). The Physician's Health S°tudy conducted at Harvard indicated that intake of cruciferous vegetables was protective against bladder cancer (RR = 0.49) (69). Reports of the association between cruciferous vegetable intake and colon cancer also indicate a linear, dose-response protective effect (74). In fact, evidence suggests that the protective effects of broccoli consumption are most pronounced among subjects with the glutathione-S-transferase null genotype (79, 87). Finally, data from Zhang and colleagues indicate cruciferous vegetable consumption was associated with reduced risk for non-Hodgkin's lymphoma among women (88). Efforts to further describe the association between cruciferous vegetable intake and cancer should be pursued in the context of large, longitudinal epidemiological studies particularly those conducted in populations where cruciferous vegetables constitute a significant portion of vegetables consumed (i.e., Japan and China).

Dietary Intervention Studies

Clinical trials focused on increasing vegetable intake are limited and only short-term feeding studies assessing mechanisms of biological activity are available using cruciferous vegetable interventions. One intervention study using brassica vegetables (broccoli, cabbage, and brussels sprouts) among postmenopausal women demonstrated a significant increase in the urinary 2-hydroxyestrone to 16-alpha-hydroxyestrone ratio, which has been shown to be inversely associated with breast cancer risk (89).

The Polyp Prevention Trial reported no reduction in recurrent polyps in response to a diet high in fruits and vegetables. The independent effect of cruciferous vegetables was not explored and it is not likely the study was adequately powered to determine a statistically significant relationship with cruciferous vegetables (90). The Women's Healthy Eating and Living Study is currently being conducted to test the hypothesis that among breast cancer survivors, a diet rich in vegetables and fruit can significantly reduce breast cancer recurrence rates (91). It will afford an opportunity to explore further the protective effects of cruciferous vegetables given preliminary evidence that cruciferous vegetable intake is increased, on average, 30% above baseline levels in intervention group subjects (Unpublished data).

CHEMOPREVENTIVE BIOLOGICAL ACTIVITY OF CRUCIFEROUS VEGETABLE CONSTITUENTS

Carcinogenesis is a multistage process developing over several years if not decades in humans. It is well recognized that a multitude of dietary constituents can act biologically to alter the carcinogenesis pathway at several points in the pathway including from the deactivation of primary carcinogens, to repair of initiated cells, to reversal of DNA damage and potentially altering cancer recurrence. Several constituents in cruciferous vegetables have been explored in experimental models, including cell culture and animal and human studies, to define and describe their chemopreventive biological activity.

Table 15.4 lists demonstrated mechanisms for chemoprevention by constituents of cruciferous vegetables. Reviews of the mechanisms of chemoprevention associated with cru-

Table 15.4. Mechanisms of Chemoprevention and Associated Phytochemicals

Chemopreventive mechanism	Cruciferous vegetable/constituent	References
Apoptosis and regulation of cell cycle	Indole-3-carbinol Cruciferous vegetable juice Sulforaphane	Shertzer 2000 (22); Bradlow 1999 (122); Chung 2000 (62); Chiao 2002 (123).
Inhibit phase I enzymes (Cytochrome P450 isoenzymes)	Dithiolthione Ascorbigen dihydroindolocarbazole, benzylisothiocyanate(BITC) Phenethylisothiocyanate (PEITC)	Greenwald 2001 (64); Moreno 1999 (124); Steinkellner 2001 (31).
Induce phase II detoxification enzymes (Glutathione-S-transferase, quinone reductase, uridine diphosphate glucuronide transferase, UDP-glucoronosyl, 1,2-dithiole-3-thiones, terpenoids)	Dithiolthiones, indoles, isothiocyanates, sulforaphane, indole-3-carbinol Brussels sprouts juice, broccoli sprout extract Wasabi	Kwak 2001 (125); Steinkellner 2001 (31); Wallig 1997 (126); Smith 2000 (96); Morimitsu 2000 (127); Brooks 2001 (100); Ye 2001 (101); Pantuck 1979 (44); Hecht 2000 (93); Prochaska 1992 (99); Hecht 1995 (92)
Inhibition of alpha-hydroxylation of nitrosamines	Indoles, isothiocyanates (by induction of GST and inhibition of cytochrome-P450 isoenzymes	Steinkellner 2001 (31)
Radical and electrophil scavenger	Indole-3-carbinol Ascorbigen	Shertzer 2000 (22)

ciferous vegetable constituents are available and attenuate the multiple yet converging evidence that these compounds, whether natural or synthetically derived, hold great promise for reducing cancer incidence (92, 93, 94).

Induction of Phase II Enzymes—Inhibition of Phase I Enzymes

Several reviews of the modulating effects of cruciferous vegetables on cancer have been recently published (23, 95, 96, 97). Dietary carcinogens must be activated to induce cancer. The ability of dietary constituents in cruciferous vegetables to inhibit phase I enzyme activation is of primary importance to their cancer chemopreventive effects. The ability of cruciferous vegetables to activate phase II drug-metabolizing enzymes was demonstrated using a controlled feeding study as early as 1979 (44). Phase II enzymes include glutathione-S-transferase, UDP glucoronosyl transferases, sulfotransferases, oxidoreductase. Phase II enzymes bind to oxygenated carcinogens making highly polar molecules that are excreted. Phase II enzymes decrease carcinogenicity by blocking carcinogen metabolic activation and enhancing carcinogen detoxification (93). More recently, a controlled feeding study in which 250 grams of cruciferous vegetables were consumed daily by males concurrently consuming cooked meat at meals showed that intake of the supplemental cruciferous vegetables induced CYP1A2 activity and significantly reduced both 2-amino-3, 8-dimethyllimidazo(4,5-f) quinoxaline (MeIQx) and 2-amino-1-methyl-6-phenylimidazol(4,5-b)pyridine (PhIP) excretion in urine (98). Evidence suggests that this response is predominantly associated with the indole content of cruciferous vegetables rather than isothiocyanates (31). Further evidence suggests that indole-3-carbinol and its nonenzymatic reaction products are among the most potent biological compounds associated with cancer prevention (22).

Data from Prochaska et al. have demonstrated in a cell culture model that phase II enzymes are inducible by 1,2-dithiolo-thiones, isothiocyanates, and indoles found in cruciferous vegetables (99). Steinkellner et al. have also demonstrated induction of cytochrome P450 1A1 and glutathione S-transferase with the addition of cruciferous vegetable juice to human HepG2 cells (31). Using isolated sulfurophane or broccoli sprout extract has also been shown to induce phase II enzyme activity in prostate cell lines (100). Ye and Zhang have also shown that the induction of phase II enzymes is dependent on the cellular accumulation of isothiocyanates and that even isothiocyanates with lower induction capacity can demonstrate a significant increase in quinone reductase and glutathione activity even when multiple doses were used (101).

Animal feeding studies using cruciferous vegetable constituents have shown variable response on drug-metabolizing enzymes including elevations in GST (102, 103), induction of CYP1A1 (104, 105, 106), increased xenobiotic metabolizing enzymes including phenacetin-O-dealkylase (107), and induction of cytochrome P450 (108). Despite the fact that dosages used in animal models far exceed those probable for human consumption, human intervention trial data do support the established biological chemopreventive mechanisms demonstrated in animal models. The cruciferous vegetables shown to induce GSTs, including π-GST, in humans are brussels sprouts and red cabbage, while broccoli and white cabbage have not consistently demonstrated this activity. A point mutation in the π-GST gene leads to decreased GST activity and is associated with several solid tumor cancers including esophageal, bladder, lung, testicular, and breast (109). Feeding studies have also demonstrated induction of CYP-450-1A2 (18).

Ideally, plant foods or constituents that selectively activate phase II metabolizing enzymes are preferable to those that induce both phase II and Phase I since Phase I enzymes have been shown to activate precarcinogens through oxidation and thus may increase cancer risk. Activation of phase II detoxifying enzymes would prevent the formation of carcinogens through this phase I activation of precarcinogens. Select phytochemicals in cruciferous vegetables, such as indole-3-carbinol, have shown dual phase enzyme activation while others induce only phase II enzymes. The specific activity of the wide variety of phytochemicals found in cruciferous vegetables has not been fully described.

Of recent interest is the association between GST polymorphisms and biological activity of isothiocyanates (ITCs). A study of lung cancer incidence among 18,244 Chinese men was conducted to determine genetic predisposition to reduced or absent enzyme activity resulting in increased ITC levels in the body. The study found a gene-diet interaction. Subjects were found to be either deficient in the enzyme (GST-MI) or not (GST-T1). Participants with detectable levels of urinary ITCs had a 40% decreased risk of lung cancer while the participants with the null genotype (GST-M1) had a 64% decrease in lung cancer risk (110). Genotypes among lung cancer versus control populations indicate that the null genotypes (GST-M1) confer enhanced chemopreventive activity of ITCs in humans possibly due to the ITCs remaining in the body longer and prolonging the protective effects (9, 110, 111). The null GST-M1 homozygous deletion has been identified in approximately 50% of the Caucasian population. Thus, the protective association between dietary intake of cruciferous vegetables and cancer may be difficult to identify in populations where the null genotype is less frequent and genotyping has not been included in statistical modeling of the data.

Inhibition of Alpha-hydroxylation of Nitrosamines

Numerous cell culture studies have demonstrated that isothiocyanates in cruciferous vegetables significantly inhibit the hydroxylation of nitrosamines thus reducing their carcinogenic potential (112, 113, 114). However, the protective effects of the indole and isothiocyanates are currently only demonstrated in animal models at doses far exceeding current human intake (115, 116).

Apoptosis and Antiproliferation

An additional mechanism by which cruciferous vegetables reduce cancer risk is related to the ability of cruciferous vegetables and the constituents thereof to induce programmed cell death and cell cycle arrest, or to inhibit the proliferation of abnormal or transformed cells. An excellent review of the topic is provided by Thornalley (30). Cell culture studies using a variety of cancer cell lines and the addition of select cruciferous vegetable composites or isolated phytochemicals help to demonstrate the impact of cruciferous vegetables on apoptosis, cell cycle arrest, and proliferation. Generally, glucosinolates have no demonstrable effect on either apoptosis or proliferation of malignant cells *in vitro*; however, select isothiocyanates do appear to show protective effects (117). For example, cell cycle arrest has been demonstrated using isothiocyanates, sulfurophane, and indoles in culture with HT29, Caco-2, and LS-174 colon cancer cell lines (118, 119, 32) as well as breast cancer cell lines (120). Interestingly, the protective effects against proliferation of transformed cells are no longer apparent once the cells proliferate to the point of confluency indicating that, at least for colon cancer, sulfurophane may be most effective in preventing the growth of cancer either at the later stages of initiation or the early stage of proliferation (119). Apoptosis has also been demonstrated in HeLa cells and is associated with increased capase 3 and c-Jun N-terminal kinase levels (121).

CHEMOPREVENTION POTENTIAL OF SELECT ISOTHIOCYANATES

Select isothiocyanates derived from glucosinolates in cruciferous vegetables, including indole-3-carbinol, pentyl- and benzyl-isothicyanates, and sulfurophane have shown promise as future chemopreventive agents.

Indole-3-carbinol

The inhibition of mammary tumors by indole-3-carbinol has been demonstrated using both estrogen-responsive and estrogen-nonresponsive cell lines. Human breast cancer cell lines that were either estrogen-responsive or estrogen-nonresponsive were treated with I3C to determine its effect. The effects of I3C were greater in the estrogen-responsive cells with a selective increase in the C-2 hydroxylation pathway and induction of cytochrome P450 1A1. This was not found in the estrogen-nonresponsive cell line (128).

Breast cancer cell lines were used to determine the effect of indole-3-carbinol on mechanisms of antitumor activity by its regulation of estrogen activity and metabolism.

I3C significantly decreased 17 beta-estradiol-activated estrogen receptor signaling. I3C down-regulated the estrogen-responsive gene expression in pS2 and cathepsin-D and up-regulated BRCA1, which exhibits multiple biological functions as a tumor suppressor. I3C and BRCA1 acted together to inhibit estrogen receptor transcriptional activity. I3C is able to alter/reduce estrogen activity through a number of mechanisms in vitro supporting the need for expanded research into this phytochemical as a potential disease modifier (129)

Indole-3-carbinol induces the isoenzyme cytochrome P450 1A1 (CYP1A1 and CYP1A2), which also alters estrogen metabolism. Estradiol produces two metabolites, 16-alpha-hydroxyestrone (16-OHE1) and 2-alpha-hydroxestrone (2-OHE1). The 16-alpha-hydroxyestrone has both genotoxic and tumorigenic effects thereby potentially increasing the risk of breast and cervical cancers. The 2-alpha-hydroxyestrone is protective. Indole-3-carbinol enhances the production of 2-OHE1 shifting the ratio of 2-alpha OHE:16alpha OHE to a more favorable ratio resulting in risk reduction (130, 131, 122).

A study by Michnovicz et al. was done on seven men who received 500 mg/day I3C for 1 week and ten women who received 400 mg/day I3C for 2 months to evaluate change in urinary estrogens. I3C was shown to alter estrogen profiles. In both men and women, urinary excretion of C-2 estrogens increased due to I3C induction of estrogen 2-hydroxylation. Urinary excretion of almost all other estrogens including estradiol, estrone, estriol, and 16-hydroxyestrone decreased suggesting that overall estrogenic exposure was decreased (131).

A second mechanism of protection associated with I3C is related to enzyme induction. Indole-3-carbinol has been shown to induce phase II enzymes, glutathione-S-transferase, quinone reductase, and uridine diphosphate glucuronide transferase, all of which have a detoxifying effect related to an increase in the excretion of carcinogenic toxins (125).

Sulforaphane

Sulforaphane has been shown to alter the development of chemically induced mammary tumors in rats through a number of mechanisms. The number of tumors that developed were reduced by 80% and the number of rats that developed tumors was decreased by about 60% (124). The formation of colon polyps in rat colons was decreased by sulforaphane (123).

DIETARY RECOMMENDATIONS

A wealth of evidence from cell culture, animal, epidemiology, and more recently, dietary intervention trials indicate that the consumption of cruciferous vegetables will likely reduce cancer risk. While the largest body of evidence is focused on breast and colon cancer, growing research supports important biological activity in other cancers including lung, prostate, and even blood-related malignancies. Although select cruciferous vegetables such as broccoli sprouts may have stronger biological activity than others, most scientists would suggest that a wide variety of cruciferous vegetables be integrated into the daily diet. Our capacity to determine associations between cruciferous vegetable intake and cancer is currently limited by the available dietary and biomarker methodology. Efforts to more accurately quantify intake and to apply biomarkers of intake to epidemiological studies must continue. Further research describing new mechanisms of biological activity beyond xenobiotic enzyme induction is warranted. In addition, exploration into the synergy among phytochemicals and nutrients in cruciferous vegetables and the role of synergistic effects on cancer chemoprevention should be defined. Finally, a primary focus on changing dietary intake toward a more plant-based diet with a sufficient quantity of cruciferous vegetables is needed. Although the 5-a-day program of the NCI is resulting in improved dietary patterns for disease prevention, behavioral research and educational interventions must complement the growing evidence-based research to ensure the health of the population is optimized.

REFERENCES

1. Terry, P., Terry, J.B., and Wolk, A., Fruit and vegetable consumption in the prevention of cancer: an update, *J. Int. Med.*, 250:280–290, 2001.

2. Steinmetz, K.A., and Potter, J.D., Vegetables, fruit, and cancer prevention: a review, *J. Am. Diet. Assoc.*, 96(10): 1027–1039, 1996.

3. World Ca Res Fund. *Food, Nutrition and the prevention of CA: a global perspective.* Washington, DC: Am Inst for Ca Research; 1997.

4. Naska, A., Vsadekis, V.G., et al, Fruit and vegetable availability among ten European countries: how does it compare with the "five-a-day" recommendation? DAFNE I and II projects of the European Commission, *Br. J. Nutr.*, 84:549–556, 2000.

5. Verhoeven, D., Verhagen, H., Glodbohm, A., Van Den Brandt, P., and VanPoppel, G., A review of mechanisms underlying anticarcinogenicity by brassica vegetables, *Chem Biol Inter*, 103: 79–129, 1997.

6. Natural Medicines Comprehensive Database, June 26, 2002.

7. Johnston, C.S., Taylor, C.A., and Hampl, J.S., More Americans Are Eating "5A Day" but Intakes of Dark Green and Cruciferous Vegetables Remain Low, *J Nutr.* 130(12): 3063–3067, 2000.

8. Nestle, M., Broccoli sprouts as inducers of carcinogen-detoxifying enzyme systems: clinical, dietary, and policy implications, *Proc. Natl. Acad. Sci. U.S.A.*, 94: 11149–11151, 1997.

9. Spitz, M.R., Duphenne, C.M., Detry, M.A., et al., Dietary intake of isothiocyanates: evidence of a joint effect with glutathione-S-transferase polymorphism in lung cancer risk, *Cancer Epidemiology, Biomarkers & Prevention*, 9: 1017–1020, 2000.

10. Seow, A., Shi, C-Y., Chung, F.-L., Jiao, D., Hankin, J., Lee, H-P., Coetzee, G.A., and Yu, M.C., Urinary Total Isothiocyanate (ITC) in a Population-based Sample of Middle-Aged and Older Chinese in Singapore: Relationship with Dietary Total ITC and Glutathione S-Transferase M1/T1/P1 Genotypes, *Cancer Epidemiology, Biomarkers & Prevention*, 7: 775–781, 1998.

11. Drewnowski, A., and Rock, C.L., The influence of genetic taste markers on food acceptance, *Am. J. Clin. Nutr.*, 62(3): 506–511, 1995.

12. Kaminski, L.C., Henderson, S.A., and Drewnowski, A., Young women's food preferences and taste responsiveness to 6-n-propylthiouracil (PROP), *Physiol Behav.*, 68(5): 691–697, 2000.

13. Drewnowski, A., Henderson, S.A., and Barratt-Fornell, A., Genetic taste markers and food preferences, *Drug Metabolism & Disposition*, 29(4 pt 2): 535–538, 2001.

14. Drewnowski, A., Henderson, S.A., Hann, C.S., Berg, W.A., and Ruffin, M.T., Genetic taste markers and preferences for vegetables and fruit of female breast cancer patients, *J. Am. Diet. Assoc.*, 100(2): 191–197, 2000.

15. Drewnowski, A., Henderson, S.A., Hann, C.S., Barratt-Fornell, A, and Ruffin, M., Age and food preferences influence dietary intakes of breast care patients, *Health Psychol.*, 18(6): 570–578, 1999.

16. Ziegler, R.G., The future of phytochemical database, *Am. J. Clin. Nutr.*, 74: 4–5, 2001.

17. Hakim I.A., Hartz V., Graver E., Whitacre R. Evaluation of a questionnaire and database for assessing dietary d-limonene intake, *Public Health Nutr.* (In press, 2002).

18. Lampe, J.W., King, I.B., Li, S., Grate, M.T., Barale, K.V., Chen, C., Feng, Z., and Potter, J.D., *Brassica* vegetables increase and apiaceous vegetables decrease cytochrome P450 1A2 activity in humans: changes in caffeine metabolic ratios in response to controlled vegetable diets, *Carcinogenesis*, 21: 1157–1162, 2000.

19. Mangels, A.R., Holden, J.M., Beecher, G.R., Forman, M.R., and Lanza, E., Carotenoid content of fruits and vegetables: an evaluation of analytic data, *J. Am. Diet. Assoc.*, 93: 284–296, 1993.

20. Prestera, T., Fahey, J.W., Holtzclaw, W.D., Abeygunawardana, C., Kachinski, J.L., and Talalay, P., Comprehensive chromatographic and spectroscopic methods for the separation of intact glucosinolates, *Anal. Biochem.*, 239: 168–179, 1996.

21. Zhang, Y., Wade, T., Prestera, T., and Talalay, P., Quantitative determination of isothiocyanates, dithiocarbamates, carbon disulfide and related thiocarbonyl compounds by cyclocondensation with 1.2-benzenedithiol, *Anal. Biochem.*, 239: 160–167, 1996.

22. Shertzer, H.G., and Senft, A.P., The micronutrient indole-3-carbinol: implications for disease and chemoprevention, *Drug metabolism & Drug Interactions*, 17(1–4): 159–188, 2000.

23. Talalay, P., and Fahey, J.W., Phytochemicals from cruciferous plants protect against cancer by modulating carcinogen metabolism, *J. Nutr.*, 131(11s): 3027S–3033S, 2001.

24. Johnson, I.T., Glucosinolates: bioavailability and importance to health, *International Journal for Vitamin & Nutrition Research*, 72(1): 26–31, 2002.

25. Shapiro, T.A., Fahey, J.W., Wade, K.L., Stephenson, K.K., and Talalay, P., Human metabolism and excretion of cancer chemoprotective glucosinolates and isothiocyanates of cruciferous vegetable. *Cancer Epidemiology Biomarkers and Prevention*, 7: 1091–1100, 1998.

26. Fahey, J.W., Zaleman, A.T., and Talalay, P., The chemical diversity and distribution of glucosinolates and isothiocyanates among plants, *Phytochemisty*, 56: 5–51, 2001.

27. McDanell, R., McLean, A.E.M, Hanley, A.B., Heaney, R.K., and Fenwick, G.R., Differential induction of mixed-function oxidase (MFO) activity in rat liver and intestine by diets containing processed cabbage: correlation with cabbage levels of glucosinalates and glucosinolate hydrolysis products, *Food Chem. Toxicol.*, 25: 363–368, 1987.

28. Kjaser, A., Glucosinolates in the Cruciferae. In: Vaughan, J.G., MacLeod, A.J., Jones, B.M.G., (Eds.), The Biology and Chemistry of Cruciferae. Academic Press, London, pp. 207–219, 1976.

29. Rodman, J.E., Divergence, convergence, and parallelism in phytochemical character: the glucosinolate-myrosinase system. In Young, D.A., Siegler, D.S. (Eds.), Phytochemistry and Angiosperm Phylogeny, Praeger, New York, pp.43–49, 1981.

30. Thornalley, P.J., Isothiocyanates: mechanism of cancer chemopreventive action, *Anti-Cancer Drugs*, 13: 331–338, 2002.

31. Steinkellner, H., Rabot, S., Freywald, C., Nobis, E., Scharf, G., Chabicovsky, M., Knasmuller, S., and Kassie, F., Effects of cruciferous vegetables and their constituents on drug metabolizing enzymes involved in the bioactivation of DNA-reactive dietary carcinogens, *Mutation Research*, 480–481: 285–297, 2001.

32. Bonnesen, C., Eggleston, I.M., and Hayes, J.D., Dietary indoles and isothiocyanates that are generated from cruciferous vegetables can both stimulate apoptosis and confer protection against DNA damage in human colon cell lines, *Cancer Research*, 61(16): 6120–6130, 2001.

33. Sang, J.P., and Truscott, R.J.W., Lipid chromatographic determination of glucosinolates in rapeseeds as desulfoglucosinolates. *J Assoc. Offic. Anal. Chem.*, 67:829, 1984.

34. Troyer, J.K., Stephenson, K.K., and Fahey, J.W., Analysis of glucosinolates from broccoli and other cruciferous vegetables by hydrophilic interaction liquid chromatography, *Journal of Chromatography A*, 919: 299–304. 2001.

35. Kushad, M.M., Brown, A.F., Kurlich, A.C., Juvik, J.A., Klein, B.P., Wallig, M.A. and Jeffery, E.H., Variation of glucosinolates in vegetable crops of Brassica oleracea, *J. Agric. Food Chem.*, 47: 1541–1548, 1999.

36. Fahey, J.W., Zhang, Y., and Talalay, P., Broccoli sprouts: an exceptionally rich source of inducers of enzymes that protect against chemical carcinogens, *Proceedings of the National Academy of Science of the USA*, 94: 10367–10372, 1997.

37. Fahey, J.W., and Stephenson, K.K., Cancer chemoprotective effects of cruciferous vegetables, *HortScience*, 34: 4–8, 1999.

38. Fenwick, G.R., Heaney, R.K., and Mullin, W.J., Glucosinolates and their breakdown products in food and food plants, *CRC Crit. Rev. Food Sci. Nutr.*, 18: 123–201, 1983.

39. Zhang, Y., Talalay, P., Cho, C.-G., and Posner, G.H., A major inducer of anticarcinogenic protective enzymes from broccoli: isolation and elucidation of structure, *Proc. Natl. Acad. Sci. U.S.A.*, 89: 2399–2403, 1992.

40. Verkerk, R., van der Gaag, M.S., Dekker, M., Jongen, and W.M.F., Effects of processing conditions on glucosinolates in cruciferous vegetables, *Cancer Letters*, 114: 193–194, 1997.

41. Loft S., Otte, J., Poulsen H.E. and Sorenson, H. Influence of intact myrosinase-treated indoleyl glucosinolates on the metabolism *in vivo* of metronidazole and antipyrine in the rat, *Food Chem Toxicol.*, 30(11):927–935, 1992.

42. Mithen R.F., Dekker M., Verkerk R., Rabot S. and Johnson I.T., The nutritional significance, biosynthesis and bioavailability of glucosinolates in human foods, *J Sci Fed.Agric.*, 80:967–984, 2000.

43. Birt, D.F., Choe, M., and Pelling, J.C., Dietary, energy, and fat effects on tumor promotion, *Cancer Research (Suppl)*, 52: 2035s–2039s, 1992.

44. Pantuck, E.J., Pantuck, C.B., Garland, W.A., Min, B.H., Wattenberg, L.W., Anderson, K.E., Kappas, A., and Conney, A.H., Stimulatory effect of Brussels sprouts and cabbage on human drug metabolism, *Clin. Pharmacol. Ther.*, 25: 88–95, 1979.

45. Verhagen, H., Poulsen, H.E., Loft, S., van Poppel, G., Willems, M.I., and van Bladeren, P.J., Reduction of oxidative DNA-damage in humans by Brussels sprouts, *Carcinogenesis*, 16: 969–970, 1995.

46. Vitisen, K., Loft, S., and Poulsen, H.E., Cytochrome P4501A2 activity in man measured by caffeine metabolism: effect of smoking, broccoli and exercise, *Adv. Exp. Med. Biol.*, 283: 407–411, 1991.

47. Nugon-Baudon, L., Szylit, O., and Raibaud, P., Production of toxic glucosinolate from rapeseed meal from intestinal microflora of rat and chicken, *J. Sci. Food Agric,.* 43: 299–308, 1998.

48. Getahun, S.M., and Chung, F-L., Conversion of glucosinolates to isothiocyanates in human after ingestion of cooked watercress, *Cancer Epidemiology, Biomarkers & Prevention*, 8: 447–451, 1999.

49. Rabot, S., Nugon-Baudon, L., Raibaud, P., and Szylit, O., Rape-seed meal toxicity in genotobiotic rats: influence of a whole human faecal flora or single human strains of *Escherichia coli* and *Bacteroides vulgatus*, *Br. J. Nutr.*, 70: 323–331, 1993.

50. Chung, F-L., Getahun, S.M, Jiao, D., and Conaway, C.C., Hydrolysis of glucosinolates to isothiocyanates in humans, *Proc. Am. Assoc. Cancer Res.*, 39: 18, 1998.

51. Rosa, E.A.S., Heaney R.K., Fenwick G.R., Portal C.A.M., Glucosinolates in crop plants, *Horticul. Rev.* 19:99–215, 1997.

52. Staack, R., Kingston, S., Wallig, M.A., and Jeffery, E.H., A comparison of the individual and collective effects of four glucosinolate breakdown products from Brussels sprouts on induction of detoxification enzymes, *Toxicol. Appl. Pharm.*, 149: 17–23, 1998.

53. Chung, F-L, Jiao, D., Getahun, S.M., and Yu, M.C., A Urinary biomarker for uptake of dietary isothiocyanates in humans, *Cancer Epidemiology, Biomarkers & Prevention*, 7:103–108, 1998.

54. Chung, F-L., Morse, M.A., Eklind, K.I., and Lewis, J., Quantation of human uptake of the anticarcinogen phenethyl isothiocyanate after a watercress meal, *Cancer Epidemiology, Biomarkers & Prevention*, 1: 383–388, 1992.

55. Jiao, D., Ho, C-T., Foiles, P., and Chung, F-L., Identification and quantification of the *N*-acetyl-cysteine conjugate of allyl isothiocyanate in human urine after ingestion of mustard, *Cancer Epidemiology, Biomarkers & Prevention*, 3: 487–492, 1994.

56. Fowke, J.H., Fahey, J.W., Stephenson, K.K., and Hebert, J.R., Using isothiocyanate excretion as a biological marker of *Brassica* vegetable consumption in epidemiological studies: evaluating the sources of variability, *Public Health Nutrition*, 4(3): 837–846, 2001.

57. Conaway, C.C., Getahun, S.M., Liebes, L.L., Pusateri, D.J., Topham, D.K., Botero-Omary, M., and Chung, F.L., Disposition of glucosinolates and sulforaphane in humans after ingestion of steamed and fresh broccoli, *Nutrition & Cancer*, 38(2): 168–178, 2000.

58. Ye, L., Dinkova-Kostova, A.T., Wade, K.L., Zhang, Y., Shapiro, T.A., and Talalay, P., Quantitative determination of dithiocarbamates in human plasma, serum, erythrocytes and urine: pharmacokinetics of broccoli sprout isothiocyanates in humans, *Clinica Chimica Acta*, 316(1–2): 43–53, 2002.

59. Liebes, L., Conaway, C.C., Hochster, H., Mendoza, S., Hecht, S.S., Crowell, J., and Chung, F.L., High-performance liquid chromatography-based determination of total isothiocyanate levels in human plasma: application to studies with 2-phenethyl isothiocyanate, *Analytical Biochemistry*, 291(2): 279–289, 2001.

60. Talalay, P., Fahey, J.W., and Zhang, Y., Broccoli sprouts: an exceptionally rich source of inducers of enzymes that protect against chemical carcinogens, *Proceedings of the National Academy of the USA*, 94(19): 10367–72, 1997.

61. Finley, J.W., Clement, Ip., Lisk, D.J., Davis, C.D., Hintze, K.J., and Whanger, P.D., Cancer-protective properties of high-selenium broccoli, *J. Agric. Food Chem.*, 49: 2679–2683, 2001.

62. Chung, F.L., Conaway, C.C., Rao, C.V., and Reddy, B.S., Chemoprevention of colonic aberrant crypt foci in Fischer rats by sulforaphane and phenethyl isothiocyanate, *Carcinogenesis*, 21(12): 2287–2297, 2000.

63. Chung, F.L., Chemoprevention of lung cancer by isothiocyanates and their conjugates in A/J mouse, *Experimental Lung Research*, 27(3): 319–330, 2001.

64. Greenwald, P., Clifford, C.K., and Milner, J.A., Diet and cancer prevention, *European Journal of Cancer*, 37: 948–965, 2001.

65. Cohen, J.H., Kristal, A.R., and Stanford, J.L., Fruit and vegetable intakes and prostate cancer risk. *J. Natl. Cancer Inst.*, 92: 61–68, 2000.

66. Gupta, p., Hebert, J., Bhonsle, R., Sinor, P., Mehta, H., and Mehta, F., Dietary factors in oral leukoplakia and submucous fibrosis in a population-based case control study in Gujarat, India, *Oral Dis.*, 4:200–206, 1998.

67. Jain, M.G., Hislop, G.T., How, G.R., and Ghadirian, P., Plant foods antioxidants and prostate cancer risk: findings from case-control studies in Canada, *Nutr. Cancer*, 34: 173–184, 1999.

68. Levi, F., Pasche, C., La Vecchia, C., Lucchini, F., and Franceschi, S., Food groups and colorectal cancer risk, *Br. J. Cancer*, 79:1283–1287, 1999.

69. Michaud, D.S., Spiegelman, D., Clinton, S.K., Rimm, E.B., Willett, W.C., and Giovannucci, E.L., Fruit and vegetable intake and incidence of bladder cancer in male prospective cohort, *J. Natl. Cancer Inst.*, 91:605–613, 1999.

70. Verhoeven, D., Godbohm, R., van Poppel, G., Verhagen, H., van den Brandt, P. Epidemiological studies on Brassica vegetables and cancer risk, *Cancer Epid Biomark Prev.*, 5:733–748, 1996.

71. Slattery, M.I., Does an apple a day keep breast cancer away?, *JAMA*, 285: 799–801, 2001.

72. Fortes C., Butler J., et al. A multi-center case-control study of diet and lung cancer among non-smokers, *Ca causes & Control*, 11:49–58, 2000.

73. Ewertz, M., and Gill, C. Dietaray Factors and Breast-Cancer Risk in Denmark. *Int. J. Cancer.* 46(5):779–784, 1990.

74. Graham, S, Dayal, H., Swanson, M., Mittelman, A., and Wilkinson, G., Diet in epidemiology of cancer of the colon and rectum, *J. Natl. Cancer Inst.*, 61: 709–714, 1978.

75. Katsouyanni, k., Trichopoulos, D., Boyle, P., Xiroouchaki, E., Trichopoulos, a., Lisseos, B., Vasilaros, S., and MacMahon, B., Diet and breast cancer: a case-control study in Greece, *Int. J. Cancer*, 38:815–820, 1986.

76. LeMarchand, L., Yoshizawa, C., Kolonel, L., Hankin, J., and Goodman, M., Vegetable consumption and lung cancer risk: a population-based case-control study in Hawaii, *JNCI*, 81:1158–1164.

77. Lin, H., Probst-Hensch, N., Louie, A., Kau, I., Witte, J., Ingles, S., Franks, H., Lee, E., and Haile, R., Glutathione transferase null genotype, broccoli, and lower prevalence of colorectal adenomas, *Cancer Epid Bio & Pre*, 7: 647–652, 1998.

78. Slattery, M.L., Schumacher, M.C., Smith, K.R., et al, Physical activity, diet, and risk of colon cancer in Utah, *Am J Epidemiology*, 128: 989–999, 1988.

79. Slattery, M.L., Kampman, E., Samowitz, W., Cann, B.J., and Potter, J.D., Interplay Between Dietary Inducers of GST and the *GSTM-1* Genotype in Colon Cancer, *Int. J. Cancer*, 87: 728–733, 2000.

80. Smith-Warner, S.A., et al., Intake of Fruits and Vegetables and Risk of Breast Cancer. A Pooled Analysis of Cohort Studies, *JAMA*, 285(6): 169–776, 2001.

81. Steinmetz, K.A., Potter, J.D., and Folsom, A.R., Vegetables, fruit, and lung cancer in the Iowa Women's Health Study, *Cancer Res*, 53: 536–543, 1993.

82. Steinmetz, K., Kushi, L., Bostick, R., Folsom, A., and Potter, J., Vegetables, fruit, and colon cancer in the Iowa Women's Health Studyl, *Am J Epidemiol*, 139:1–15, 1994.

83. Terry, P., Wolk, A., Persson, I., and Magnusson, C., Brassica vegetables and breast cancer risk., *J.Am. Med. Assoc.*, 286: 2975–2977, 2001.

84. Voorrips, L.E., Goldbohm, R.A., Verhoeven, D.T., et al., Vegetable and fruit consumption and lung cancer risk in the Netherlands Cohort Study on diet and cancer, *Cancer Causes Control*, 11:101–115, 2000.

85. Ewertz, M., Machado, S.G., Boice, J.D. Jr., and Jensen, O.M., Endometrial cancer following treatment for breast cancer: a case control study in Denmark, *British Journal of Cancer*, 50(5): 687–692, 1984.

86. Kolonel, L.N., Hankin, J.H., Whittemore, A.S., Wu, A.H., Gallagher, R.P., Wilkens, L.R., John, E.M., Howe, G.R., Dreon, D.M., West, D.W., and Paffenberger, R.S., Jr., Vegetables, fruits, legumes and prostate cancer: a multicenter case-control study, *Cancer Epidemiol. Biomark. Prev.*, 9: 795–804, 2000.

87. Probst-Hensch, N.M., Tannenbaum, S.R., Chan, K.K., Coetzee, C.A., Ross, R.K., and Yu, M.C., Absence of the glutathione S-transferase M1 gene increases cytochrome P4501A2 activity among frequent consumers of cruciferous vegetables in a Caucasian population, *Cancer Epidemiology Biomarkers & Preventions*, 7: 635–638, 1998.

88. Zhang, S.M., Hunter, D.J., Rosner, B.A., Giovannucci, E.L., Colditz G.A., Speizer, F.E., and Willett, W.C., Intake of fruits, vegetables and related nutrients and the risk of non-Hodgkin's lymphoma among women, *Cancer Epidemiol. Biomark. Prev.*, 9:477–485, 2000.

89. Fowke, J.H., Longcope, C., and Hebert, J.R., Brassica vegetable consumption shifts estrogen metabolism in healthy postmenopausal women, *Cancer Epidemiology Biomarkers Prev.*, 9: 773–779, 2000.

90. Shatzkin, A., Lanza, E., Corle, D., et al. Lack of Affect of a Low-Fat, High-Fiber Diet on Recurrence of Colorectal Adenomas. Polyp Prevention Trial Study Group, *N.E.J.M.*, 342:1149–1155, 2000.

91. Pierce J.P., Rock, C.L., Flatt, S. W., Newman, V., Faerber S., Gilpin E.A., Hollenbach K.A., Thomson C.A., Ritenbaugh C.R., Marshall J.R. Can We Promote a Major Change in Dietary Pattern to Study its Effect on Cancer? Evidence from the WHEL Study., *Controlled Clin Trials* (in press, 2002).

92. Hecht, S.S., Chemoprevention by isothiocyanates, *J. Cell. Biochem.*, (suppl.) 22: 195–209, 1995.

93. Hecht, S.S., Chemoprevention by modifiers of carcinogen metabolism. In: *Phytochemicals as Bioactive Agents* (Bidlack, W.R., Omaye, S.T., Meskin, M.S., and Topham, D.K.W., eds.) 43–74. Technomic Publishing Co., Lancaster, PA., 2000.

94. Jeffrey, E., and Jarrell, V., Cruciferous Vegetables and Cancer Prevention. In: Handbook of Nutraceuticals and Functional Foods (Wolinsky, I., ed.). Pp. 169–192. CRC Press, New York, New York, 2001.

95. Smith, T.J., Mechanisms, of carcinogenesis inhibition by isothiocyanates, *Expert Opinion on Investigational Drugs*, 10(12): 2167–74, 2001.

96. Smith T.J., and Yang, C.S., Effect of organosulfur compounds from garlic and cruciferous vegetables on drug metabolism enzymes, *Drug Metabolism & Drug Interactions*, 17(1–4): 23–49, 2000.

97. Hecht, S.S., Inhibition of carcinogenesis by isothiocyanates, *Drug Metabolism Reviews*, 32(3–4): 395–411, 2000.

98. Murray, S., Lake, B.G., Gray, S., Edwards, A.J., Spingall, C, Bowey, E.A., Williamson, G., Boobis, A.R., and Gooderham, N.J., Effect of cruciferous vegetable consumption on heterocyclic aromatic amine metabolism in man, *Carcinogenesis*, 22: 1413–4120, 2001.

99. Prochaska, H.J., Santamaria, A.B., and Talalay, P., Rapid detection of inducers of enzymes that protect against carcinogens, *Proc. Natl. Acad. Sci.*, 89: 2394–2398, 1992.

100. Brooks, J.D., Paton, V.G., and Vidanes, G., Potent induction of phase 2 enzymes in human prostate cells by sulforaphane, *Cancer Epidemiology, Biomarkers & Prevention*, 10(9): 949–954, 2001.

101. Ye, L., and Zhang, Y., Total intracellular accumulation levels of dietary isothiocyanates determine their activity in elevation of cellular glutathione and induction of Phase 2 detoxification enzymes, *Carcinogenesis*, 22(12): 1987–1992, 2001.

102. Benson, A.M., and Baretto, P.B., Effects of Disulfiram, diethyldithiocarbamate, bisethylxanthogen and benzyl isothiocyanate on glutathione transferase activities in mouse organs, *Cancer Res.*, 45: 4219–4223, 1985

103. Boogards, J.J.P., van Ommen, B., Falke, H.E., Willems, M.I., and van Bladeren, P.J., Glutathione S-transferase subunit induction patterns of Brussels sprouts, allyl isothiocyanate and goitrin in rat liver and small mucosa: a new approach for the identification of inducing xenobiotics, *Food Chem. Toxicol.*, 28: 81–88, 1990.

104. Bonnesen, C., Stephenson, P.U., Anderson, O., Sorensen, H., and Vang, O., Modulation of cytochrome P-450 and glutathione S-transferase isoform expression in vivo by intact and degraded indolyl glucosinolates, *Nutr. Cancer*, 33: 178–187, 1999.

105. He, Y.H., Friesen, M.D., Ruch, R.J., and Schut, H.A., Indole-3-carbinol as a chemopreventive agent in 2-amino-1-methyl-6-phenylimidazo[4.5-b]pyridine (PhIP) carcinogenesis: inhibition of PhIP-DNA adduct formation, acceleration of PhIP metabolism and induction of cytochrome P-450 in female F344 rats, *Food Chem. Toxicol.*, 38: 15–23, 2000.

106. Renwick, A.B., Mistry, H., Barton, P.T., Mallet, F., Price, R.J., Beamand, J.A., and Lake, B.G., Effect of some indole derivatives on xenobiotic metabolism and xenobiotic induced toxicity in cultured rat liver slices, *Food Chem. Toxicol.,* 37: 609–618, 1999.

107. Kore, A.M. Jefferey, E.H., and Wallig, M.A., Effects of isothiocyanato-3-(methylsulinyl)-propane on xenobiotic metabolizing enzymes in rats, *Food Chem. Toxicol.,* 31: 723–729, 1993.

108. Wortelboer, H.M., de-Druif, C.A., van-Iersel, A.A., Voordhoek, J., Blaauboer, B.J., van-Bladeren, and Falker, H.E., Effects of cooked Brussels sprouts on cytochrome P-450 profile and phase II enzymes in liver and small intestine mucosa of rats, *Food Chem. Toxicol.,* 30: 17–27, 1992.

109. Taningher, M., Malacarne, D., Izzotti, D., Ugolini, A., and Parodi, S., Drug metabolism polymorphisms as modulators of cancer susceptibility. *Mutat. Res.,* 436: 227–261, 1999.

110. London, S.J., Yuan, J.M., Chung, F.L., et al., Isothiocyanates, glutathione-S-transferase M1 and T1 polymorphisms, and lung-risk: a prospective study of men in Shanghai, China, *Lancet,* 536: 724–729, 2000.

111. Zhao, B., Seow A., Lee, E.J.D., et al., Dietary isothiocyanates, glutathione S-transferase-M1, T1 polymorphisms and lung cancer risk among Chinese women in Singapore, *Cancer Epidemiology Biomarkers & Prevention,* 10: 1063–1067, 2001.

112. Chung, F., Wang, M., Hecht, S., Effects of Dietary Indoles and Isothiocyanates on N-nitroso-dimethylamine and 4-(methylnitrosamino)-1-(pyridyl)-1-butanone alpha hydroxylation and DNA-methylation in Rat Liver, *Carcinogenesis,* 6:539–543, 1985.

113. Smith, T., Guo, Z., Guengerich, F., Yang, C., Metabolism of 4-(methylnitrosamino)-1-butanone (NNK) by human cytochrome P450 1A2 and its inhibition by phenetyl isotiocyanate, *Carcinogenesis,* 17(4): 809–813, 1996.

114. Hamilton, S., and Tee, R., Effects of Isothiocyanates on the Metabolism of 4-(methylnitrosamino)-1-(3-pyridyl)-1-butanone (NNK) and benzo(a)pyrene by Hamster and Rat Liver Microsomes, *Anticancer Res.,* 14:1089–1094, 1994.

115. US NTIS PB report, Evalutation of the health aspects of mustard as food ingredients, *Food Am. Soc. Exp. Biol.,* 254: 528, 1975.

116. Kassie, F., and Knasmuller, S., Genotoxic effects of allyl isothiocyanate (AITC) and phenetyl isothiocyanate (PEITC), *Chem. Biol. Interact.,* 127: 163–180, 2000.

117. Nastruzzi, C., Cortesi, R., Espositio, E., Menegatti, E., Leoni, O., Iori, R., and Palmieri, S., *In Vitro* cytotoxic activity of some glucosinolate-derived products generated by myrosinase hydrolysis, *J. Agric. Food Chem.,* 44: 1014–1021, 1996.

118. Hasegawa, T., Nishino, H., and Iwashima, A., Isothiocyanates inhibit cell cycle progression of HeLa cells at G2/M phase, *Anticancer Drugs,* 4: 273–275, 1993.

119. Musk, S.R.R., Stephenson, P., Smith, T.K., Stening, P., Fyfe, D., and Johnson, I.T., Selective toxicity of compounds naturally present in food toward the transformed phenotype of human colorectal cell line HT29, *Nutr. Cancer,* 24: 289–298, 1995.

120. Cover, C.M., Hsieh, S.J. Tran, S.H., et al., Indole-3-carbinol inhibits the expression of cyclin-dependent kinase-6 and induces a G1 cell cycle arrest of human breast cancer cells independent of estrogen receptor signaling, *J. Biol. Chem.,* 273: 3838–3847, 1998.

121. Yu, R., Jiao, J.-J., Duh, L.-L., Tan, T.-H., and Kong, A.-N.T., Phenethyl isothiocyanate, a natural chemopreventive agent, activates c-Jun N-terminal kinase 1, *Cancer Res.,* 56: 2954–2959, 1996.

122. Bradlow, H.., Sepkovic, D., Telang, N., Osborne, M. Multifunctional aspects of the action of indole-3-carbino as an antitumor agent. *Annals of the New York Academy of Sciences.* 889:204–213, 1999.

123. Chiao, J.W., Chung, F.L., Kancherla, R., Ahmed, T., Mittelman, A., and Conaway, C.C., Sulforaphane and its metabolite mediate growth arrest and apoptosis in human prostate cancer cells, *International Journal of Oncology*, 20(3): 631–636, 2002.

124. Moreno, R., Kent, U., Hodge, K., and Hollenberg, P., Inactivation of cytochrome P450 2E1 by benzyl isothiocyanate, *Chem. Res. Toxicol.*, 12: 582–587, 1999.

125. Kwak, M., Egner, P., Dolan, P., Ramos-Gomez, M., Groopman, J., Itoh, K., Yamamoto, M., and Kensler, T., Tole of phase 2 enzyme induction in chemoprotection by dithiolethiones, *Mutation Research*, 305(15):480–481, 2001.

126. Wallig, M., Kingston, R., Staack, R., and Jeffery, E., Induction of rat pancreatic glutathione S-transferase and quinone reductase activities by a mixture of glucosinolate breakdown derivatives found in brussels sprouts, *Food and Chem Toxicology*, 36:365–373, 1998.

127. Morimitsu, Y., Hayashi, K., Nakagawa, Y., Horio, F., Uchida, K., and Osawa, T. Antiplatelet and anticancer isothiocyanates in Japanese domestic horseradish, wasabi, *Biofactors*, 13(1–4):271–276, 2000.

128. Tiwari, R.K., Guo, L., Bradlow, H.L., Telang, N.T., and Osborne, M.P., Selective responsiveness of human breast cancer cells to indol-3-carbinol, a chemopreventive agent, *J. Natl. Cancer Inst.*, 86(2): 126–131, 1994.

129. Meng, Q., Yuan, G., Goldberg, I., Rosen, E., Auborn, K., and Fan, S. Indole-2carbinol is a negative regulator of estrogen receptor-alpha signaling in human tumor cells, *J. Nutr.*, 130:2927–2931, 2000.

130. Telang, N.T., Katdare, M., Bradlow, H.L., Osborne, M.P., and Fishman, J., Inhibition of proliferation and modulation of estradiol metabolism: novel mechanisms for breast cancer prevention by the phytochemical indole-3-carbinol, *Proceedings of the Society for Experimental Biology & Medicine*, 216)2): 246–52, 1997.

131. Michnovicz, J., Aldercreutz, H., and Bradlow, H., Changes in levels of urinary estrogen metabolites after oral indole-3-carbinol treatment in humans, *J. Natl. Cancer Inst.*, 89(10):718–723, 1997.

16

Breast Cancer Prevention

**Brent P. Mahoney
and Paula Inserra**

OVERVIEW

One in nine women in the United States will develop breast cancer in her lifetime. More than 180,000 women each year will be diagnosed with breast cancer this year. Half of these women will present with advanced disease and only half of these women will be curable, yielding greater than 44,000 deaths a year. In the United States, breast cancer is the second leading cause of cancer mortality among women behind lung cancer. Although early detection, both with mammography and physical examination, has improved therapeutic outcome, this disease still exacts a heavy toll on society. A diagnosis of breast cancer brings with it fear, apprehension, and uncertainty as well as the physical and emotional burden of surgery, radiation, and chemotherapy for which it has been aptly said the cure may be worse than the disease. Hence, although further improvements in early detection may save lives, preventing this disease altogether is highly preferable.

The specific goal of reducing one's risk for developing breast cancer can be achieved by both avoiding activities or exposures that increase an individual's risk and by incorporating activities or exposures into one's life that reduce one's risk. Our cues for finding agents that increase our risk for developing breast cancer can be taken from the fields of both carcinogenesis and cancer epidemiology, whereas our cues for finding agents that reduce our risk for developing breast can be taken from the fields of cancer chemoprevention and cancer epidemiology.

BREAST CANCER EPIDEMIOLOGY

The epidemiologic evidence has shown us that only 5 to 10% of breast cancer cases are the result of a dominant heritable trait (Radford and Zehnbauer 1996). Namely, mutations in the BRCA1, BRCA2, P53, and ATM genes have been implicated as being causative (Miki et al. 1994, Zhang et al. 1998, Wooster et al. 1995, Bertwistle and Ashworth 1998, Newman et al. 1996, Malone et al. 1998). The fact that 90 to 95%of breast cancer arises spontaneously gives us great hope that improved breast cancer prevention can result in a dramatic impact upon the incidence and mortality rates of this disease. Breast cancer development is strongly associated with environmental factors common to Western civilization. This assertion is supported by the observation that Asian women have a four- to sevenfold lower incidence of breast cancer in their native country's as opposed to those raised in the United States (Deapen et al. 2002). Breast cancer incidence increases with age and this supports the multihit hypothesis for the genesis of breast cancer. A dose-dependent relationship has been shown to exist between breast cancer and radiation exposure (Aisenberg et al. 1997). The same relationship has been shown to exist with chemical carcinogens in animal models. Ironically, cigarette smoking has not been shown to be associated with breast cancer and this relationship has been extensively studied. This implies that chemical carcinogenesis plays a small role in the development of breast cancer. In fact, the only common chemical carcinogen shown to increase a woman's risk for developing breast cancer has been alcohol. Moderate and heavy alcohol consumption does increase a woman's risk for developing breast cancer. It should also be noted that the radiation exposure a woman receives from a mammographic examination is very low and not likely to contribute to the disease unless a genetic predisposition to breast cancer exists that disables a cell's DNA repair mechanisms, such as an ATM knockout mutation (Zheng et al. 2002). Along these lines, it is likely that radiation exposure late in life will have little effect on the development of breast cancer unless the dose is exceedingly high. This is due to the window of susceptibility for breast cancer induction being early in life owing to the disease's lengthy natural history. In summary, when we look at genetic and common nonhormonal environmental factors, we can conclude that the majority of breast cancers arise spontaneously and are not hereditary and that physical and chemical (nonhormonal) carcinogenesis seems to play only a small role in the development of the disease. Specifically, moderate and heavy alcohol consumption should be avoided. As with other forms of cancer prevention, cancer risk is most effectively reduced when prevention is employed early in life when the cancers are being initiated and/or are in the early stages of tumor promotion. Hence, for breast cancer this is likely to be in the teens, twenties, and thirties.

HORMONES AND BREAST CANCER

Further review of the epidemiologic literature reveals a strong association between breast cancer risk and hormonal factors. Both early menarche and late menopause are associated with an increased risk for developing breast cancer. Additionally, both null and late parity are associated with an increased risk of breast cancer. Postmenopausal obesity, but not premenopausal obesity owing to the effect of stored lipids on hormone levels, increases a woman's risk for breast cancer. Premenopausal obesity is associated with anovulation and decreased progesterone levels whereas postmenopausal obesity results in elevated estrogen levels in the blood.

Breast-feeding has also been shown to reduce one's risk for developing breast cancer. This correlates strongly with anovulation (Beral et al. 2002). High dietary fat intake has also been associated with an elevated risk for developing breast cancer. Mechanistically high dietary fat may act to promote breast cancer development in many different ways by its effects on inflammatory cytokines and steroid hormone synthesis, or by modulating other hormonal factors. Among these possibilities, clearly the steroid hormone rationale remains the most plausible. Unopposed estrogens used in early hormone replacement therapy are also associated with increased incidence of breast cancer. Later formulations where estrogen was balanced with progesterone are also, but to a lesser extent, associated with breast cancer (Rossouw et al. 2002, Fletcher 2002). From these observed associations, a unifying theme emerges, that is to say that increased estrogen exposure or possibly, more correctly, a hormonal imbalance where estrogens predominate seems to be strongly associated with the development of breast cancer (Fentiman 2001). It can also be directly concluded that one can lower the risk for developing breast cancer by consuming a low-fat diet and avoiding exogenous estrogen exposure most commonly found in hormone replacement therapy. Moreover, obesity in childhood is associated with early menarche, and this is associated with increased breast cancer risk and hence should be avoided.

PHARMACOLOGIC APPROACHES TO BREAST CANCER PREVENTION

In Western society, hormonal imbalance with a predominance of estrogen may result from increased dietary fat intake, intake of exogenous estrogens, and exposure to environmental estrogens among others. Effective pharmacological approaches to breast cancer prevention have targeted the estrogen receptor of breast cancer cells. Initially, selective estrogen receptor blockers, such as tamoxifen, and more recently raloxifene, have been used (Pappas and Jordan 2001, Vogel et al. 2002). Alternatively, potent selective third-generation aromatase inhibitors, such as anastozole, letrozole, and exemestane, have come on the market. These drugs act to inhibit the synthesis of estrogen, thus depleting the body's stores (Dixon 2002). Anastozole lacks the side effects of less-selective aromatase inhibitors, such as aminoglutethimide. These approaches are so powerful that they are also effectively utilized in the treatment of breast cancer, in some cases as the sole chemotherapeutic agent. The aforementioned selective estrogen receptor blocking agents have yielded 57 and 75% reductions in the relative risk of developing breast cancer in patients on relatively short trials of these respective agents (Harper-Wynne et al. 2002). These agents are quite potent and although relatively well tolerated are not without side effects. These agents may be inappropriate for women who do not have a strong predisposition toward developing breast cancer (i.e., previous breast cancer, a diagnosis of atypical breast hyperplasia, or a hereditary breast cancer syndrome). Specifically, lower doses of these drugs may be effectively employed for breast cancer chemoprevention in the future among healthy individuals. The effectiveness of low doses of these agents in breast cancer chemoprevention could be optimized by long-term treatment and intervention at an early time in life when the cancers are in an early stage of their development.

Until further work in this area is done, it cannot be recommended that healthy individuals embark upon utilizing these agents for the purpose of chemoprevention. In the meantime, bioactive substances in soy and other plant products are proposed to have activities similar to the aforementioned drugs, with reduced side effects. These plant products, namely, isoflavonoids and other phytoestrogens, are potential breast cancer chemopreventive agents and their further study is currently a hot area of research.

DIETARY CHEMOPREVENTIVE STRATEGIES

Phytoestrogens are plant steroids, which have structural similarity to estrogen. Phytoestrogens may interact with estrogen receptors and, depending on the phytoestrogen, it may activate, block, or act as a partial agonist (Adlercreutz 2002). The net effect of all of this activity at the sight of the estrogen receptor is a modulating effect, which is achieved by competitively blocking more potent estrogens, like estradiol, from interacting with the receptor. In doing this, the partial agonist activity of these compounds results in reduced side effects compared to more potent agents like tamoxifen. Additionally, isoflavonoids inhibit estrogen biosynthesis and alter the metabolism of estrogens (Kumar et al. 2002). The studies looking at supplemental isoflavonoids and other phytoestrogens as breast cancer chemopreventive agents have shown mixed and largely ineffective results (Sirtori 2001). Alternatively, diets rich in soy products and isoflavonoid-containing foods have shown a significant reduction in relative risk of breast cancer. This effect may be owed to nonflavonoid compounds also present in soy (Lu et al. 2001). Overall, there are inconsistent data regarding the likely estrogenic and antiestrogenic effects of soy on breast tissue (Sirtori 2001). The current literature strongly supports the notion that research needs to be done with specific phytoestrogens that have highly specific and desirable activities such as the isoflavonoid genistein. Genistein has been shown to suppress steroid hormone levels in premenopausal women and exert an anti-mammary-tumor effect in animal model systems presumably by inhibiting aromatase activity (Mizunuma et al. 2002). Soy food products, as well as other plant foods rich in phytoestrogens, may have some value in reducing one's risk of developing breast cancer, but there is no compelling evidence to support the use of supplemental isoflavonoids, at least in current formulations, as chemopreventive agents. This is likely a consequence of their lack of specificity and highly variable activity.

While gross vitamin deficiency syndromes such as beriberi are rare in the Western world, the majority of people are walking around with suboptimal levels or marginal deficiencies of vitamins that are critical for proper cellular function and differentiation. Suboptimal levels of folic acid, B6, and B12, which are necessary cofactors for cellular methylation reactions, are a risk factor for the development of breast cancer as well as cardiovascular disease (Fletcher and Fairfield 2002). Additionally, meat intake does not show a correlation with increased risk for developing breast cancer but a rich intake of fruits and vegetables is inversely correlated with breast cancer rates (Dos Santos Silva et al. 2002, Biesalski 2002).

A ROLE FOR INFLAMMATORY PROSTAGLANDIN BLOCKADE

NSAIDs are nonsteroidal anti-inflammatory drugs for which aspirin or salicylic acid, the willow tree bark extract, is the prototype. NSAIDs have been convincingly shown to reduce the relative risk for developing breast cancer (Moran 2002, Cotterchio et al. 2001, Sansom et al. 2001, Mcikova-Kalicka et al. 2001, Leris and Mokbel 2001, Sharpe et al. 2000). NSAIDs have also been shown to reduce the risk of developing many other common cancer types as well, most notably, colon cancer, where the relative risk reduction is greater than 50% (Akhmedkhanov et al. 2001, Langman et al. 2000). Some breast cancer cells have been shown to overexpress COX-2 and the resultant inflammatory cytokine milieu has been shown to cause cell growth and tumor promotion (Inano and Onoda 2002, Giercksky 2001). Low-dose aspirin treatment has many benefits, including a reduced risk for heart disease and a reduction in risk for many common cancer types. Aspirin, and potentially other NSAIDs, are therefore highly recommended for chemoprevention of breast cancer, as well as for general health and longevity promotion for women who do not develop adverse reactions.

Alternatively, omega-3 fatty acids, found in flaxseed and fish oils, have a similar effect on cytokine profile to that of NSAIDs. These also have proven anti-inflammatory abilities by virtue of inhibiting series-2 prostaglandin synthesis. Fish oil supplementation has also been shown to have direct cytotoxic effects on breast cancer cells (Hardman et al. 2001). Omega-3 fatty acids have been shown to upregulate the expression of tumor suppressor genes BRCA1 and BRCA2 in the breast cancer cell line (Bernard-Gallon et al. 2002, Kachhap et al. 2001). Additionally, omega-3 fatty acids have been shown to down-regulate expression of protein kinase A and C (oncogenes) in breast cancer cells (Moore et al. 2001). Moreover, omega-3 fatty acids have been shown to decrease critical factors that result in tumor angiogenesis and hence limit tumor growth rate (Mukutmoni-Norris et al. 2000). These various factors may in part explain the growth suppressive and apoptotic effects of omega-3 fatty acids on breast tumors (Stoll 2002). High levels of omega-3 fatty acids in breast adipose tissue were found to confer a potent protective effect against breast cancer development (Maillard et al. 2002). Although randomized placebo controlled trials have not been done with omega-3 fatty acids as a potential breast cancer chemopreventive agent, these studies are certainly warranted. Moreover, the other health benefits that are associated with omega-3 fatty acid consumption including reduced cardiovascular disease, reduced inflammatory disease, and lower cancer incidents at multiple sites makes it easy to recommend increasing omega-3 fatty acid consumption.

THE PINEAL HORMONE MELATONIN AND BREAST CANCER— BUILDING EVIDENCE

Melatonin has also been implicated as a potential chemopreventive agent against the development of breast cancer. Women who work night shifts have lower levels of melatonin and higher incidence of breast cancer (Kenny 2002, Malone 2002). Plasma melatonin levels inversely correlate with breast cancer incidence (Kajdaniuk et al. 2002). The logical extension of this hypothesis that blind people have significantly lower risk of breast cancer has also been proven (Rohr and Herold 2002). Moreover, melatonin has been shown to be directly cytotoxic to breast cancer cells in culture (Cos et al. 2002, Yuan et al. 2002, Nowfar et al. 2002). Melatonin is normally secreted by the pineal gland and is thought to regulate circadian rhythms (Coudert 2002). Melatonin directly suppresses the hypothymus-pituitary-gonadal axis. This suppression may lower and normalize steroid hormone levels, which plays a role in breast cancer development (Rohr and Herold 2002). Additionally melatonin directly inhibits estrogen receptor transactivation and cAMP levels in breast cancer cells (Keifer et al. 2002). Hence, melatonin has a logical rationale, an epidemiologic association and strong in vitro evidence for being a preventive agent against the development of breast cancer. Large prospective studies are lacking but certainly warranted. Melatonin has minimal side effects and this would lend it toward being an ideal chemopreventive agent if its efficacy were clearly proven.

CONCLUSION

Physical activity is a fundamental part of a healthy lifestyle and is strongly associated with reduced risk of cardiovascular disease and improved serum lipid profile, namely elevated HDL levels. High levels of physical activity have also been shown to reduce the incidence of breast cancer in elderly women (Breslow et al. 2001). Hence, physical activity in addition to dietary modifications can be recommended for reducing one's breast cancer risk.

REFERENCES

Adlercreutz, H. (2002) Phyto-oestrogens and cancer. Lancet Oncol. 2002 Jun;3(6):364–73.

Aisenberg, AC, et al. (1997) High risk of breast carcinoma after irradiation of young women with Hodgkin's disease. Cancer 79:1203.

Akhmedkhanov, A, Toniolo, P, Zeleniuch-Jacquotte, A, Kato, I, Koenig, KL, Shore, RE. (2001) Aspirin and epithelial ovarian cancer. Prev Med 33(6):682–7.

Beral, V, et al. (2002) Evidence from randomised trials on the long-term effects of hormone replcement therapy. Lancet 360: 942–944.

Bernard-Gallon, DJ, Vissac-Sabatier, C, Antoine-Vincent, D, Rio, PG, Maurizis, JC, Fustier, P, Bignon, YJ. (2002) Differential effects of n-3 and n-6 polyunsaturated fatty acids on BRCA1 and BRCA2 gene expression in breast cell lines. Br J Nutr 87(4):281–9.

Bertwistle, D, Ashworth, A. (1998) Functions of the BRCA 1 and BRCA 2 genes. Curr Opin Genet Dev 8:14.

Biesalski, HK. (2002) Meat and cancer: meat as a component of a healthy diet. Eur J Clin Nutr 56 Suppl 1: S2–11.

Breslow, RA, Ballard-Barbash, R, Munoz, K, Graubard, BI. (2001) Long-term recreational physical activity and breast cancer in the National Health and Nutrition Examination Survey I epidemiologic follow-up study. Cancer Epidemiol Biomarkers Prev 10(7):805–8.

Cos, S, Mediavilla, MD, Fernandez, R, Gonzalez-Lamuno, D., Sanchez-Barcelo, EJ. (2002) Does melatonin induce apoptosis in MCF-7 human breast cancer cells in vitro? J Pineal Res 32(2):90–6.

Cotterchio, M, Kreiger, N, Sloan, M, Steingart, A. (2001) Nonsteroidal anti-inflammatory drug use and breast cancer risk. Cancer Epidemiol Biomarkers Prev 10(11):1213–7.

Coudert, B. (2002) Circadian concepts in normal and neoplastic breast. Chronobiol Int 19(1):221–35.

Deapen, D, Liu L, Perkins C, Berstein L, Ross RK. (2002) Rapidly rising breast cancer incidence rates among Asian-American women. Int J Cancer 99(5):747–50.

Dixon, JM. (2002) Exemestane: a potent irreversible aromatase inactivator and a promising advance in breast cancer treatment. Expert Rev Anticancer Ther 2(3):267–75.

Dos Santos Silva, I, Mangani P, McCormick V, Bhakta D, Sevak L, McMichael AJ. (2002) Lifelong vegetarianism and risk of breast cancer: a population-based case-control study among South Asian migrant women living in England. Int J Cancer 99(2):238–44.

Fentiman, IS. (2001) Fixed and modifiable risk factors for breast cancer. Int J Clin Pract 55(8):527–30.

Fletcher, RH, Fairfield, KM. (2002) Vitamins for chronic disease prevention in adults: clinical applications. JAMA 287(23)3127–29.

Fletcher, SW, Colditz, GA. (2002) Failure of estrogen plus progestin therapy for prevention. JAMA 288(3):318–321.

Giercksky, KE. (2001) COX-2 inhibition and prevention of cancer. Best Pract Res Clin Gastroenterol 15(5):821–33.

Hardman, WE, Avula CP, Fernandes G, Cameron IL. (2001) Three percent dietary fish oil concentrate increased efficacy of doxorubicin against MDA-MB 231 breast cancer xenografts. Clin Cancer Res 7(7):2041–9.

Harper-Wynne, C, Ross G, Sacks N, Salter J, Nasiri N, Iqbal J, A'Hern R, Dowsett M. (2002) Effects of the aromatase inhibitor letrozole on normal breast epithelial cell proliferation and metabolic indices in postmenopausal women: a pilot study for breast cancer prevention. Cancer Epidemiol Biomarkers Prev 11(7):614–21.

Inano, H, Onoda, M. (2002) Prevention of radiation-induced mammary tumors. Int J Radiat Oncol Biol Phys 52(1):212–23.

Kachhap, SK, Dange, PP, Santani, RH, Sawant, SS, Ghosh, SN. (2001) Effect of omega-3 fatty acid (docosahexanoic acid) on BRCA1 gene expression and growth in MCF-7 cell line. Cancer Biother Radiopharm 16(3):257–63.

Kajdaniuk, D, Marek, B, Kos-Kudla, B, Zwirska-Korczala, K, Ostrowska, Z, Buntner, B, Szymszal, J. (2002) Does the negative correlation found in breast cancer patients between plasma melatonin and insulin-like growth factor-I concentrations imply the existence of an additional mechanism of oncostatic melatonin influence involved in defense? Med Sci Monit. (6):CR457–61.

Keifer, T, Ram, PT, Yuan, L, Hill, SM. (2002) Melatonin inhibits estrogen receptor transactivation and camp level in breast cancer cells. Breast Cancer Res Treat 71(1): 37–45.

Kenny, C. (2002) Breast cancer: Night shift nurses at risk. Nurs Times 97(43):9.

Kumar, NB, Cantor, A, Allen, K, Riccardi, D, Cox, CE. (2002) The specific role of isoflavones on estrogen metabolism in premenopausal women. Cancer 94(4):1166–74.

Langman, MJ, Cheng, KK, Gilman, EA, Lancashire, RJ. (2000) Effect of anti-inflammatory drugs on overall risk of common cancer: case-control study in general practice research database. BMJ 320(7250):1642–6.

Leris, C, Mokbel, K. (2001) The prevention of breast cancer. Curr Med Res Opin 16(4):252–7.

Lu, LJ, Anderson, KE, Grady, JJ, Nagamani, M. (2001) Effects of an isoflavone-free soy diet on ovarian hormones in premenopausal women. J Clin Endocrinol Metab 86(7):3045–52.

Maillard, V, Bougnoux, P, Ferrari, P, Jourdan, ML, Pinault, M, Lavillonniere, F, Body, G, Le Floch, O, Chajes, V. (2002) N-3 and N-6 fatty acids in breast adipose tissue and relative risk of breast cancer in a case control study in Tours, France. Int J Cancer 98(1):78–83.

Malone, KE, et al. (1998) BRCA1 mutations and breast cancer in the general population. Analyses in women before age 35 years and in women before age 45 years with first degree family history. JAMA 279:922.

Malone, RE. (2002) Night shifts and breast cancer risk: policy implications. J Emerg Nurs 28(2):169–171.

Mcikova-Kalicka, K, Bojova, B, Adamekova, E, Mnichova-Chamilova, M, Kubatka, P, Ahlersova, E, Ahler, I. (2001) Preventive effect of indomethicin and melatonin on 7, 12-dimethybenz-a-anthracene-induced mammary carcinogenesis in female Sprague-Dawley rats. A preliminary report. Folia Biol (Praha) 47(2):75–9.

Miki, Y, et al. (1994) A strong candidate for breast and ovarian cancer susceptibility gene BRCA1. Science 266:66.

Mizunuma, H, Kanazawa, K, Ogura, S, Otsuka, S, Nagai, H. (2002) Anticarcinogenic effects of isoflavones may be mediated by genistein in mouse mammary tumor virus-induced breast cancer. Oncology 62(1):78–84.

Moore, NG, Wang-Johanning, F, Chang, PL, Johanning, GL. (2001) Omega-3 fatty acids decrease protein kinase expression in human breast cancer cells. Breast Cancer Res Treat 67(3):279–83.

Moran, EM. (2002) Epidemiological and clinical aspects of nonsteroidal anti-inflammatory drugs and cancer risks. J Environ Pethol Toxocol Oncol 21(2):193–201.

Mukutmoni-Norris, M, Hubbard, NE, Erickson, KL. (2000) Modulation of murine mammary tumor vasculature by dietary n-3 fatty acids in fish oil. Cancer Lett 150(1):101–9.

Newman, B, et al. (1996) Frequency of breast cancer attributable to BRCA1 in a population-based series of American women. JAMA 279:915.

Nowfar, S, Teplitzky, SR, Melancon, K, Kiefer, TL, Cheng, Q, Dwived, PD, Bischoff, ED, Moro, K, Anderson, MB, Dai, J, Lai, L, Yuan, L, Hill, SM. (2002) Tumor prevention by 9-cis-retinoic acid in the N-nitroso-N-methylurea model of mammary carcinogenesis is potentiated by the pineal hormone melatonin. Breast Cancer Res Treat 72(1):33–43.

Pappas, SG, Jordan VC. (2001) Raloxifene for the treatment and prevention of breast cancer? Expert Rev Anticancer Ther 1(3):334–40.

Radford, DM, Zehnbauer, BA. (1996) Inherited breast cancer. Surg Clin North Am 144:205.

Rohr, UD, Herold, J. (2002) Melatonin deficiencies in women. Maturitas 41(suppl 1):s85–104.

Rossouw, JE, et al. (2002) Risk and Benefits of Estrogen Plus progestin in healthy postmenopausal women: Principal results from the women's health Initiative Randomized Controlled Trial. JAMA 288(3):321–333.

Sansom, OJ, Stark, LA, Dunlop, MG, Clarke, AR. (2001) Suppression of intestinal and mammary neoplasia by lifetime administration of aspirin in Apc(Min/+) and Apc(Min/+), Msh2(-/-) mice. Cancer Res 61(19):7060–4.

Sharpe, CR, Collet, JP, McNutt, M, Belzile, E, Boivin, JF, Hanley, JA. (2000) Nested case-control study of the effects of non-steroidal anti-inflammatory drugs on breast cancer risk and stage. Br J Cancer 83(1):112–20.

Sirtori, CR. (2001) Risks and benefits of soy phytoestrogens in cardiovascular diseases, cancer, climacertic symptoms and osteoporosis. Drug Saf 24(9):665–82.

Stoll, BA. (2002) N-3 fatty acids and lipid peroxidation in breast cancer inhibition. Br J Nutr 87(3):193–8.

Vogel, VG, Costantino, JP, Wickerham, DL, Cronin, WM, Wolmark, N. (2002) The study of tamoxifen and raloxifene: preliminary enrollment data from a randomized breast cancer risk reduction trial. Clin Breast Cancer 3(2):153–9.

Wooster, R, et al. (1995) Identification of the breast cancer susceptibility gene BRCA2. Nature 378:789.

Yuan, L, Colins, AR, Dai, J., Dubocovich, ML, Hill, SM. (2002) MT(1) melatonin receptor overexpression enhances the growth suppressive effect of melatonin in human breast cancer cells. Mol Cell Endocrinol 192(1–2):147–56.

Zhang, H, et al. (1998) BRCA 1, BRCA 2, and DNA damage response: collision or collusion? Cell 92:433.

Zheng, T, Holford, TR, Mayne, ST, Luo, J, Owens, PH, Zhang, W, Zhang, Y. (2002) Radiation exposure from diagnostic and therapeutic treatments and risk of breast cancer. Eur J Cancer Prev 11(3):229–35.

Index

Page references in *italics* refer to figures or tables.

Lightning Source UK Ltd.
Milton Keynes UK
UKOW01n0828180614

233595UK00001B/13/P

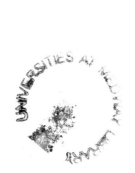